Themes and Per ~~~~~~~ ~~~~~~~
in Nursing

SECOND EDITION

Edited by

Keith Soothill,

Lancaster University, UK

Christine Henry,

University of Central Lancashire, UK

Kevin Kendrick,

Liverpool John Moores University, UK

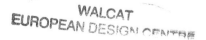

CHAPMAN & HALL

London · Weinheim · New York · Tokyo · Melbourne · Madras

Published by Chapman & Hall, 2–6 Boundary Row, London SE1 8HN, UK

Chapman & Hall, 2–6 Boundary Row, London SE1 8HN, UK

Chapman & Hall GmbH, Pappelallee 3, 69469 Weinheim, Germany

Chapman & Hall USA, 115 Fifth Avenue, New York NY 10003, USA

Chapman & Hall Japan, ITP-Japan, Kyowa Building, 3F, 2-2-1 Hirakawacho, Chiyoda-ku, Tokyo 102, Japan

Chapman & Hall Australia, 102 Dodds Street, South Melbourne, Victoria 3205, Australia

Chapman & Hall India, R. Seshadri, 32 Second Main Road, CIT East, Madras 600 035, India

Distributed in the USA and Canada by Singular Publishing Group Inc., 4284 41st Street, San Diego, California 92105

First edition 1992

Second edition 1996

© 1996 Keith Soothill, Christine Henry and Kevin Kendrick

Typeset in 10/12pt Times by Mews Photosetting, Beckenham, Kent

Printed in Great Britain

ISBN 0 412 64220 4   1 56593 4666 (USA)

A catalogue record for this book is available from the British Library

Library of Congress Catalog Card Number: 96-83042

∞ Printed on permanent acid-free text paper, manufactured in accordance with ANSI/NISO Z39.48-1992 and ANSI/NISO Z39.48-1984 (Permanence of Paper).

Contents

Contributors

Stephen Ackroyd is an organizational consultant and Senior Lecturer in the Management School, Lancaster University

Paul Bagguley is Lecturer in the School of Sociology and Social Policy, University of Leeds.

Ruth Balogh is Honorary Senior Research Associate, Centre for Health Services Research, University of Newcastle.

Jon Barry is Lecturer, Department of Mathematics and Statistics, Lancaster University.

George Butler is Principal Lecturer at the University College of St Martin and Research Student in the Centre for Professional Ethics, University of Central Lancashire.

Ruth Chadwick is Head of Centre for Professional Ethics and Professor of Moral Philosophy, University of Central Lancashire.

Tom Chapman is Director of the Centre for Health Research and Evaluation, Edge Hill University College.

Helen Fields is Nursing Officer (Education), National Health Service Executive.

Brian Francis is Assistant Director, Centre for Applied Statistics, Lancaster University.

Norma Fryer is Senior Lecturer in the Department of Midwifery Studies, University of Central Lancashire.

Emily Griffiths was formerly a District Nursing Sister, now a full-time mother.

Elizabeth Hanson is Assistant Professor and Clinical Research Associate in the Faculty of Nursing, University of Manitoba, Winnipeg, Canada.

Christine Henry is former Head of the Centre for Professional Ethics, University of Central Lancashire.

J. Stuart Horner is Director of Public Health, North West Lancashire Health Authority and Fellow of the Centre for Professional Ethics, University of Central Lancashire.

Martin Johnston is Senior Lecturer in Ethics, Department of Health and Nursing Studies, University of Central Lancashire.

Kevin Kendrick is Senior Lecturer in Philosophy and Health Care Ethics, Liverpool John Moores University.

Mairi Levitt is Research Assistant in the Centre for Professional Ethics, University of Central Lancashire.

Lesley Mackay is Honorary Senior Research Fellow, Department of Applied Social Science, Lancaster University.

Glenys Pashley is Senior Lecturer in the Department of Social Work, Faculty of Health, University of Central Lancashire.

Moira Peelo is Honorary Research Associate, Department of Applied Social Science, Lancaster University.

Jane Pritchard is Research Assistant and Research Student in the Centre for Professional Ethics, University of Central Lancashire.

Barbara Shailer is Deputy Head of Wolfson School of Health Sciences, Thames Valley University, Berkshire and Research Student in the Centre for Professional Ethics, University of Central Lancashire.

Jeanne Siddiqui is Head of midwifery education and Countess of Chester Health Park, School of Nursing and Midwifery, Chester College of Higher Education.

Keith Soothill is Professor of Social Research in the Department of Applied Social Science, Lancaster University.

Pauline Weir is Clinical Practice Development Nurse at the Royal Liverpool University Hospital.

Catherine Williams is Senior Lecturer in the Department of Primary Health Care, University College of St Martin, Lancaster.

David Worthington is Lecturer in Management Science, The Management School, Lancaster University.

Preface to the second edition

The delivery of effective healthcare is a major priority for the nursing profession and nurses must therefore confront issues related to all aspects of health and healthcare reform. A priority has been to develop appropriate texts which will not only complement the rapid changes in nursing education, but also encourage confidence in appraisal and allow students of nursing and the qualified practitioner to sensitively utilize their critical skills.

The transfer of nursing education to the higher education sector is occurring in different ways on a national and international level. This shift emphasizes a variety of changes, such as new opportunities in nursing and midwifery career structures, the advancement in nursing research, professional practice and accountability. Certainly the world of nursing is changing rapidly and since the first edition new issues have emerged or, in some cases, old issues are now being taken more seriously. A major focus is now on ethics and nursing and we have developed a new section in this second edition entirely devoted to *Applied Ethics in Nursing Practice*. This material fits comfortably between revised sections which focus on *Perceptions and Frameworks for Practice* and *Managing and Delivering Care*.

Acknowledgments

Many people have assisted, both directly and indirectly, in bringing the second edition of this collaborative project to fruition. To everyone we extend our thanks. We hope that everybody who has supported us in their various ways feels that the venture has been worthwhile.

Keith Soothill
Christine Henry
Kevin Kendrick

List of tables and figures

PART I

Perceptions and Frameworks for Practice

Perceptions of nursing, both from within the profession and by those viewing it from the outside, are crucial ingredients in understanding the present standing of nurses. What soon becomes evident is the complexity of the messages being conveyed. Nursing is in a state of flux: important shifts are currently taking place and even more fundamental shifts are perhaps on the horizon.

Previous work on nursing has tended to consider the profession in isolation but, whatever else they do, nurses must interact with a whole range of other professional groups as well as the lay persons who are their patients. A crucial area where much difficulty is experienced is in the relationship between doctors and nurses which is, in brief, both complicated and contradictory. Thus, for example, nurses may sometimes find that the behaviour of doctors leaves a lot to be desired and yet nurses often greatly value the approval of doctors. Failure to understand or appreciate their distinctive roles as well as recognizing the difficulties under which the other works may adversely affect patients, both directly and indirectly.

In Chapter 1 Lesley Mackay focuses on the different perceptions which these two – still essentially gendered – occupations hold of each other. While it is a fact that in hospitals the jobs that nurses and doctors do often overlap, it is surprising, therefore, that the descriptions of the 'good nurse' and the 'good doctor' given by doctors and nurses are so different. Part of the explanation seems to lie in the way doctors and nurses contrast the content of the work they do. Many doctors seem to have unflattering attitudes towards the work of nurses; and nurses' demands for patient-orientated doctors appear to go unheard. Curiously, nurses and doctors, it seems, are seeking a mirror image of their own skills in their ideal doctors and nurses.

However, there are dangers in considering nursing as a whole and Moira Peelo, Brian Francis and Keith Soothill (Chapter 2) point out how their work shows that nurses are not a homogeneous group; instead nurses have differing attitudes both to the NHS and to nursing. These authors' use of a probabilistic clustering technique known as latent class analysis identified four groups with very different perceptions of nursing. In fact, they maintain that the demand for higher pay for nurses has provided a narrow focus for widely expressed concern about the National Health Service in recent years. They argue that, to meet the nursing demands of the future, we need to come to terms with meeting the needs of *each* of these various groups of nurses.

The contribution by Christine Henry (Chapter 3) focuses on conceptions of the nature of persons and indicates how philosophical approaches may be helpful in seeking to understand what is meant by the concept of the person. This discussion is a prerequisite before Henry goes on to suggest that a better comprehension of the concept is necessarily central for good healthcare. The ethical and educational implications of the various conceptions lead to some recommendations for the education of nurses, doctors and teachers.

Glenys Pashley (Chapter 4) focuses on psychiatric nurse educators' and practitioners' conceptions of mental illness. Her study emphasizes that nurses utilize a commonsense view and reflects the need to enhance the curriculum further to include more integrated knowledge from psychology, sociology and the law.

Curriculum issues feature significantly in the contribution of Tom Chapman and Helen Fields (Chapter 5). While noting that knowledge underpinning the nursing professional's education programmes must move away from a biomedical focused model, they emphasize the need for a more integrated and flexible knowledge base that enhances and substantiates a 'caring' rather than a 'curing' profession. While interpersonal and therapeutic skills are important educational strategies for the Project 2000 curriculum, developing such skills are a continuous curriculum challenge.

Recent changes in nurse education will obviously influence not only the perceptions of nursing but aspects of professional practice and accountability. Ruth Balogh (Chapter 6) discusses performance indicators and professional accountability relating to nurse education and clinical practice. She remarks that, in the past, schools of nursing have had a rather ambiguous status; hence the need for radical changes in nurse education. The changes ought to clarify the perceptions we have of nursing and what nursing education should be in the future. Balogh gives an overview of professional accountability which outlines performance and quality. However, in being concerned with not just measuring the output of qualified practitioners but also with the ethical dimension that underpins professional accountability for future practitioners, Balogh's contribution leads appropriately into Part II, which focuses more directly on ethical issues.

<table>
<tr><td>

Nursing and doctoring: where's the difference?
</td><td>

1
</td></tr>
</table>

Lesley Mackay

INTRODUCTION

In recent research into nurses recruitment and wastage, the relationship between doctors and nurses was often reported to be unsatisfactory (Mackay, 1989; Hayward *et al.*, 1991). Nurses, and in particular junior nurses, spoke of being ignored by doctors. Some doctors would not even look at a student nurse or an enrolled nurse. When these doctors wanted information, only a staff nurse or a sister would do. It became apparent that patient care must suffer when communication between doctors and nurses could not take place because one of them did not have enough stripes on her cap. Not only does patient care suffer but valuable time and energy is wasted looking and then waiting for the 'right' nurse to talk to. When communication between members of the healthcare team is poor, everyone suffers. Interprofessional relationships between all members of the healthcare team are important. But none is more important than the one between nurses and doctors.

Despite the critical importance of interprofessional relationships in hospitals, it is an area which has received surprisingly little attention in the UK (but see Porter, 1991, 1992; Busby and Gilchrist, 1992). Yet it is through the 'sieve' of the hospital that all healthcare professionals proceed. The relationships encountered within the hospital are likely to be replayed or at least reflected in the relationships between healthcare workers in the community.

At Lancaster University we carried out research into interprofessional relationships between doctors and nurses in hospitals. Funding was received from the Economic and Social Research Council to carry out the investigation. Once the pilot survey had been conducted and our ideas were

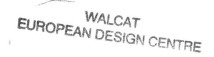

clarified, we conducted fieldwork in five locations in Scotland and England which have included teaching and non-teaching hospitals. As little systematic research has been undertaken in this area, our investigation was very exploratory in nature. Our aims were to provide a 'map' of the working relationships between nurses and doctors: the difficulties and the successes in day-to-day working relationships.

Interviews with 25 nurses and 25 doctors were conducted at each location. The nurses interviewed were staff nurses or sister/charge nurses. The doctors were house officers, senior house officers, registrars, senior registrars and consultants. We chose to concentrate on five main specialties: general medicine, general surgery, psychiatry, medicine for the elderly and intensive care. In keeping with the exploratory nature of the research, we used semi-structured interviews.

IDEAL TYPES

In previous research into nurse recruitment and wastage (Mackay, 1989), we asked nurses about their conceptions of the 'good nurse'. From nurses at the top to nurses newly embarking on nursing, there was broad agreement on the attributes of the good nurse. We wished to investigate this area further. How did the description of a doctor's ideal nurse compare with that of a nurse? What was the 'good doctor' like? Did nurses and doctors have similar views on their ideal doctor?

Nurses' and doctors' views regarding ideal types of the good nurse and the good doctor are built up from a variety of sources. The socialization that takes place during training ensures that the views of the newcomers soon come to reflect those of older colleagues. In our previous research we found a surprising similarity between the views of first-year nursing students and nursing officers on the attributes that made a 'good nurse'. (For an interesting discussion of socialization, see Conway, 1983; see also Soothill and Bradby, 1993. And for a personal view of the socialization of a doctor, see Marinker, 1974; see also Allen, 1988.) Personal experience and knowledge are combined with stereotypes from the mass media. (Kalisch and Kalisch (1986) report on the way in which nurses are portrayed in the electronic media; see also Holloway in Chapter 2. Karpf (1988) discusses the media portrayal of doctors.)

The notion of a 'good nurse' and a 'good doctor' is implicit in many of the opinions and attitudes of doctors and nurses. The notion serves as a benchmark for their own and the other group's behaviour at work. To some extent, it is a standard against which members of one's own and the other group are measured. We asked both nurses and doctors to describe 'the good nurse' and 'the good doctor'. For ease of reporting only, nurses will be referred to as female and doctors as male. (It is worth noting, however, that although half of all medical students are now female this has not yet altered the assumption of nurses in general conversation that doctors are male.)

The good nurse: the nurses' view

For nurses, the 'good nurse' is caring and sensitive to the needs of patients. The aspects emphasized by nurses centre on the way a nurse relates to her patients: the need to be genuine, understanding, patient and kind. The good nurse will listen carefully and communicate well. She will be approachable and have time to talk. At the same time the good nurse has to be assertive and to remain calm whatever the circumstances. For the most part, the attributes of the good nurse are personal characteristics. While such attributes can be developed they cannot be learned. (Gamarnikow (1978) points to the similarities between the 'good nurse' and the 'good woman'.)

The emphasis nurses place on 'character' may be a reflection of the continuing influence of Florence Nightingale. (For an appreciation of her influence, see Baly, 1986.) Nightingale emphasized the importance of the personal character of the nurse rather than training or skills. In her view, the good nurse was kind, compassionate and patient. Such a nurse is born not made. (For discussions of the dynamics regarding the image of the nurse, see Ehrenreich and English, 1973: 36; and Salvage, 1985: 18ff.) As the good nurse cannot be 'made', the value set on training and the development of skill is not great. I have argued elsewhere that nurses do not sufficiently value their training and the skills they develop (Mackay, 1989).

The good nurse: the doctors' view

For doctors, the 'good nurse' is competent at her job: she knows about her patients, she will anticipate problems and she will use her initiative. While it is important for a good nurse to be sensitive to the needs of patients, it is even more important for her to act as a first line of defence for doctors. The good nurse will act as the doctor's 'eyes and ears' on the ward in his absence and on whom they can rely. And doctors are often absent from the ward. The good nurse will be willing and able to contribute information towards patient management. At the same time, the good nurse will ensure that doctors are not 'pestered' unnecessarily or thoughtlessly. Doctors are in a position of considerable dependence on the judgments of nursing staff as, for example, in deciding when to summon the doctor.

The good nurse: differences of opinion

An important difference in the descriptions of the good nurse given by doctors and nurses is that relating to 'skill'. Although some nurses mention the need for the good nurse to be competent and good at her job, the emphasis is on character rather than skills. For medical staff, character is secondary to competence. Competence means that a nurse knows when a patient needs attention; she can take decisions; she knows what she is doing and the ward runs smoothly. At the same time, competence comes through experience and knowledge. It is an attribute which can be acquired. Thus while nurses appear to maintain a belief that nurses are 'born not made', doctors value the skills acquired through training. It is worth noting in passing that nurses, in explaining why they took up nursing, frequently say that it is 'something I always wanted to do'. Doctors, on the other hand, often mention that they entered medicine because they had the requisite number and grades of 'A'-levels or that they were encouraged to enter medicine by their schools. In other words, nurses' reasons for their career choice tend to focus on some idea of vocation, while doctors' choices focus on academic attainment.

It is noteworthy that doctors emphasize the skill aspect, the learned component, of work activity. After all, they go through extensive training in which the level of their knowledge and skill become all-important. (The differences in professional training, and funding for that training, may act as an additional barrier to positively valuing the skills of colleagues (Hennessy, 1994).)

Primarily, doctors are trained as scientists. A glance at any prospectus for a British medical school will illustrate the importance of the scientific perspective. An emphasis on the scientific is made at the expense of an emphasis on a sense of vocation. For admission to medical school, academic attainments appear to be all-important. (This comment does need qualifying in the light of Johnson's (1991) research which has shown that type of school and medical family connections are particularly important in selecting medical students.) It appears that relative little scrutiny is given to the personal characteristics of potential doctors. From the prospectuses of UK medical schools it also appears that during their training few doctors receive more than a token input regarding interpersonal relationships. Yet it is on these interpersonal relationships that nurses place so much weight. There appears to be a fundamental difference in the orientations of those who recruit and train in medicine and nursing.

Given the processes of socialization, it is not surprising that both doctors and nurses emphasize the attributes which are valued within their own occupation. Correspondingly, nurses and doctors attach less value to the attributes valued in the other occupation.

The good doctor: the nurses' view

Nurses evaluations of the 'good doctor' centre repeatedly on the way patients are treated. The good doctor does not rush patients: he will spend time talking with them and he will listen carefully to what they have to say. He will take time to tell patients what is being planned for them with regard to their treatments. The good doctor also needs to be a listener: to nursing staff as well as to patients. Indeed, the good doctor seeks, and listens to, advice from nurses. He consults nurses, treating them as equals; he is receptive to their opinions. A few nurses – but they are a minority – mention the need for a doctor to be competent and to know what he is doing. Again, for nurses, the emphasis is on interpersonal skills rather than on skills as a medical practitioner. (That is not to say that nurses tolerate a bad or incompetent doctor.)

The good doctor: the doctor's view

Doctors' evaluations of the good doctor focus mainly on the level of skill. Above all, the good doctor should be competent at his job. At the same time he should be inquisitive, decisive and not too 'businesslike' with patients. Similarly, the good doctor should be approachable and willing to spend time with patients.

The good doctor: a comparison

In comparing the views of nurses and doctors, there was a clear difference in the priorities regarding the good doctor. Nurses emphasized doctors' 'approach' to patients; doctors emphasized the skills required. Although nurses very much value the doctor who seeks their advice and uses their experience, this aspect was only occasionally mentioned by doctors.

Nurses and doctors particularly value attributes in the other group which are valued within their own occupation. Yet if these ideas were achieved and doctors, say, were to increase the importance they accorded to interpersonal skills, it would negatively affect nurses' claims to having a distinctive competence which sets them apart, and as being worthy of respect, from doctors.

The attributes valued by doctors and nurses underline a difference in perception as to priorities in hospital healthcare. It is a difference which has also been found to exist among nursing and medical students (Ryan and McKenna, 1994). Nurses, on the one hand, emphasize 'getting to know the patient as a person', while doctors emphasize 'getting to the root of the problem' with the aim of correctly and speedily diagnosing 'the problem'. While the medical profession focuses on the biophysical, nursing focuses on the illness, 'a concept referring to the broader subjective experiences and practical difficulties faced by patients' (Campbell-Heider and Pollock, 1987). The medical profession would argue, quite rightly, that the primary concern of the patient is the diagnosis and cure of the problem for which the patient was admitted. Nursing staff would argue, again quite rightly, that in order to effectively treat a patient, many different aspects of the patient ought to be taken into consideration. The tension between the two perspectives is highlighted in decisions as to when to stop the 'active treatment' of patients (see Mackay, 1993). Thus, nurses often say that doctors want to pursue treatment 'to the bitter end', while they would prefer some patients to be left to die in peace and with dignity. Doctors say they have a duty to do everything they can to save life and that nurses do not have to bear the final responsibility for patients' lives.

THE DIFFERENCE BETWEEN WHAT NURSES AND DOCTORS DO

The doctors and nurses we interviewed were asked to 'describe the difference between what a nurse does and what a doctor does'. The question was aimed at obtaining descriptions of the relationship between nursing and medicine. The question essentially asks for a contrast to be made between the roles. And to state the obvious, it is a question that emphasizes differences rather than similarities. This is an important point because in many areas the tasks of nurses and doctors, especially junior doctors, overlap.

This task overlap between (junior) doctors and nurses is not often mentioned when doctors and nurses are asked to describe the differences in their work. On the few occasions that the blurring of roles between nurses and doctors was mentioned, it was primarily from doctors and nurses working within psychiatry.

The difference: the doctors' view

Doctors' descriptions of the difference focus on the central role that doctors see themselves as occupying: doctors give the orders; doctors diagnose and prescribe; doctors have the final say. Nurses are seen by doctors as obeying the doctor's orders, administering the treatment and undertaking 'basic care'. Primarily, these doctors are describing a power relationship. The doctor has the power: he prescribes, he initiates, he decides and he orders.

The difference: the nurses' view

In the nurses' descriptions of the difference, they use the same words as the doctors. For example, 'doctors decide what nurses are going to do'; 'they [doctors] decide what needs doing and we do it'; 'doctors prescribe and nurses carry it out'. As with the doctors' descriptions, there is an explicit acceptance of a power relationship: the one gives orders, the other follows them. Campbell-Heider and Pollock comment: 'Nurses accept the notion that only a physician can diagnose a health problem; they rely on the physician for decision-making and reflect passive-dependent behaviors; the doctor is reinforced as the "captain"; and the whole process is so subtle that the rationale for this behavior is actually distorted' (1987: 423).

The difference: a comparison

The caring role and the practical role which nurses carry out is often mentioned by both doctors and nurses. But doctors make little mention of the close relationship that nurses enjoy with patients, while nurses quite often refer to this aspect. Thus, nurses will refer to 'looking after the whole patient' or being 'involved with everything to do with the patient'. Some nurses describe themselves as being 'the patient's advocate' but this role was not mentioned by the doctors. (For a summary of the arguments relating to this role, see Castledine, 1981; and for some dilemmas in the advocacy role, see Ellis, 1992.) At the same time, nothing about the doctor's relationship with the patient was ever mentioned by either nurses or doctors.

The nurse's role is often viewed in extremely limited terms by doctors. Thus nurses look after the 'basic functions' of patients; give patients their food; wash them. Some doctors emphasize the importance of the basic work, pointing out that nurses give continual, 24-hour care and have an intimate contact with their patients that doctors lack. Yet again and again, the lack of decision-making power is implicit in the doctors' comments. Nurses 'act out what we say'; 'administer the prescribed treatment'; 'facilitate our work'. The nurse's role here is one of support, not one of equivalence. Only occasionally does a doctor refer to teamwork in describing the difference between what nurses and doctors do.

The stark division between doctors' ordering and nurses' obeying is less clear-cut for those nurses who see their role as prescribing nursing care. In the view of these nurses, nursing has a distinct area of expertise which is not under the direction of the medical profession. (The presence of two conflicting ideologies in nursing – nurses as autonomous professionals and nurses as subordinates to doctors – has been commented on elsewhere; see Devine, 1978.) Doctors did not mention any such distinct or discrete area of competence of nursing staff.

DISCREPANCIES BETWEEN THE TWO QUESTIONS

The descriptions of the good nurse and doctor contrast with the perceptions of differences between what nurses and doctors do. The good nurse who uses her initiative is simultaneously seen by some doctors simply as being involved in carrying out basic care. The doctor who describes nurses as doing bedpans and washing patients also wants the good nurse to 'pick up what he's missed'. Doctors who emphasize the centrality of their own diagnostic role and their direction of the activities of nursing staff at the same time want the good nurse to be 'capable of assessing patients'. Thus, in response to one question, there is a denial of the need for nurses to be skilled, yet in response to the second question, the high value placed on a skilled nurse is asserted. Why? One possible answer is in the great disparity in pay, status and career prospects of doctors in comparison with nurses. Thus, doctors may need to defend that disparity by maintaining the high level of skills required by doctors and the relatively low level of skill required to be a nurse. Yet in the actual working situation, the reality is that doctors depend extensively on nurses for information. Nurses who lack skill and expertise are likely to cause doctors a great deal of additional and unnecessary work.

Nurses are aware of undertaking diagnoses as when, for example, they are taking decisions about calling a doctor to see a patient. Doctors are aware of this aspect of the nurses' role but its importance is played down. There is an acceptance, say, that nurses undertake a basic assessment of patients, but less attention is given to the 'intuitive' decision taken by a nurse to call a doctor because the patient is 'not right'. (The experience required in reaching 'intuitive' decisions appears not to be recognized by doctors and is insufficiently recognized by nurses.) Nevertheless, these diagnoses are essentially interim diagnoses only. (That they can contribute to saving life is another matter.) There is a widespread recognition among nurses (and doctors) that doctors take the final and ultimate decisions and responsibility for the care of patients. (The dominance of doctors can be illusory; see Stein, 1967; Hughes, 1988. But see also Mackay, 1993, 1994.)

Some nurses, while describing the directing and ordering role of doctors, also see the good doctor as one who treats nursing staff as equals and/or who is prepared to work as part of a team. It is difficult to see how a group which is seen to bear the final responsibility for patients can realistically be expected to treat a group which carries out their orders as equal. It is also difficult to see the current relationship between doctors and nurses as being other than unequal. After all, the majority of these nurses and doctors attest to the decision-making role of the medical profession and the need for nurses to carry out doctors' orders. However, this is not to say that these nurses see themselves in the role of 'handmaiden'. Indeed, such a label is abhorred by most nurses (Mackay, 1993), although they recognize the existence of that perception among doctors (Ryan and McKenna, 1994: 120).

It seems that both doctors and nurses, in describing the good nurse and the good doctor respectively, set out an ideal which mirrors their own activities. Yet in describing the differences in the work roles, the work of nurses is simplified by doctors. Similarly, the unilateral decision-making role of doctors is emphasized. At the same time the division between nurses and doctors is enlarged, in denial of the interdependent nature of the relationship between doctors and nurses. The need for the nurse to act as 'the eyes and the ears' of the doctor, for her to undertake some level of diagnosis and for her to make decisions and initiate action are ignored in the contrasts between roles. It seems that when pressed, doctors seldom make reference to ideas of teamwork or of working together as equals.

This may change. For example, the mounting pressures on all healthcare workers are likely to mean changes in work content and working practices (see, for example, Hurst, 1992; Morley, 1992). Similarly, when the Project 2000 changes in nurse training have worked their way through the system, the attitudes of both nurses and doctors to the role and capabilities of the nurse may alter. Such optimism may be misplaced. Nurses are still the most passive members of the healthcare team according to the leader of the Royal College of Nursing (*Nursing Times*, 1992). And even at the most senior levels of medicine and nursing, there is a lack of cooperation – so much so that the General Medical Council and the United Kingdom Central Council have never even managed to issue a joint statement (Castledine, 1993).

CONCLUSION

Essentially, the questions about the good doctor and nurse and the difference between what they do have probed the attitudes of nurses and doctors to one another. It is worth noting that many of the difficulties and conflicts which doctors and nurses report in everyday working relationships centre on the attitudes displayed to one another. The difficulties reported regarding attitudes may well be a reflection of the contradictory nature of these attitudes. It seems that nurses want doctors to exhibit the characteristics of the good nurse and doctors want nurses to exhibit the characteristics of the good doctor.

The comments about the good nurse and the good doctor are perhaps more revealing of the subjects whose opinions were sought than of the objects they described. Nurses and doctors are sensible in setting a high value on their own skills. However, in seeking to find a reflection of one's own skills in the work of another group, there is an implicit denial of that other group's contribution. Doctors are not as good at their interpersonal skills as nurses. Nurses are not diagnosticians or decision-makers on treatment. Each group has its own sphere of competence, to which greater recognition needs to be given by the other. As one doctor and one nurse pointed out, neither can work on their own.

Perhaps some of the tensions encountered in working together could be overcome if the special contribution each group has to make was sufficiently recognized.

REFERENCES

Allen, I. (1988) *Doctors and Their Careers*, Policy Studies Institute, London.

Baly, M. E. (1986) *Florence Nightingale and the Nursing Legacy*, Croom Helm, London.

Busby, A. and Gilchrist, B. (1992) The role of the nurse in the medical ward round. *Journal of Advanced Nursing*, **17**(3), 339–46.

Campbell-Heider, N. and Pollock, D. (1987) Barriers to physician–nurse collegiality: an anthropological perspective. *Social Science and Medicine*, **25**(5), 421–5.

Castledine, G. (1981) The nurse as the patient's advocate – pros and cons. *Nursing Mirror*, 11 November, **153**(20), 38–40.

Castledine, G. (1993) Doctors and nurses: dangerous liaisons. *British Journal of Nursing*, **2**(8), 428.

Conway, M. E. (1983) Socialization and roles in nursing. *Annual Review of Nursing Research*, **1**, 183–208.

Devine, B. A. (1978) Nurse-physician interaction: status and social structure within two hospital wards. *Journal of Advanced Nursing*, **3**, 287–95.

Ehrenreich, B. and English, D. (1973) *Witches, Midwives and Nurses: a History of Women Healers*, Feminist Press, New York.

Ellis, P. (1992) Role of the nurse advocate. *British Journal of Nursing*, **1**(1), 40–3.

Gamarnikow, E. (1978) The sexual division of labour: the case of nursing, in *Feminism and Materialism*, (eds A. Kuhn and A. Wolpe), Routledge & Kegan Paul, London, pp. 96–123.

Hayward, A.J., Will, V.E., MacAskill, S. and Hastings, G.B. (1991) *Retention within the Nursing Profession in Scotland*, University of Strathclyde, Department of Marketing, Glasgow.

Hennessy, D. (1994) The new NHS: challenges and opportunities for medical and nursing education. *Health Trends*, **26**(1), 7–10.

Hughes, D. (1988) When nurse knows best: some aspects of nurse/doctor interaction in a casualty department. *Sociology of Health and Illness*, **10**(1), 1–22.

Hurst, K. (1992) Changes in nursing practice 1984–1992. *Nursing Times*, **88**(12), 18 March, 54.

Johnson, M.L. (1991) A comparison of the social characteristics and academic achievement of medical students and unsuccessful medical school applicants. *British Journal of Medical Education*, **5**(4), 260–3.

Kalisch, P.A. and Kalisch, B.J. (1986) A comparative analysis of nurse and physician characters in the entertainment media. *Journal of Advanced Nursing*, **11**, 179–95.

Karpf, A. (1988) In *Doctoring the Media*, Routledge, London.

Mackay, L. (1989) *Nursing a Problem*, Open University Press, Milton Keynes.

Mackay, L. (1993) *Conflicts in Care: Medicine and Nursing*, Chapman & Hall, London.

Mackay, L. (1994) The patient as pawn in interprofessional relationships, in *Interprofessional Relations in Health Care* (eds K. Soothill, L. Mackay and C. Webb), Edward Arnold, London.

Marinker, M. (1974) Medical education and human values. *Journal of the Royal College of General Practitioners*, **24**, 445–62.

Morley, B. (1992) Role of the night nurse practitioner. *British Journal of Nursing*, 1(14), 719–21.

Nursing Times (1992) Hancock says profession has little status. *Nursing Times*, **88**(35), 26 August, 9.

Porter, S. (1991) A participant observation study of power relations between nurses and doctors in a general hospital. *Journal of Advanced Nursing*, **16**(6), 728–35.

Porter, S. (1992) Women in a women's job: the gendered experience of nurses. *Sociology of Health and Illness*, **14**(4), 510–27.

Ryan, A.A. and McKenna, H.P. (1994) A comparative study of the attitudes of nursing and medical students to aspects of patient care and the nurse's role in organizing that care. *Journal of Advanced Nursing*, **19**, 114–23.

Salvage, J. (1985) *The Politics of Nursing*, Heinemann, London.

Soothill, K. and Bradby, M. (1993) The chosen few. *Nursing Times,* **89**(13), 36–40.

Stein, L. (1967) The doctor–nurse game. *Archives of General Psychiatry*, **16**, 699–703.

2 | NHS nursing: vocation, career or just a job?

Moira Peelo, Brian Francis and Keith Soothill

INTRODUCTION

There has been intense interest in the attitudes of nurses to conditions of work and much speculation about why they leave the National Health Service. The tradition of expecting one explanation of nurses' feelings about their work is a long one: the standard expectation has been that nursing is a vocation, with implications of altruism and feminine, selfless care (Lorentzon, 1990). The dominance of this model over our thinking about nursing makes it hard to see that there has probably always been diversity within the nursing population when it comes to motivation, both between nurses and within individuals over time. By the 1980s, much discussion of nurses leaving the NHS concentrated on the issue of pay and more recently, the debate has focused on changes within the NHS. This chapter simply describes data which illustrates the naïvety of the 'one-explanation' account of nurses' feelings about their work.

The crucial point to recognize is that nurses are not an homogeneous group, a simple fact often overlooked by politicians, managers, unions and the media. Politicians are suddenly introduced to the problems of nursing without knowledge or interest in the subtleties of the issues; managers try to introduce working practices which encourage conformity rather than diversity; unions seek the common interests which bind their members together; and the media want a straightforward message which appeals to the sensibilities of their readers. For the rest, however, the picture is much more complex: even among nurses, what are seen as issues for some nurses are not mentioned by others and vice versa. Until we begin to understand the varying demands, interests and needs within the nursing profession and the complex patterns of nurses' concern, we cannot understand why nurses continue to leave the profession.

Concern about nurses' conditions, pay, status and duties is not new: 19th century reformers wished to attract trained personnel into hospitals but some, like Mrs Bedford Fenwick, were concerned that high pay might attract the wrong sort of recruit (Leeson and Gray, 1978). The move away from untrained, lower-class nurses to more genteel recruits highlighted tension between nursing as an extension of a domestic role, on the one hand, with emphasis on hygiene as well as motherly care; and, on the other, a desire for professional status which made the carrying out of duties usually performed by lower domestic servants problematic (Gamarnikow, 1978). Florence Nightingale, we are told, viewed these non-nursing duties as character-building, but not all shared her opinion in a period that saw attempts to get nurses registered and hence officially recognized (Leeson and Gray, 1978). Nightingale also favoured training nurses in obedience, with moral restraints and an emphasis on vocation, much as nuns might describe their religious calling; vocation coupled with carrying out hard, physical tasks resulted in a model of nursing that Abbott and Wallace (1990) have described as 'the selfless sacrifice of the nurse to the needs of the patient' (p. 21). Today, tension remains between the view of nursing as a truly caring 'vocation' and notions of professionalism, seen to be mutually exclusive approaches or at least as problematic companions: concern for the emotional as well as the physical well-being of patients has traditionally been a part of a nursing vocation, whatever other technical skills and knowledge are required. Downe (1990) has written that the pursuit of a skills-based professional status for nurses is dangerous if it does not also ensure better care for clients, since this unmeasurable element reflects a state of 'being' a nurse which is an essential ingredient rather than a sign of weakness.

What was not in doubt in the 19th-century nursing reforms was the subsidiary role of nursing to medicine: Witz (1985), in describing the struggle for the registration of midwives, illustrated how such changes in nursing coincided with the striving of doctors for professional dominance of medicine. Game and Pringle (1983) have called the division of labour in the health sector 'a sexual division in its most blatant form' (p. 94) in both the nursing/female, medicine/male model and in its actual work ethos and practices. Gamarnikow (1978) described the sexual division of labour as 'a patriarchal ideological structure in that it reproduces patriarchal relations in extra-familial labour processes' (p. 121), and nursing illustrates this with its emphasis on 'the interconnections between femininity, motherhood, housekeeping' (p. 121). Yet, in spite of the equation of nursing with these values and attributes, recruitment into nursing is seen as an issue concerning young women, and a caption to a press photo of two nurses tells all: 'Crisis in care ... up to half of all girl school leavers will have to become nurses to meet the demands of the 21st century; (*The Guardian*, 30 July 1988). While adolescent girls, according to Martin and Roberts (1984), do see their futures as dominated by family and domestic commitments, they often 'expect to return after having a family' (p. 60) to paid employment. At the very least, one might expect this sector to have most experience in accommodating the needs of its older female employees. However, Game and Pringle have described how, in spite of evidence that, in Australia, large percentages of nurses are married women with children, hours of work are particularly difficult to combine with family life.

Evidence of variety in nurses, their needs, concerns, ages and motivation, then, may have been frequently overlooked but it is not a new phenomenon. At a time when the emphasis was on bad pay, Mackay (1988a) attempted to widen the terms of the debate by indicating that the lack of career prospects also plays a significant part in why nurses leave the NHS. Mackay (1988b) has shown that nurses were extremely dissatisfied: nurses reported that they were very frustrated, for they simply did not have the time to look after their patients properly. They recognized they were failing to meet their own standards of care. These were the nurses' perceptions and they felt that it should be to staffing levels above all else that local managers – who were not in a position to offer extra pay – should first turn their attention. Mackay (1988c) also focused on the misuse of nurses and reminded us that the *Briggs Report on Nursing* (1972) found fairly high levels of misuse of nurses regarding 'non-nursing chores'. Mackay (1993) has predicted that Project 2000 may well encourage short-term solutions to staffing problems to become institutionalized, as task are divided between graduate and less-qualified nurses, with the latter carrying out more menial tasks. Many are now beginning to recognize that nurses will have to be used more carefully and their talents nurtured if there are not enough to go around – or, more seriously, not enough money to employ a sufficient number. In brief, we must now attend to their concerns. We maintain that a more sophisticated statistical approach enables us to recognize the range of differing expectations held by nurses and the variety of demands they make of nursing. These issues need to be recognized and addressed if a nursing workforce is to be satisfactorily maintained.

DATA COLLECTION AND INITIAL ANALYSIS

In our demonstration project[1] a random sample of one in three nurses in post in a district health authority in the north of England was taken in

---

[1] The original study began in 1985 and this sample was drawn in July 1986. Mackay's (1986) work largely focuses on the qualitative study while this chapter demonstrates the value of a detailed analysis of the questionnaire responses.

July 1986 and a questionnaire was posted to their home address. We surveyed a wide range of posts: from students and pupil nurses up to and including sisters and charge nurses. After one follow-up letter, a total of over 60% of nurses responded to the questionnaire, providing a group of 435 persons who were still in post at the time of the study.

Standard questionnaire items on age, sex, post, marital history and residence were included as well as a section on life events and a bank of attitudinal questions on nursing and the NHS. Following Mercer (1979), we asked nurses to rate the importance (on a five-point scale later collapsed to a four-point scale for subsequent analysis) of each of 11 improvements which would encourage trained nurses to stay in the NHS. We also asked the sample to identify reasons (from a checklist of ten reasons) which might cause them to leave nursing, and followed up with additional questions in which we asked the nurses for their attitudes to matters of salary (much too high, too high, about right, too low or much too low), promotion prospects (very good, quite good, not very good or poor), career opportunities (sufficient or not sufficient), community care (strongly approve, approve, indifferent, disapprove or strongly disapprove) and whether absenteeism was thought to be a problem (yes, no or sometimes). In total, there were 26 attitudinal items

Searching for one major factor which causes nurses to leave would provide an inaccurate and simplistic picture, for as respondents came to sort out the reasons which might affect their decision to leave, the picture was diverse. In fact, none of the ten reasons attracted more than 35% of the sample stating it as a likely reason while, conversely, none attracted less than 5%. When one comes to personal motivation for possible leaving, it is the diversity of reasons which merits attention.

When analysing frequencies, the temptation to look for one causal factor can be great: for example, in our series of questions both replicating the work of other studies and introducing new areas of interest, the topic of pay emerged in various guises: 76% thought the present level of salary for nurses 'too low' or 'much too low'; over 94% per cent regarded increased salaries as 'important or very important' as an improvement necessary to encourage trained nurses to stay (with 62% of these answering 'very important'). Indeed, 'increased salaries' was the reason given as 'important' or 'very important' most often from among the list provided. But when the respondents were asked what might cause *them* to leave nursing, 'dislike of nursing pay' was no longer the dominant reason given.

However, as Table 2.1 shows, while no single item constitutes a main cause for leaving, the responses are by no means totally random. Table 2.1 summarizes the responses of our stayers' sample to the various attitudinal items, cross-classified by current age. Here some patterns begin to emerge. Of those under 25 years, having a baby, a dislike of nursing pay or a possible preference for nursing outside the NHS emerged as the three

Table 2.1 Attitudes to nursing and current age

Attitude	Age group				
	Under 25 %	25–29 %	30–39 %	over 40 %	All nurses %
1 What might cause you to leave nursing?					
1(a) Marriage	7.1	4.1	5.7	3.9	5.3
1(b) Baby	61.9	47.4	24.4	7.8	35.4
1(c) Partner moving jobs	24.8	28.9	24.4	11.8	22.5
1(d) Looking after children	31.0	34.0	22.0	7.8	23.7
1(e) Looking after dependants	15.0	23.7	20.3	28.4	21.6
1(f) Wanting a rest from paid work	2.7	9.3	9.8	9.8	7.8
1(g) Dislike of nursing work	9.7	9.3	7.3	2.9	7.4
1(h) Dislike of nursing pay	37.2	32.0	27.6	10.8	27.1
1(i) Wanting to get out of nursing	18.6	24.7	23.6	7.8	18.9
1(j) Prefer nursing outside NHS	34.5	16.5	16.3	10.8	19.8
2 What improvements are necessary to encourage trained nurses to stay? (Response: very important)					
2(a) Relaxation of discipline	8.0	3.1	4.9	2.0	4.6
2(b) Better promotion possibilities	37.2	47.4	32.5	28.4	36.1
2(c) Increased salaries	71.7	69.1	61.0	46.1	62.1
2(d) Regular training opportunities	46.9	48.5	52.8	52.9	50.3
2(e) More auxiliary help	19.5	20.6	15.4	25.5	20.0
2(f) More flexible hours	11.5	21.6	30.9	36.3	25.1
2(g) Special responsibility pay	35.4	43.3	48.0	43.1	42.5
2(h) Shorter working week	6.2	6.2	16.3	16.7	11.5
2(i) Split time between hospital and community	5.3	6.2	7.3	13.7	8.0
2(j) More nursing accommodation	11.5	17.5	8.1	22.8	14.5
2(k) Crèche/nursing facilities	34.8	46.9	46.3	35.6	41.0
3. Additional attitudinal questions					
3(a) Present level of salary? (Too low or much too low)	95.5	80.4	72.4	58.0	76.8
3(b) Does nursing offer sufficient career opportunities (Yes)	50.0	36.5	36.4	41.2	41.1
3(c) Do you consider the promotion prospects for someone like yourself? (Quite good or very good)	38.4	25.8	32.0	22.0	29.9
3(d) Do you see absenteeism among nurses as being a problem?	57.7	62.9	59.3	55.9	58.9
3(e) How do you feel about the present moves to community care? (Disapprove or strongly disapprove.)	7.2	15.5	11.4	22.6	13.8
Sample size	113	97	123	102	435

most predominant reasons given as possibly causing them to leave nursing. The likelihood of these reasons being offered declined markedly with age. A new set of possibilities for leaving rose to prominence among those aged 40 or over: nearly one-third saw looking after dependants as a possible reason most frequently stated. However, closer attention to Table 2.1 shows that the possibility of having a baby as a reason decreases markedly with age and looking after dependants increases markedly with age; looking after children, however, as a possible source for leaving is fairly constant at all age groups apart from the oldest. So taking these examples in turn, suitable maternity-leave arrangements might interest younger nurses, day centres for elderly dependents may be helpful to older nurses, while crèche/nursing facilities may well appeal to nurses of all age groups (this is reflected in the responses on crèche/nursing facilities in Table 2.1 – row 2(k)).

Attitudes apparently related to age are fascinating but hazardous and cross-sectional data can be misleading. It is dangerous to interpret this effect as a change of attitude as a nurse proceeds through a career path. For example, while one can accept on biological grounds that the chances of a nurse being likely to leave to have a baby will decrease markedly when she is over 40, one cannot have similar confidence that the 35% who were under 25 and said they might leave nursing owing to a possible preference for nursing outside the NHS will change their attitude towards nursing outside the NHS as they grow older. In other words, it seems unlikely that when they are aged 40 years or over only 11% will be attracted by the possibility of nursing outside the NHS. (When it comes to that point in time with this cohort, many more may have exercised their option of working outside the NHS before reaching 40, and the percentage in the group that remain may be similar to 11%.)

The current cohort of those aged under 25 will have spent all their years in nursing since the Conservative government came to power in 1979 and in an era when the growth of private medical care has been actively encouraged and the concept made more generally acceptable. In short, the social and political context when the attitudes of our young nurses in the study were being formed was very different from the older nurses in the study. Hence, one can see the dramatic shift in the attitude of those aged under 25 when 35% say they may prefer nursing outside the NHS and those aged 25 and over when only 13% take a similar attitude. So while Table 2.1 tends to suggest that attitudes to the NHS seem to be associated with age reached, we feel that caution should be exercised in making such a ready connection that attitudes may change with age.

One way of examining these possibilities is to assume that there are groups of nurses with differing attitudes to the NHS and nursing, and that the proportion of these groups differ in each age. We investigate this possibility by looking for clusters of nurses with relatively similar responses to the attitude items.

THE CLASSIFICATION AND ITS RESULTS

Various authors over the last 20 years have suggested a wide variety of algorithms for determining patterns in data. Gordon (1981) is one of many to suggest that many methods currently in use have no strong statistical basis, making it difficult to determine the number of groups. Latent class analysis provides solutions to a number of difficulties of standard cluster analysis. First, the number of different groups or types of activity may be assessed by examining the 'goodness of fit' of the various solutions (two group, three group, etc.) to the data: this is formally measured by the 'deviance' which is based on the likelihood function. Second, the analysis gives a set of probabilities (referred to here as response probabilities) which provide information on the importance of each response in each question in distinguishing between the groups. Formally stated, each response probability is: the probability of an individual in a particular group giving a particular response to a particular item. Finally, latent class analysis does not give a rigid assignment of individuals to groups but instead provides a set of 'posterior probabilities' for each individual, giving the individual probability of assignment to or membership of each group. Thus an individual has a probability of belonging to a number of groups and this is often a more realistic assumption to make.

Latent class analysis has been used extensively in sociological applications (Clogg, 1979). One example is the classification of a survey population into groups based on their responses to a questionnaire designed to measure prejudice toward black Americans (Tuch, 1981). The algorithmic approach used here follows Aitkin, Bennett and Hesketh (1981a) who re-analysed data from the *Teaching Styles and Pupil Progress* study of Bennett (1976), which produced a classification of teachers into a number of teaching styles. The algorithm used by Aitkin, Bennett and Hesketh (1981a) was extended by Hinde to deal with multinomial responses and with missing data. It was subsequently used in a study on the Welsh language background of children (Baker and Hinde, 1984). We used the same computer algorithm, which is written in the statistical programming language GENSTAT. No attempt is made here to describe latent class analysis in detail, as other authors (Lazarsfeld and Henry, 1968; Aitkin, Anderson and Hinde, 1981b; Everitt, 1984) have produced detailed treatments.

Williams, Soothill and Barry (1991) rightly argue that this means of analysis is no predictor of the likelihood of individual nurses leaving the NHS: prediction of behaviour is a research aim of positivist social scientists and not a necessary part, of itself, of the intentions of statistical modellers. Ackroyd (1993) has argued cogently that knowing something of nurses' feelings about their work does not explain their attachment to a job or whether or not an individual might leave it. Ackroyd's work illustrates how, to understand the relationships between expressed emotions and behaviour, a wider theoretical construct beyond the latent class analysis of data is needed, one which allows for the complexity of situation and feelings to be encompassed.

Four groups of nursing attitudes were identified by this analysis (the statistical information is provided in the Appendix on page 30). An advantage with probabilistic clustering procedures is that the technique does not attempt to shoehorn nurses into groups, but allows for the possibility that some nurses will be difficult to assign to the groups found and may have equal probabilities of belonging to a number of groups. Instead, the analysis gives us probabilities for each nurse to belong to each of the four groups and we can therefore attempt to classify our sample of nurses into the four groups by looking for high probabilities of belonging to a particular group. We adopted a criterion of assigning a nurse to a group if the nurse's probability of belonging to that group is greater than 0.75. On that assumption, the four-group solution produces the assignment of nurses in the sample to the groups shown in Table 2.2.

Table 2.2 The four-group solution: assignment of nurses to groups

Group	1	2	3	4	unclassified
Number of nurses	79	77	82	123	74

We now examine the four-group solution in greater detail. Table 2.3 shows the response probabilities for this classification. Major differences between the probabilities can be identified. For example, there is a probability of 0.60 that Group 4 nurses will give 'baby' as a reason for leaving nursing, compared with a probability of 0.13 of Group 1 nurses giving the same reason. Group 2 nurses have a probability of 0.70 of giving 'dislike of nursing pay' as a reason for leaving nursing, compared with substantially lower probabilities in the other three groups. Group 3 nurses have a high probability (0.74) of seeing 'more flexible hours' as very important to encourage trained nurses to stay, compared with low probabilities for the other three groups.

We can continue this process and attempt to produce a description of each of the four groups produced by the clustering procedure. Although the groups are defined in terms of probabilities of giving answers to certain questions, we can think of these probabilities in terms of expected proportions of nurses giving a particular answer if a hypothetical sample of nurses of the group under examination had been taken. We can therefore adopt a straightforward approach and treat high probabilities as being indicative of concerns specifically raised by each of the groups.

Table 2.3 Response probabilities for each group – four-group solution

Attitude	Group 1	Group 2	Group 3	Group 4
1 What might cause you to leave nursing?				
1(a) Marriage	0.02	0.08	0.02	0.08
1(b) Baby	0.14	0.43	0.14	0.60
1(c) Partner moving jobs	0.09	0.38	0.16	0.26
1(d) Looking after children	0.02	0.30	0.08	0.45
1(e) Looking after dependants	0.14	0.22	0.15	0.31
1(f) Wanting a rest from paid work	0.10	0.12	0.07	0.04
1(g) Dislike of nursing work	0.00	0.21	0.15	0.31
1(h) Dislike of nursing pay	0.12	0.70	0.16	0.16
1(i) Wanting to get out of nursing	0.15	0.46	0.16	0.05
1(j) Prefer nursing outside NHS	0.19	0.34	0.13	0.15
2 What improvements are necessary to encourage trained nurses to stay? (Response: very important)				
2(a) Relaxation of discipline	0.00	0.09	0.08	0.04
2(b) Better promotion possibilities	0.16	0.58	0.60	0.26
2(c) Increased salaries	0.34	0.84	0.84	0.58
2(d) Regular training opportunities	0.29	0.59	0.84	0.44
2(e) More auxiliary help	0.11	0.24	0.50	0.10
2(f) More flexible hours	0.10	0.20	0.74	0.12
2(g) Special responsibility pay	0.12	0.60	0.85	0.32
2(h) Shorter working week	0.04	0.14	0.35	0.04
2(i) Split time between hospital and community	0.04	0.05	0.28	0.03
2(j) More nursing accommodation	0.09	0.22	0.30	0.07
2(k) Crèche/nursing facilities	0.19	0.46	0.63	0.43
3. Additional attitudinal questions				
3(a) Present level of salary? (Too low or much too low)	0.73	0.96	0.70	0.70
3(b) Does nursing offer sufficient career opportunities (Yes)	0.37	0.19	0.38	0.82
3(c) Do you consider the promotion prospects for someone like yourself? (Quite good or very good)	0.12	0.06	0.29	0.65
3(d) Do you see absenteeism among nurses as being a problem?	0.58	0.71	0.68	0.53
3(e) How do you feel about the present moves to community care? (Disapprove or strongly disapprove.)	0.26	0.24	0.22	0.05

Group 1 Nursing come what may

Curiously, there are no matters which specifically concern nurses classified as Group 1 more than any of the other three groups. Of the total
body of nurses in the sample, these are the ones who see the fewest
problems in nursing at present; furthermore, they are also nurses who
see less in their own situation, such as having a baby, their partner
moving jobs, looking after children and so on, which is likely to cause
them to leave nursing. Whatever may happen, they seem to be saying
that they will be staying in nursing. Nursing pay is not likely to drive
them away into other work; indeed, while the probability of giving the
answers 'too low'; or 'much too low' for the level of salary being paid
to nurses at that time is still high (0.73), they have a low probability
(0.34) of answering 'very important' when salary is considered as an
improvement to encourage nurses to stay. It seems little will deter them
from continuing in nursing and, further, they make few new demands
on the system. Compared with other nurses, they do not bemoan the
pay, the poor promotion possibilities or the lack of training opportunities, etc. Quite simply, nursing is their life whatever its trials and
tribulations.

Group 2 Nursing, but for how much longer?

These nurses disproportionately felt they were more likely to leave nursing for a wide variety of reasons. The strongest differences can be seen on
the responses of disliking nursing work and pay, or just simply wanting to
get out of nursing. The likelihood of preferring nursing outside the NHS
was also higher than for the other groups. However, they also seemed
likely to leave for other external factors, such as having a baby, looking
after children or looking after dependants. They feel that improvements
are necessary in promotion, salaries and training, but are less likely than
Group 3 to rate other improvements as being 'very important'. If this
group has a single source of disillusionment, it is pay, with the highest
probability among the groups of rating their own salary as inadequate.
Hence, these can be identified as nurses seeking a well-paid occupation
and perhaps rapidly coming to the conclusion that NHS nursing is not for
them.

Group 3 Nursing: battling it out

This group is characterized by its low probabilities of giving reasons for
wanting to leave nursing and in this respect is somewhat similar to Group
1 nurses. However, their attitude to the improvements' questions tells a
different story. This group has extremely high probabilities of seeing a

wide range of improvements as 'very important', from increased salaries to issues such as a shorter working week and increased responsibility pay. Their responses indicated they were particularly concerned about the level of nursing pay and all the trappings that transform a mundane job into a career, such as training opportunities, promotion possibilities, special responsibility pay and more auxiliary help. Group 3 nurses are also unlikely to leave because of family reasons. This does not mean that they would not have children but they did not wish to leave paid employment to look after them. Hence they, more than any of the other three groups, feel that crèche/nursing facilities are among the improvements necessary to encourage trained nurses to stay. They now find themselves in nursing and like it; they want it to be uninterrupted and rewarding. On the whole they seem likely to be stayers, but, unlike Group 1, they remain extremely concerned about the pay and conditions of the nursing profession.

Group 4 Nursing, 'just a job'

This is another quite distinct group in which there is a much more ready response to factors and demands external to nursing. These are the nurses who, it seems, are more likely to leave as a result of marriage, having a baby, their partner moving jobs, looking after children or looking after dependants. For them, nursing largely seems to offer sufficient opportunities and there is a much greater satisfaction about 'the promotion prospects for someone like yourself'. They do not express concern about flexible hours, nursing accommodation, etc. as a way of encouraging trained nurses to stay. Crèche facilities have less interest for them than for Group 3, for many probably intend to give up work to care for their children. They also express serious concern about the pay and so if it is 'just a job', it needs to be paid satisfactorily. They are certainly much less concerned with the problem of career opportunities and have probably thought much less about alternative kinds of work. However, one suspects that, if the private health sector outside the NHS was thought to pay well, then this group of nurses would be among those tempted to move. In brief, these nurses are interested in well-paid nursing jobs but recognize that they may leave nursing because of family commitments.

DISCUSSION

As Everitt (1974) has said, cluster-analysis techniques provide methods of breaking complex data sets into manageable groups. We have seen that latent class analysis provides a model-based approach for investigating the number of groups and provides a picture of the attitudinal response of such groups. Our evidence indicates that nurses are not an homogeneous group, but hold very different expectations from nursing. This outcome has serious implications for recruitment policy, as it implies the futility of a one-solution strategy as an approach to staffing.

Our statistical analysis of a random sample of nurses from one district health authority suggested that four groups may be the most appropriate way of understanding their responses to a set of attitudinal items. The most frequent constellation of attitudes (28%) resulted in primarily seeing 'nursing as a job' (Group 4). The remaining groups split evenly with just under one-fifth of the sample in each group. Hence, it is obviously misleading to consider the nursing profession as an homogeneous group or even having one major group with a dominant set of attitudes. Once these groups have been established, we are then able to build up group profiles by examining the characteristics of nurses who have been assigned to a particular group. Analysed this way, we are able to retain the complexity inherent in the sample, rather than making assumptions about the sample and any subsets. For example, it is possible to cross-classify the group variable by a number of descriptive variables (such as age, marital status, number of children at home, specialty, etc.) and by further attitudinal variables not included in the original analysis. These variables help to provide background information, but this kind of analysis in no way validates the groups; so, for example, it is perfectly possible for people of similar profiles in relation to age and marital status to be assigned to different groups by virtue of their attitudes.

Building up group profiles makes clear that this method of analysis reveals levels of complexity which should not be ignored. Age, for example, emerged as an important difference between the groups. So Group 1 nurses ('Nursing come what may') were more likely to be aged 30–39 or 40+ than to be aged 25–29; Group 2 ('Nursing, but for how much longer?') nurses were more likely to be aged 30–39 or younger, but were unlikely to be 40+; Group 3 ('Battling it out') also included many aged 30–39 plus those of 40+; over 40% of Group 4 nurses ('Nursing, just a job') were under 25, with a further 20% under 30.

In what ways these age differences between groups matter is both more complex and lends itself to more interpretations than might, at first, be imagined. This cohort have grown up and trained in a period in which opportunities for nurses outside the NHS have expanded, and must seem to be realistic options. The job market has, in this respect, altered. Also, the expectation of marriage and childrearing breaks, in this predominantly female profession, echoes the hairdressers in Attwood and Hatton's study (1983), whose expected 'life' as a hairdresser was five years before taking the anticipated break. These 'lifecycle' events, however, did not exclude a return to hairdressing, but were a prelude to working in the less glitzy, glamorous salons. As such, the hairdressing industry perceived these young women as failures in not following a specific and expected route; their nursing counterparts may also return to non-NHS jobs, nursing homes or other private work rather than disappear completely from the nursing scene.

Dex (1988) has illustrated that 'there are considerable variations between women, not just by age and lifecycles, but according to their experience, education and prospects' (p. 148) which influence the attitudes of women to work. Brown (1976) has also argued for a need to understand 'the ways in which the labour market operates' (p. 39) and the constraints set upon the worker, to further our understanding of the 'relationship between "structure" and "consciousness"' (p. 40), rather than looking at workers' perceptions alone. In nursing, Firth and Britton (1989) have highlighted some situational elements in professional 'burnout', notably that supportive action by managers could reduce absenteeism. The complex relationships between the daily experience of working life and the longer-term expectations of nursing are illustrated by Clifton (1990), who has written of the ways in which management styles and goals can cut across a nurse's commitment to caring for the whole patient rather than mechanistically carrying out tasks.

In this study, in addition to generational and cyclical aspects of age, it became apparent that there are situational aspects which need to be borne in mind. Group 4 nurses, containing a high proportion of students, were the least qualified; they perceived nursing as offering sufficient training opportunities. By comparison, Groups 2 and 3 contained high proportions of midwives and mental health nurses; their responses indicate levels of discontent over the ways in which their qualifications and experience are used. We have already seen that both groups were likely to view special responsibility pay as a necessary incentive to retain trained staff (see Table 2.3). Group 1 nurses, who were more content than Groups 2 and 3, contained a high proportion of the sample's community nurses. Another aspect of the relationship between situation and age was highlighted by Group 3: they were highly likely to be combining childrearing with an occupation to which they were committed, yet apparently found the conditions of work difficult and unrewarding. Perhaps not surprisingly, they saw crèche and nursery facilities as important provisions which might encourage trained nurses to stay. This particular set of concerns is at odds with the traditional picture of a nurse as young and single; a picture, incidentally, which Vicinus (1985: 118) shows us to be inappropriate even a century ago when nurses faced the expectation of early retirement and so took the option of private nursing, which provided 'better pay and longer working life'.

We have indicated that there are currently considerable divergencies in attitudes towards nursing among nurses and there is little chance of a longitudinal study to clarify what is actually happening. These attitudes are complex and appear to reflect interaction between conditions of work with an individual's personal circumstances, expectations and experience. As these nurses clearly differ in their situations, ages and workplaces it becomes harder to talk of 'nurses' as one group. Whittaker and Olesen (1964) describe how the legend of Florence Nightingale, widely accepted as the culture-heroine of the nursing profession, has many faces and functions. The differing faces of this legend reflect prevailing ideologies in nursing and each generation claims something specific from the Florence Nightingale legend as its own: 'To those asked to accept and incorporate change [the legend] shows a face which reflects the very change desired.To some women it projects the face of traditional womanhood, to others it shows how traditional femininity could be combined with a career' (Whittaker and Olesen, 1964: 130). From this analysis, we would argue that it is unwise to attempt to delineate one model of nursing in the NHS. In order to recruit and maintain the necessary workforce, we must recognize that there are different attitudes within nursing and come to terms with the different needs they reflect.

ACKNOWLEDGMENT

We are grateful to the Leverhulme Trust for providing financial support for the above research.

GLOSSARY

Algorithms A set of mathematical calculations to carry out a statistical or mathematical technique.

Attitudinal questions A set of questions on a questionnaire which ask the respondent for their opinions on various issues.

Clustering methods A set of statistical techniques which attempt to classify individuals into groups, and where the individuals within a group are more similar in some respect than individuals from different groups.

Cross-sectional data Information which is collected on one occasion at the same date or in the same time period for a number of individuals.

This is usually contrasted with longitudinal data, where information on the same individual is collected over time, on more than one occasion.

Deviance A number which measures the 'goodness of fit' of a statistical model to the data. In our example, the statistical model is the assumption of a certain number of groups. The deviance decreases as the number of groups increases, until a perfect fit is obtained when every individual belongs to their own individual group.

Fit To estimate mathematically a set of numbers based on a set of assumptions about the structure of the data. In our example, the set of numbers are probabilities and the assumptions are the number of different groups which are present in the sample.

Five-point scale In response to an attitudinal question, the respondent will have a choice of one of five categories in which to record their view on the question topic. The categories often measure agreement or disagreement to a statement, and, if so, will usually be ordered, with category 1 representing the most extreme category of disagreement, and category 5 the most extreme category of agreement. Other scales are also used.

Frequencies Counts of numbers of individuals (i.e. not proportions, percentages, or measurements).

GENSTAT A statistical computer package or program.

Homogeneous group A group with similar opinions and behaviour patterns.

Latent class analysis A statistical technique for carrying out probabilistic clustering. Literally, classes or groups which are not observed but which are latent or hidden in the data.

Likelihood function A mathematical formula which represents the probability of observing the data which was actually observed under a set of assumptions (on the number of groups).

Monte Carlo testing Also often referred to as simulation, the technique uses random numbers to generate sets of data assuming a particular hypothesis (for example 'there are three groups present in the data'), then uses those sets of data to examine the effect of assuming different assumptions (for example 'there are four groups present in the data').

Multinomial responses Responses to a single question which are categorized into more than two groups.

Probabilistic clustering A method of clustering which, rather than giving an absolute assignment of individuals to groups, instead provides probabilities for an individual to belong to each of the groups.

Probability A probability is a measure of how likely an event is to occur. Probabilities always lie between zero and one inclusive.

REFERENCES

Abbott, P. and Wallace, C. (1990) Social work and nursing: a history, in *The Sociology of the Caring Professions,* (eds P. Abbott and C. Wallace), The Farmer Press, London.

Ackroyd, S. (1993) Towards an understanding of nurses' attachments to their work: morale amongst nurses in an acute hospital. *Journal of Advances in Health and Nursing Care*, **2**(3), 23–45.

Aitkin, M.A., Bennett, S.N. and Hesketh, J. (1981a) Teaching styles and pupil progress: a reanalysis. *British Journal of Educational Psychology*, **51**, 170–86.

Aitkin, M.A., Anderson, D.A. and Hinde, J.P. (1981b) Statistical modelling of data on teaching styles. *Journal of the Royal Statistical Society*, Series A,. **144**, 419–61.

Attwood, M. and Hatton, F. (1983) Getting on, gender differences in career development: a case study in the hairdressing industry, in *Gender, Class and Work*, (eds E. Gamarnikow, D.H.J. Morgan, J. Purvis and D.E. Taylorson), Heinemann, London.

Baker, C. and Hinde, J. (1984) Language background classification. *Journal of Multilingual and Multicultural Development*, **5**, 43–56.

Bennett, S.N. (1976) *Teaching Styles and Pupil Progress*, Open Books, London.

Brown, R. (1976) Women as employees: some comments on research in industrial sociology, in *Dependence and Exploitation in Work and Marriage*, (eds D.L. Barker and S. Allen), Longman, London.

Clifton, B. (1990) Who's helping who … ? *Health Matters*, Issue 4, June, p. 18.

Clogg, C. (1979) Some latent structure models for the analysis of likert type data. *Social Science Research*, **8**, 287–301.

Dex, S. (1988) *Women's Attitudes Towards Work*, Macmillan, London.

Downe, S. (1990) A noble vocation. *Nursing Times* 3 Oct, vol. 86, no. 40, p. 24.

Everitt, B.(1974) *Cluster Analysis*, Heinemann/SSRC, London.

Everitt, B. (1984) *An Introduction to Latent Variable Models*, Chapman & Hall, London.

Firth, H. and Britton, P. (1989) 'Burnout', absence and turnover amongst British nursing staff. *Journal of Occupational Psychology*, **62**, 55–9.

Gamarnikow, E. (1978) Sexual division of labour: the case of nursing in *Feminism and Materialism*, (eds A. Kuhn and A.Wolpe), Routledge & Kegan Paul, London.

Game, A. and Pringle, R. (1983) *Gender At Work*, Pluto Press, London.

Gordon, A.D. (1981) *Classification*, Chapman & Hall, London.

Lazarsfeld, P.F. and Henry, N.W. (1968) *Latent Structure Analysis*, Houghton Miffin, Boston.

Leeson, J. and Gray, J. (1978) *Women and Medicine*, Tavistock, London.

Lorentzon, M. (1990) Professional status and managerial tasks: feminine service ideology in British nursing and social work in *The Sociology of the Caring Professions* (eds P. Abbott and C. Wallace), The Falmer Press, London.

Mackay, L. (1988a) Career women. *Nursing Times,* 9 March, vol. 84, no. 10.

Mackay, L. (1988b) The nurses nearest the door. *The Guardian*, 13 January.

Mackay, L. (1988c) No time to care. *Nursing Times*, 16 March, vol. 84, no. 11.

Mackay, L. (1989) *Nursing A Problem*, Open University Press, Buckingham.

Mackay, L. (1993) *Conflicts in Care: Medicine and Nursing*, Chapman & Hall, London.

Martin, J. and Roberts, C. (1984) *Women And Employment: A Lifetime Perspective*, HMSO, London.

Mercer, G.M. (1979) *The Employment of Nurses*, Croom Helm, London.

Tuch, S.A. (1981) Analysing recent trends in prejudice towards blacks: insights from latent class models. *American Journal of Sociology*, **87**, 130–42.

Vicinus, M. (1985) *Independent Women: Work and Community for Single Women 1850–1920*, Virago Press, London.

Whittaker, E. and Olesen, V. (1964) The faces of Florence Nightingale: functions of the heroine legend in an occupational sub-culture. *Human Organisation*, vol. 23, **2**, 123–30.

Williams, C., Soothill, K. and Barry, J. (1991) Nursing: just a job? Do statistics tell us what we think? *Journal of Advanced Nursing*, **16**, 910–19.

Witz, A. (1985) *Midwifery And Medicine*, Lancaster Regionalism Group, Working Paper 13.

APPENDIX 1

Examination of the deviances for various numbers of groups from one to five provide us with evidence to determine the number of groups of attitudes present. If the observed deviance reductions shown in Table 2.4 are greater than the largest of 19 simulated deviance reductions, then there is evidence that these reductions in deviance are unlikely to have occurred by chance, and thus evidence for the higher number of groups. Table 2.4 shows that there are large reductions in deviance from the one to the two-group, from the two- to the three-group solutions and from the three-group to the four-group solutions. Monte Carlo testing procedures allow us to determine the importance of these deviance reductions by generating random data with the characteristics of the sample assuming a certain number of groups, then carrying out a latent class analysis on this data assuming that there is a further group present. In this way, we can simulate deviance reductions for comparing three groups over two groups, four groups over three groups, etc. We can see from the table below that there is strong evidence for the existence of two groups over one group, for three groups over two groups, and for four groups over three groups. The evidence for five groups is less strong, as the deviance reduction is close to the simulated test value, and we do not consider the five-group solution further.

Table 2.4 Deviances for the classification problem

Number of groups	Deviance	Deviance difference	Largest of 19 simulated differences
1	17957		
		396	118.4
2	17563		
		270	123.0
3	17293		
		201	123.2
4	17092		
		125	124.7
5	16967		

| 3 | # Conceptions of the nature of person by doctors, nurses and teachers |

Christine Henry

CONCEPTIONS OF THE NATURE OF PERSONS

First it is essential to seek some understanding of what is meant by the concept of the person and who legitimately can be counted as a person before emphasizing the idea that a better comprehension is necessarily central for good healthcare.

The concept of the person with some of its uses stand for what humans essentially are, and more than one answer to the question of what constitutes a person can be given. Nevertheless, it may be helpful to identify three possible models that are useful in understanding the concept of the person. The three models are only tentative conceptual schemes and must not be viewed as definitions of the person. However, each model will allow for diversity in perspectives, with the underpinning assumption that each model is insufficient in itself. The concept of the person defies definition in the formal and descriptive sense. Further, it is claimed by some philosophers to be a primitive concept and difficult to analyse.

The moral/evaluative model of the person

A moral conception of the person is put forward by Abelson (1977), who claims that the term 'person' is normative and evaluative like the term 'good'. Abelson also remarks that we do not have any established criteria for applying person status. In other words, it is open to us whether we ascribe person status or not, and neither logic nor language can give the answer to who should and who should not be given the title 'person'. Even when we observe the behaviour of others, although we may find grounds for person ascription it is not logically conclusive because behaviour does not entail such status. Further, Abelson states that the ascription of personhood does not rest entirely on respect for human beings. It is possible that the mental defective and the very small infant can be given semi-person status and this does happen within the healthcare field. Similarly, recent history reflects the reality of a whole race of people being deprived of full person status – for example, the treatment of the Jewish people in Nazi Germany. Abelson argues that the term 'person' is an open-ended evaluative term and therefore empirically unanalysable. However, he claims that the individual person is a subject of psychological and moral predicates and therefore independent of biological classification. If this is the case, then it is possible from this moral and evaluative model to ascribe person status to non-humans. The term 'person' is therefore not a natural concept and defies biological classification.

Not only is the term difficult to define in formal ways but it is a term that is viewed as species neutral. Abelson remarks that in everyday language there may be some confusion between the two terms 'person' and 'human'. The term 'person' is viewed as purely normative whereas the term 'human' is semi-normative and descriptive. The term 'human' will convey a limited reference to the species and at the same time refer to characteristics of humans.

The latter semi-normative elements involve the characteristics that are values. The term 'human' can be used interchangeably with the term 'person' in everyday commonsense ways (for example, 'Well, she's only human after all'). This indicates that being human is valued in that we are not machine-like or perfect in a formal or descriptive sense. Abelson suggests that in our everyday use we often imply that the terms 'human' and 'person' are the same or have the same meaning.

This model emphasizes value and a moral sense of the term 'person'. Harris (1985) remarks that a person will be any being capable of valuing its own existence. Although it is not as simple as Harris claims, it implies that there does not appear to be any sort of necessary truth that all persons are human beings. Midgley (1983) also remarks that other animals beside ourselves may value their own existence and from this point of view are capable of being a person. This supports Abelson's claim that the concept of the person is open-ended and evaluative like the term 'good'. Shoemaker and Swinbourne (1984) support the idea that the animal is the form in which the person is physically realized at a given time. Locke (1632–1704) remarks that human beings in one sense are animals and he distinguishes between the identity of a person and that of a man; holding the former does not involve the identity of an animal (Henry, 1986).

The formal traditional model of persons

Why is it that some human beings are identified as having only semi-person status? This may relate to a more formal model of the person influenced by a number of Western traditional philosophers. One of the criticisms levelled at Midgley's statement that other animals may value their own existence is its attribution of the features of a special kind of consciousness and features of rationality to other animals. These special features are particularly attributed to the human mind and have been viewed as person features and what differentiates ourselves as human beings from other sentient beings. Further, it may be one of the reasons why, in commonsense terms, the severely mentally handicapped, the very young infant, the confused elderly and the patient on a life-support machine are not viewed as persons in the full sense of the term. Not only do traditional philosophical views influence the conceptions of the nature of persons, but also the type of education that is given can reflect traditional values and the need for attributing defining features in order to categorize, recognize or make sense of individuals and their situation.

Hampshire (1959) claims that persons are distinguishable from other sentient beings because they are capable of putting their thoughts into words. A person must be able to communicate in general but also let their intentions be known. Strawson (1959) supports this by claiming that we do not ascribe psychological concepts such as memory, motivation or intention to other animals. However, Midgley disagrees and claims that we have no right to diminish the inner lives of the rest of creation. Further, in commonsense everyday terms we often do attribute psychological features to other animals who share our lives and with whom we have a special relationship (for example our family dog). In this sense Midgley supports and advocates a value perspective which is more open-ended and links to a commonsense view rather than the formal traditional or ideal model.

Dennett (1979) presents some possible themes or features that have been identified as necessary but not sufficient conditions of personhood and may summarize an idea/formal model of the person. He claims that we require an intelligent, conscious, feeling agent to coincide with a moral notion of a person who is accountable, having rights and responsibilities. He claims that the notion of a conscious, feeling agent is a necessary if not sufficient condition of moral personhood. Dennett outlines a further six themes identifying other necessary but not sufficient conditions of personhood. Dennett's six familiar themes are useful for seeing different ways in which an individual might identify person features. Further, the themes may be used as distinguishing features between persons and non-persons. However, the danger arises when only one model of the conception of the nature of persons is used. It is therefore essential to remember that even the formal model must remain an open-ended list of features and be taken as an ideal model only, that we can approximate to the idea anyhow, and that there must be caution in attempts at defining persons by attributing identifiable features.

Dennett suggests that the first and most obvious condition is that persons are seen as rational beings. This theme indicates that reason involves a higher-order notion of knowledge, language and intelligence. Second, states of consciousness are attributed and psychological features such as intentions are predicated to these states. The third theme depends on whether something counting as a person rests on a particular stance being adopted towards it. In other words, individuals are treated in a certain way and to some extent this is part of being a person. This theme involves a social element. A reminder of how Nazi Germany treated a group of people as non-persons reflects how it is possible to influence the treatment and care of people in the healthcare field simply by taking a particular stance towards individuals: i.e. by treating them as persons or by treating them as things or non-persons. Dennett remarks that the first three themes are mutually dependent: i.e. the person is rational, intentional and a subject (not object) of a particular stance. These three themes are a necessary but not sufficient proviso for the fourth theme of reciprocity, which implies that a being who has a personal stance taken towards it must be capable of reciprocating in some way. This fourth theme is in turn a necessary but not sufficient condition of communication. This fifth theme of communication is a necessary condition of Dennett's sixth and final theme. Persons are distinguishable from other sentient beings by being conscious in a special way. Self-consciousness is a condition for persons being moral agents.

These themes of Dennett's can be identified as a common cluster of person features. However, Dennett's themes may be viewed as an ideal feature list for the nature of persons, which would be difficult or impossible to apply in certain cases.

The social commonsense model of persons

An alternative way of understanding the concept of the person links closely with a commonsense view. Teichman (1972) states that in commonsense terms we treat humanity as the deciding mark for the ascription of person status. Teichman, like Abelson, suggests that in ordinary use the word 'person' and the extension of the term 'human being' give the impression of being identical. She observes that the only natural persons we actually meet in real life are human beings, although she acknowledges it is logically possible for another variety of natural persons to exist on other planets, i.e. non-human persons.

An extension of this viewpoint could be the inclusion of other animals on this planet that are strikingly like us (i.e. like us psychologically, with intentions and so on). What is important from Teichman's point of view is that the intention (meaning and application) of the word 'person' allows for this possibility. Teichman's view is not only social but involves the idea of the term being meaningfully applicable. Further, any meaningfully socially constructed view is not descriptive but involves values and an element of open-endedness. Teichman emphasizes the fellowship or relationship within the social context. However, Teichman points out that the notion of having a particular kind of body, whether misshapen or unusual but recognizably human, rules out parrots, dolphins and chimpanzees, although the latter in some ways are similar to human beings. She emphasizes an alternative view of a social and human commonsense model of the person. This perspective is restricted to the human persons if we use the term 'human being' as a starting point. Further, there may be a self-creating element with the term that rises out of our own interpretative (phenomenological) world. This latter point links to the idea of what is meaningful to ourselves when ascribing person status.

Teichman's view relates to Wittgenstein's approach in that language (in the human context) is essentially social. The meaning of the word is to be found not in logical analysis but in its use within a particular language game to which it belongs. These language games are not just a matter of words and use but also include feelings, gestures, attitudes and skills. These complex related elements compose a particular 'form of life'. A form of life is part of our interpretative world. For example, Wittgenstein claimed that other animals have different forms of life and if a lion could speak we would not understand him. The language used in each game overlaps, sharing the same words but having different meanings. Application of Wittgenstein's view can be illustrated crudely in the use of the word 'human'. For example, in a particular language game between medical biologists it may be specifically used to mean biological membership of a species, whereas a group of nurses or general practitioners may use the term 'human' to mean the same as 'person' when talking about the patient or client. The same word is used in each language game but has a different meaning (Henry, 1986). The two terms 'human' and 'person' can also come together in some language games but act differently in others. The major focus of this model concerns everyday functions of language, the use of which can be associated with a human commonsense view of the world, which in broad terms considers the social context to be important. Once again this model, like the previous models, cannot offer a definition of the nature of persons and is not sufficient on its own.

The three models offer different viewpoints but hopefully can coexist with other more varied perceptions and help to push back the boundaries of understanding to show how confusions can arise with the conceptions of the nature of persons that are held by health professionals. The conceptions that we have will, in turn, influence the way we treat and care for individuals within the healthcare system.

The next section focuses on a small research study of doctors', nurses' and teachers' conceptions of the nature of persons.

THE RESEARCH APPROACH AND RESULTS

The major research project from which this small study is taken was concerned with commonsense conceptions of the nature of persons among children, adolescents and adults. While the main study focused on social cognitive developmental psychology, a rich source of data emerged concerning ethical and professional issues, particularly with the doctors, nurses and teachers who formed the sample of adults in the study. While the number of adult respondents was small (24 adults), it is important to point out that not only were the adult group part of a main study but also that the research was qualitative by nature of its originality, with its emphasis on exploratory procedures rather than the formulation of generalizations. Further, the author takes a philosophical stance in that research of this nature not only allows for further exploratory research to be carried out at a future date and therefore lays down a foundational framework in which to proceed, but it also contributes to the body of knowledge that will expand levels of understanding of perceptions of ourselves as professionals.

Specific attention was paid to two aspects: (a) the criteria for person/non-person distinctions, including temporal phases in personhood: namely the nature of origins (i.e. birth) and cessation (i.e. death); and (b) the content of persons and the meaning of person predicates: for example, features of the mind (i.e. consciousness, rationality, self-reflection and, to some extent, emotion).

The major form of collecting data was the semi-structured interview, although other methods such as a semantic differential rating scale were used as support. The transcribed interviews were subjected to a detailed content analysis from which categories were devised and ordered into frequency response tables. This was to give an overview of the similarities and differences in responses to the conceptions of the nature of persons held within and between groups., A clustan computer format yielded a cluster analysis on the two areas of person/non-person distinctions and content and features applied to persons.

Given the framework of both philosophical aspects inherent in the conceptualization of the nature of persons and the initial lack of previous research, it was thought desirable that the investigation should explore aspects of person conceptions initially from a cognitive developmental point of view, particularly with the children and adolescents, and from an ethical and educational point of view with the adult group. The latter exploratory study will be the focus of this final section. The author felt that expressing views on the conceptions of the nature of persons demanded a more personal approach and the semi-structured interview was seen as appropriate. While it was recognized that there were several disadvantages relating to interviews (such as the limit on the number of respondents, sources of error relating to the interviewer, the instrument itself and overall reliability and validity), these factors can be and were partially overcome by minimizing subjectivity and bias from the interviewer, respondent and the substantive content of the questions. As Valentine (1982) remarks, the problems raised by taking introspective reports are no more serious than the problems raised by other methods. In fact, no one method of collecting data guarantees certainty.

Doctors', nurses' and teachers' conceptions of the nature of persons

Generally, from a philosophical standpoint younger children in the main study did not differentiate between the two terms 'human' and 'person'. The term 'human', as Teichman suggested, was therefore used as a starting point for the acquisition of a concept of the person. However, the older groups, including the adults, showed a more qualitative distinction between persons and non-persons utilizing more rational constructs in their conceptions, and variations in the conceptions were evident.

Persons and non-person distinctions

The general hypotheses from the main study concerned cognitive developmental psychology. Nevertheless, certain important areas implicit within the hypotheses relate closely to concerns for doctors, nurses and teachers. The research involved representations or images of the person and attempted to tease out construals in this conceptual field that are often taken for granted within the healthcare domains.

Through the process of growing older, the individual may have more variable experience, be influenced by the learning environment and therefore become less bound by context. The adult group's conceptions of persons, particularly in the distinctions between persons and non-persons, not only use more abstract and inferential constructs but also approximate towards a more ideal/formal model of the person.

The doctors, nurses and teachers highlighted the fact that abstract features should be attributed to persons. This sort of concept acquisition can be dependent on their own experiences, which are more variable, and therefore influenced by the learning environment. It was apparent that the adult group used more psychological attributes to distinguish between persons and non-persons.

The doctors, nurses and teachers emphasized that the beginnings of persons (i.e. origins) were variable, although an innate potentiality for persons (before birth) had a preference overall. This could cause some confusion in relation to abortion and embryonic research. There was also a divided preference for views of the ending of persons in constructs for finite and infinite lifespans relating to the conceptions of death of persons.

There is obvious variation in response to the adults for divided preferences, like birth and pre-birth categories, which may reflect aspects of variation in interpretation and individual experiences.

Features and content of persons

The doctors, nurses and teachers show variation in their conceptions of the nature of mind. The variations indicate experience and individual preferences, although overall they show a preference for dualistic conceptions (mind being non-material and body being material). However, the doctors in particular show a preference for the mind conceived as brain, mind as aspects of the brain and mind as sum of parts. These constructs may be influenced by their education and training and indicate a sophisticated monistic and materialistic viewpoint. The adult group particularly reflected Dennett's (1979) ideal type of model in that there was a high response to features of rationality, consciousness and self-awareness, treated as a person and symbolic language.

Teichman (1985) remarks that an attempted analysis of the concept of the person cannot be taken for granted in that it will to some extent be guided by ordinary use. However, particularly in relation to content, the doctors, nurses and teachers did not necessarily adhere to this view. The group had a tendency to approximate towards an ideal/formal model for features and content attributed to persons. Teichman suggests that it is usually only philosophy students who add features such as self-consciousness and rationality to persons. The highly selected sample of adults were chosen from the professional fields of medicine, nursing and teaching. Therefore to some extent their conceptions may have been influenced by their education and training. This in turn may highlight the Western traditional philosophy that influences formal higher education.

There was little use of the ethical or moral model of the conceptions of the nature of persons within the adult group. The moral view not only relates to viewing the person as a non-biological term but also demands some thinking in ethical terms. Further, in professional life the doctors, nurses and teachers must utilize this rather abstract and moral viewpoint. This emphasizes the importance of an ethical curriculum for the professionals.

More knowledge is explored in thinking about the self and others, utilizing as a starting point the discussion of the three tentative models within a new curriculum. In doing this, more direction is given to how we may behave and treat others. Underpinning this is also the basic tenet of Wittgenstein in that meaning is within use. In other words, how we use a particular term like 'person' will reflect the meaning we give to it. There is a need to consolidate some of our thinking about the nature of persons because of the moral and social issues involved in the practice of healthcare and the essential central concern for respect for persons.

ETHICAL AND EDUCATIONAL ISSUES

Obviously the conceptions of the nature of persons have more than one interpretation. For instance, on the one hand it may mean that each person is rational and self-conscious; on the other hand, each individual can be ascribed person status on the understanding that neither logic nor language will solve the problem for us as to who should or should not be counted as a person. The first interpretation relates to attributing features to each individual, and the doctors, nurses and teachers had a tendency to do this. In some ways it is restrictive and not useful for moral or social issues. The moral and social aspects are involved in how we view others in the world and in the decisions and actions we take. The second interpretation is more open and can be linked to the commonsense model and will also involve as a consequence respect for persons. What is important through education is to sort out some of the confusions that arise in ascribing person status to ourselves and others who we care for and the moral issues involved in treatment of non-persons as well as persons who share our world. It seems that there are no clear natural dividing lines between some non-persons and persons – for example the six-month-old fetus. While it would be silly to give votes to oysters, just as it would be silly to call them persons, it is the borderline cases that cause us problems (Russell, 1974). Perhaps it is worth noting that the commonsense model gets out of. the tricky position of distinguishing between ourselves and other animals by referring to a human identifiable shape or differences in forms of life (e.g. if a lion could speak we would not understand him). The formal or ideal feature list could exclude other animals by not attributing major person features to them such as intentions or self-consciousness. However, this is rather a dangerous form of application because the feature list is open-ended and ought not to be applied in absolute terms. The moral/evaluative model makes it possible to ascribe the term 'person' to non-humans, perhaps including other animals that share our world. If it is meaningful then it is possible to have non-human persons. However, there are contradictions within and between these selective models.

In examining the conceptions of the nature of persons for this particular group of doctors, nurses and teachers, several questions arise in relation to the ethics of care. Does the distinction between persons and non-persons depend on whether the term 'person' is meaningfully applicable or not? The fetus is human and a potential member of a rational species, a potential person: but is it a person? (Rational species is different from biological membership: see Teichman, 1985). Can it be inferred that the severely defective infant, the madly insane, the confused elderly individual and the individual on a life-support system are in some way exempt from some very important elements of personhood? These are important questions to ask when considering the perspectives which nurses have about the individual in their care. Consider the situation within an intensive care unit where a young person has an intact brain stem but the upper parts of the brain have been irrevocably traumatized. This presents a position where the major physical functions of heartbeat, breathing and excretion can be maintained because the brain stem has remained viable. However, because the upper part of the brain is severely damaged it means that cognitive processes such as thoughts, feelings and emotions may no longer be expressed. This situation can cause a great deal of anxiety not just for nurses but also for relatives.

Historically, death was signified by the stopping of the heart and the eventual putrefaction of the body. There is no such definitive process today. Consider the position of relatives who can see monitors which record heartbeat and breathing. Further, the body is still warm to touch and the individual's cheeks may have colour in them. All these traits illustrate the presence of life. Despite this fact, the relative will never again experience those special elements expressed by their loved one which made them unique as a person. They will never hear laughter, share a joke or experience the joy or pain of a relationship which has been such an important part of living.

This is not an abstract scenario; it is something which nurses may often have to face. It is therefore important that we examine the various threads involved in understanding personhood. Is the young patient with brain damage still a person, despite losing the facility to express important cognitive elements so central to personhood? There can be no doubt that an intact brain stem will maintain bodily functions, but we have to ask whether or not there is more to being a person than merely having a biological realm? Respect ought to be attributed to the young person by the nurses and therefore a moral definition of personhood is maintained. Further, the relatives may clearly attribute personhood to their loved one simply because it is meaningful to do so, in that they have known and experienced a relationship with them. All these issues graphically illustrate the importance of examining our understanding of personhood in the light of everyday nursing practice. This is why ethical and philosophical analysis needs to play a central role in the education process for health professionals.

Part of the ethical curriculum for doctors, nurses and teachers should include the exploration and discussion of the conceptions of the nature of persons. Downie and Telfer (1980) point out that natural science explanations of the world are based on conceptions of things. However, within the healthcare domains it is essential to explore forms of knowledge more appropriately matched to conceptions of care and subsequently persons. Persons are not things unless we choose to avoid giving them person status (as in Nazi Germany). Reflecting on the new forms of knowledge needed in the professionals' curriculum may encourage a more healthy respect that can enhance the care and treatment of persons in the healthcare system.

GLOSSARY

Cognitive Relating to the faculty of knowing and perceiving things.

Consciousness The mind's capacity to reflect upon itself. It is analogous with the psychological concept of perception.

Dualistic In philosophical terms this usually relates to the notion that the mind and the body are to be viewed as two separate entities. The philosopher who is thought to have first developed this theme was René Descartes.

Empirical Developing and reinforcing knowledge through observation and experiment.

Monistic This is the complete opposite of dualism; it holds the basic tenet that minds and bodies do not differ in their intrinsic nature. This ties in with contemporary ideas concerning holism.

Person Beings who are capable of making choices and then acting upon those decisions. Persons also possess a reflective awareness usually referred to as 'self-consciousness'.

Rationality Possessing the ability to reason.

Semantic differential A research tool which analyses the different meanings and interpretations that language may hold.

Sentient The ability to sense and feel the world around us.

REFERENCES

Abelson, R. (1977) *Persons: A Study in Philosophical Psychology*, Macmillan, London.

Dennett, D. (1979) *Brainstorms*, Harvester Press, Sussex.

Downie, R. and Telfer, E. (1986) *Caring and Curing*, Methuen, London.

Hampshire, S. (1959) *Thought and Action*, Chatto & Windus, London.

Harris, J. (1985) *The Value of Life*, Routledge & Kegan Paul, London.

Henry, I.C. (1986) The conceptions of the nature of persons amongst children, adolescents and adults, Unpublished PhD thesis, Leeds University.

Midgley, M. (1983) *Animals and Why They Matter: A Journey Around the Species Barrier*, Penguin, Harmondsworth.

Russell, B. (1974) *History of Western Philosophy*, Allen & Unwin, London.

Shoemaker, R. and Swinbourne, S. (1984) *Personal Identity*, Basil Blackwell, Oxford.

Strawson, P.F. (1959) *Individuals*, Methuen, London.

Teichman, J. (1972) Wittgenstein on persons and human beings, In *Understanding Wittgenstein*, Royal Institute of Philosophy Lectures, London, pp. 133–48, Macmillan.

Teichman, J. (1985) The definition of person. *Journal of the Royal Institute of Philosophy*, **60**, 175–85.

Valentine, E. (1982) *Conceptual Issues in Psychology*, Allen & Unwin, London.

4 | Professional conceptions of mental illness and related issues

Glenys Pashley

Psychiatric health professionals are generally in the position of having to treat and care for persons who have been labelled as mentally ill. For this reason it was thought useful to examine just how such professionals conceive of the term 'mental illness'. The term is difficult to define, perhaps even unanalysable. The boundaries of mental illness are a persistent point of debate: it is seen as a myth, as being analogous to physical illness or disease, as maladaptive behaviour, as the result of incongruent thoughts and beliefs or conflicting unconscious desires, as a divided self-concept or as a complex social product that has ultimately formed the basis for psychiatry. Underlying such criteria there seems to be a preconception of what the person is. Indeed, different theories make different assumptions about the person which, in turn, lead to different perspectives of mental illness.

The knowledge base underpinning and supporting the concept of mental illness is not one of a single image but of a range of complex, ambiguous and often incommensurable fragments of knowledge drawn from history, philosophy, science, psychiatry, psychology, sociology and the law. It is not surprising then that confusion and disagreement reign regarding what is to count as mental illness and that the boundaries of mental illness are inexact. In order to arrive at a clearer understanding of the term 'mental illness', a multidisciplinary perspective is demanded which takes into account not only the fragmented, formal and descriptive knowledge base, but also the idiosyncratic and shared commonsense knowledge that individual psychiatric health professionals bring to their role. Central to this commonsense aspect will be the person's beliefs, attitudes and values, the influence of the social context, the meaning and use of language and experience in a social world which necessarily contributes to the person's individual ways of perceiving and under-standing. Indeed, Szasz, as cited by Bentall and Pilgrim (1993), has drawn to our attention the psychiatric prejudice underlying the causes of mental illness and the role of values in psychiatric decision-making.

To explore how a number of psychiatric health professionals conceived of mental illness, 25 psychiatric nurses and ten psychiatric nurse tutors completed a Semantic Differential Scaling Booklet and an open-ended interview.

THE SEMANTIC DIFFERENTIAL

The Semantic Differential (S/D) consisted of 11 bipolar adjectives which respondents had to apply to three different types of individuals. The bipolar adjectives focused on the following terms: personhood status, bad, feelings, intelligent, punishment, responsible, good, treatment, rational, sane and therapy. The types of individuals were: a mentally ill individual, a schizophrenic individual and an individual with a destruc-tive personality. The S/D was constructed on the basis of a five-point scale. The raw score of 1 was taken to mean that respondents thought, say, the mentally ill individual was rational, a score of 2 would indicate that such an individual was probably rational, a score of 4 was taken to suggest that a mentally ill individual was probably not rational and a score of 5 was taken to mean that such an individual was thought to be definitely not rational. Where respondents had a raw score of 3 this was interpreted that they were unsure, simply did not know or wanted to say it would depend on other influencing factors. For discussion purposes, the respondents were separated into four groups: male nurses (12), female nurses (13), male tutors (7) and female tutors (3). The findings from the S/D could have been quantitatively and statistically analysed but it was thought, given the abstract and complex nature of the concepts and terms involved, that a more meaningful understanding would be gained through a qualitative and interprative approach. Therefore, a rather broad, global and generalized interpretation of the response was made.

The mentally ill individual

The mentally ill individual was attributed with full personhood status and was seen as definitely having feelings. They were generally perceived to be good rather than bad. It is important to note, however, that these terms presented a degree of difficulty for some respondents; for example, 12 respondents could not decide whether this type of individual was bad or not and 27 respondents could not judge whether they were good or not. It is likely that these respondents who were more cautious with their judgments and generalizations wanted to say it would depend on other factors and circumstances. These other influential factors may relate to the professional's own experience, in the sense that they have found mentally ill individuals to be bad at times and good at other times. An interesting point which emphasizes the ambiguity in meaning and use of language is that the term 'bad' is not always seen as the opposite of 'good'; for example, 19 respondents conceived of the mentally ill individual as being definitely not bad, but only four respondents thought this type of individual to be definitely good. Interestingly, it was the male and female nurses rather than the tutors who were the most reluctant and cautious in judging the terms 'good' and 'bad'. This relates, perhaps, to the fact that these professionals have the most direct contact with mentally ill individuals and are, therefore, in a position of constantly interacting with individuals who may behave in a good and/or bad manner. However, the meaning and use of language here is important; what one nurse or tutor may mean by the terms 'good' and 'bad' behaviour may not have the same meaning for another nurse or tutor. Further, the meaning that individual respondents attach to such terms will be influenced by beliefs, attitudes, values and the social context in which the behaviour occurs and experience. The S/D does not specify the meaning or use for respondents; it rests with each individual to create their own meaning and use, given the context the S/D provides. Such attributed meaning and use will probably change in the new context of the interview situation where respondents can discuss their ideas in more depth and introduce their own influential circumstances.

The feature of intelligence as applied to the mentally ill individual reflected another problem area for respondents. Although 20 respondents viewed this type of individual to be intelligent or probably intelligent, 15 felt unable to judge and recorded a raw score of 3. This level of indecision may be a consequence of the concept of intelligence itself being controversial and dependent on several other cognitive processes for a clearer understanding: for example, thought, memory and problem-solving. The female nurses were particularly cautious in attributing this feature to the mentally ill individual.

The features of rationality and sanity were difficult for respondents to judge. No respondents conceived of this type of individual to be completely rational and sane, or completely not rational and not sane; the majority recorded a raw score of 3. The concepts of rationality and sanity are complex, not only in terms of their meaning and interpretation but also in the sense that recognition rests on subjective inferences, values, beliefs, attitudes, commonsense and more formal knowledge and experience. The *Concise Oxford Dictionary* (1987) defines rational as being 'endowed with reason, reasoning; sensible, sane, moderate, not foolish or absurd or extreme'. However, Berenson (1981) remarks that a misguided dichotomy exists between what is to count as rational and irrational, and that the dichotomy has its roots in a belief that what is rational involves logical thought and what is irrational entails illogical emotion. It is likely that respondents judging the features of rationality and sanity as they understand them applying to the mentally ill individual have in mind the notion of thought disorder. What is important to remember is that thought processes are unobservable and can only be inferred from an individual's actual behaviour. The questions arise: is thought accurately reflected in behaviour? and are the observers of that behaviour correct in their interpretation? This is where the centrality of the meaning and use of language, experience and commonsense knowledge can influence our judgments about others.

The attribution of responsibility to the mentally ill individual, like the feature of being rational and sane or not, was a difficult area for respondents to assess. Generally speaking, the majority of respondents recorded a raw score of 3, suggesting that they could not decide because it was seen to be dependent on other factors. The mentally ill individual was thought of as not deserving to be punished; rather, they should be medically treated or receive some form of psychological therapy. There was a preference by all groups in favour of therapy over and above any type of medically oriented treatment.

The schizophrenic individual

The schizophrenic individual was attributed with full personhood status by all individual respondents, except one male nurse. It is difficult to offer any explanation for this viewpoint; perhaps at best it can be assumed that his experience of individuals who have been labelled schizophrenic has left some lasting impressions and doubts as to the nature of their being. The schizophrenic individual, like the mentally ill individual, was definitely thought to have feelings. Similarly, the schizophrenic individual generated problems for respondents when faced with attributing the feature of intelligence. Although 22 respondents viewed this type of individual as intelligent or probably intelligent, 13 were unable to decide and, therefore, recorded a raw score of 3. The schizophrenic individual, like the mentally ill individual, was generally seen to be good rather than bad. However, there was a broad agreement among all groups of respondents that the schizophrenic individual is slightly less bad and slightly more good than the mentally ill individual.

The schizophrenic individual was generally conceived to be less rational and less sane than the mentally ill individual. Indeed, three respondents viewed the schizophrenic individual as being totally not rational, whereas no respondents had seen the mentally ill individual to be completely not rational. The assumption can be made that respondents may have seen the schizophrenic individual to be less rational and sane because of their professional knowledge of the characteristics often held to be typical of schizophrenia: for example, thought disorder, delusions, hallucinations and withdrawal from reality. These characteristics, to some extent, can all be associated with the terms 'rationality' and 'sanity'. However, these terms presented a problem for respondents to attribute to the schizophrenic individual; the majority were unsure or felt it would be dependent on other factors.

The feature of responsibility as attributed to the schizophrenic individual was virtually identical to the degree of responsibility levied at the mentally ill individual; in fact, for both types of individuals, 21 respondents recorded a raw score of 3, thus reflecting their difficulty in attributing this feature generally. On a commonsense level this seems consistent, since within the meaning of the terms 'schizophrenic' and 'mental illness' there is much room for overlap. However, given that respondents had claimed the schizophrenic individual to be slightly less rational and sane than the mentally ill individual, it could have been anticipated that the schizophrenic individual would be thought to be relatively less responsible, assuming that respondents hold individuals to be responsible on the basis of how rational and sane they are. This was not the case. The majority of respondents did not judge the schizophrenic individual to be less responsible; in fact, the male tutors perceived this type of individual to be more responsible than the mentally ill individual. It is difficult to explain this conception on the basis of the completed S/D, which leaves respondents no room for self-explanation. Hence the need for the interview, which allowed respondents to discuss these issues in more depth.

Punishment was generally seen to be slightly less appropriate for the schizophrenic individual than for the mentally ill individual, if, indeed, it was thought appropriate at all. Just as therapy was deemed to be slightly more suitable for the mentally ill individual, treatment was thought to be slightly more suitable for the schizophrenic individual. This fits with the theoretical belief that schizophrenia is a physical illness or dysfunction which can be treated by physical means. The female nurses were the one group who readily reflected this view, while the male nurses and male and female tutors appeared to see more value in both treatment and therapy.

The individual with a personality disorder

The individual with a personality disorder, like the schizophrenic individual, was attributed with full personhood status by all the respondents except for one female tutor who found she could not judge this feature. The feature of feelings did, to a limited extent, differentiate the individual with a personality disorder from the other two types of individuals.

Generally speaking, this type of individual was seen to have fewer feelings than either the mentally ill or the schizophrenic individual.

However, given that individuals with a personality disorder are usually thought to display more heightened and intense feelings than, say, a mentally ill individual, there seems to be an element of inconsistency. Perhaps one possible but tentative explanation for this may relate to the way in which respondents interpret the term feelings. The feelings often associated with personality disorders are: disturbed, violent, self-destructive, impulsive and restless. The feelings often associated with mental illness are: depression, void of emotion and an inability to express emotions. This could be seen to reflect a 'hard' and 'soft' categorization of feelings; the implication being that the individual with a personality disorder is thought by the respondents to have less soft feelings, rather than less feelings *per se*.

The concept of intelligence appeared to be another feature that differentiated the individual with a personality disorder from the mentally ill and the schizophrenic individual. Respondents generally viewed this type of individual to be less intelligent, or found it difficult to attribute any degree of intelligence than they did for either of the other two types of individuals. Respondents also found great difficulty in attributing the features of bad and/or good to the individual with a personality disorder, although the general tendency was to perceive this individual as bad rather than not bad, and as not good rather than good. In effect, this type of individual was thought to be more bad and less good than either the mentally ill or the schizophrenic individual.

The features of rationality and sanity as they were applied to the individual with a personality disorder presented respondents with some difficulty. The general opinion, however, was that this type of individual was more rational and sane than either the mentally ill or the schizophrenic individual. Given this broad trend it follows that respondents might see this type of individual as being more responsible than either of the other two types of individuals. This viewpoint was supported by the respondents in the sense that the majority perceived this type of individual to be responsible or probably responsible for their behaviour. Most respondents were in some doubt as to whether the individual with a personality disorder should be punished, although punishment was generally thought to be more appropriate for this type of individual than it was for either the mentally ill or the schizophrenic individual.

Medical treatment for the individual with a personality disorder was seen to be far less suitable than it was for the mentally ill or the schizophrenic individual. However, the range of scores was diverse, reflecting that respondents had mixed feelings about this issue. Conversely, psychological therapy was seen to be far more suitable for this type of individual than medical treatment. Both the male and the female nurses strongly supported this view, unlike the male and female tutors who thought it to be less appropriate. One possible explanation here is that the nurses, who are constantly using therapy in their everyday work experience, may appreciate its value for a range of different types of individuals far more than do the tutors, who do not have the same and current level of practice and experiential knowledge.

Much of the meaning that respondents had in mind when completing the S/D remains untapped because of the way in which respondents are limited by the research tool itself; it is somewhat mechanistic in the sense that respondents simply tick a box representing the numbers 1 to 5 in order to indicate their viewpoint. This allows the respondents no room for explaining why they put their tick where they did. However, as an introductory research methodology it has proved most useful and identified several important factors regarding conceptions of mental illness. It expects respondents to make value judgments regarding the attribution of features or properties to different types of individuals. Some respondents appeared to do this with relative ease whereas other respondents were more cautious with their judgments. How easy or cautious respondents are is likely to be influenced by professional knowledge and experience, social, cultural and personal beliefs, attitudes and opinions. The attribution of features to the different types of individuals very much relies on experience; for example, a psychiatric nurse working in a regional secure unit is likely to have experienced 'bad' behaviour by mentally ill individuals or individuals with a personality disorder to a greater extent than psychiatric nurses working on a ward where patients are being rehabilitated for transition into the community. The notion of experience also involves commonsense knowledge; for example, some respondents may not have had direct contact with or have any formal knowledge of personality disorders, but still have a conception of what for them represents an individual with a personality disorder. On the basis of this common sense knowledge, respondents make value judgments and attribute features. However, respondents who scored 3 on the S/D may well not have been prepared to make such value judgments because there are so many unknown influential factors.

A final and important point to note is that the attribution of particular features to the different types of individuals reflects that a sliding scale appeared to be in operation. For example, the individual with a personality disorder was seen to be more bad, to have fewer feelings, to be less intelligent, and to be more rational, sane and responsible than either the mentally ill or the schizophrenic individual. However, it is worth reiterating that many respondents were unsure about several of these features, essentially because of the complexity of such terms.

The S/D was used as a research tool for simply introducing respondents to the broad and particular concepts perceived by the researcher as being relevant to the term 'mental illness'. It was seen as a means eliciting the subjective and initial responses to such ideas, as a way of discovering in broad and general terms any possible areas of uncertainty, confusion, similarity and difference, and where more in-depth discussion was required. The open-ended interview certainly enhanced this in-depth discussion and also allowed the respondents to introduce their own ideas and concepts and the issues which they felt were central to the term 'mental illness'. The amount and richness of information generated by the interview was extensive, and it is only possible within this chapter to focus selectively on particular terms, concepts and issues that complement some of the broad generalizations derived from the S/D.

THE INTERVIEW

All 35 respondents participated in an in-depth interview which was tape-recorded and later transcribed. A post-coded classification system was developed in order to enhance the qualitative interpretation and understanding of conceptions of mental illness and related issues. As James (1977) remarks, a qualitative interpretation provides 'perspective, insight and understandable decryption'. The information that emerged from the respondents' statements was interpreted on the basis of four themes incorporating 27 categories and sub-categories.

Theme 1 Broad conceptions of mental illness, was concerned with how respondents viewed three major aspects of the concept of mental illness, namely, the causes of mental illness, the social influences upon becoming mentally ill and the broad, loosely defined features that generally distinguish a mentally ill individual. The following eight 'A' categories comprise this first theme:

A1 Physical causes;
A2 Multiplicity of causes;
A3 Defined by society/culture;
A4 Involves the labelling process;
A5 Effects of institutionalization;
A6 Behavioural problems;
A7 Disorders of thinking;
A8 Emotional problems.

Theme 2 Psychological features of the mentally ill individual, was more specific with regard to the physical and psychological features of mental illness. It was concerned with respondents' conceptions of how mentally ill individuals think, feel and behave and, given these perceived features, whether this type of individual ought to be held responsible for this behaviour or not. The following ten 'B' categories represent this second theme:

B 1   Odd/bizarre behaviour;
B 1.1 Lack of coping skills;
B1.2 Difficulties in communicating;
B 2   Degree of rationality dependent on severity of illness;
B2.1 Lack of insight/awareness;
B2.2 Mentally ill people see themselves as rational;
B 3   Extreme/exaggerated/inappropriate emotions;
B3.1 Emotional thought disorder;
B 4   Degree of responsibility dependent on severity of illness;
B4.1 Degree of responsibility dependent on degree of rationality.

Theme 3 Treatment for the mentally ill individual, focused on the issue of how such an individual ought to be treated and cared for, and was composed of the following four 'C' categories:

C 1   Drugs overprescribed;
C 1.1 Drugs as a means of control/suppress symptoms/mask causes;
C 1.2 Drugs supportive to therapy/multidisciplinary approach;
C 2   Use of psychological therapies only.

Theme 4 Punishment for the mentally ill individual, concerned whether or not punishment is an appropriate course of action to be taken against this type of individual. The following five 'D' categories represent this fourth theme:

D 1 Punishment dependent on degree of responsibility;
D 2 Punishment dependent on degree of rationality;
D 3 Should be punished like any other offender;
D 4 Punishment not seen as beneficial to any mentally ill individual;
D 5 Other labels used for punishment.

It is worth noting that a small number of respondents supported a medical perspective of mental illness in the sense that the cause of mental illness/schizophrenia was seen to be physical (A1), and that behavioural problems (A6) and disorders of thinking (A7) could be controlled through the use of drugs, a physical form of treatment. For example, one psychiatric nurse tutor remarked, 'Psychotic illnesses are much more organically based' and a psychiatric nurse claimed, 'I think you need drugs if the symptoms are very bad to get the person to a state where you can work therapeutically. You need to suppress the physical symptoms.'

There are two points in particular worthy of mention here. First, there are sound ethical reasons for using drugs if they can break the cycle of stress or depression for the person. Second, there are less sound reasons for using drugs if they are used to control and manipulate the person so that they are in a state whereby the health practitioner can work therapeutically. There seems to be an underlying assumption that if the person's symptoms are masked or suppressed, then the real self or person becomes available for therapy. The use of drugs may have effects which health professionals are unaware of and, therefore, the real self or person may likewise be suppressed due to the effects of drugs; hence, therapy may be of little value either before or after treatment.

Those respondents who supported a medical/physical perspective of mental illness/schizophrenia tended to equate the mind with the brain and to use the two terms interchangeably. Rose (1987) would corroborate this unity of the two terms 'mind' and 'brain' and advocate that any event or activity which can be described in biological brain language must also have a description in psychological mind language. However, there is an important way in which the languages of the mind and brain are incommensurable; the information content of a person's speech does not translate into statements about molecules or cells, even though both speech and molecules are aspects of the same unitary phenomenon. Speech carries sets of meanings which are influenced by social, cultural, economic, religious and experiential factors, and which are not reducible to biological parts. Further, conceptions of mental illness involve conceptions of what is normal; norms are not biologically based, they entail interpersonal agreement, shared meanings, assumptions, beliefs and evaluative judgments about what is acceptable behaviour and acceptable ways of thinking in different societies and cultures.

A number of respondents conceived of mental illness/schizophrenia as being defined by society (A3), as involving the effects of labelling (A4 and A5), that difficulties in interpersonal communication prevail (B1.2) and that the causes of mental illness can include a multitude of social as well as biological and psychological factors (A2). There is a sense in which some respondents adopted an eclectic perspective of mental illness because all aspects of an individual's experience were held to be possible causes of mental illness/schizophrenia. However, implicit within the eclectic perspective is a strong emphasis on social viewpoint which argues that mental illness is socially constructed, that the meaning and use of language are important and that the wider social influences are contributory factors. The social perspective also reminds us that all symptoms and behaviour have to be considered as taking place within a social context; it is here the boundary between what is normal and abnormal is determined. For Bentall and Pilgrim (1993) the causes of variation in abnormal behaviour are multiple 'and include biological, personal and social variables, but judgments about how these variations are to be evaluated are always socially negotiated and may vary across time and place'.

Some respondents conceived of mental illness/schizophrenia very much in behavioural terms (A6) and supported the notion of odd behaviour (B1), lack of coping skills (B1.1) and difficulties in communication (B1.2) as features of mental illness which can, perhaps, be treated through behavioural therapy. For example, a psychiatric nurse remarked, 'The main difference is in the way the behaviour manifests itself … it's usually more unpredictable, it can't be defined in normal terms'. The emphasis here seems to rest on the actions of the individual; either they are appropriate, acceptable and conform to society's expectations and norms or they do not. If the actions of the individual are not socially acceptable, this raises the question of whether they ought to be changed and, if change is recommended, then ought this to be brought about through treatment, therapy and/or punishment? Further, who decides that a change in behaviour is necessary? For some respondents, punishment can serve to change behaviour into something more socially acceptable and/or make the individual realize they have done something wrong (D3). According to a psychiatric nurse, 'Occasionally if you get a very undesirable behaviour and you want to stop it or change it, then punishment can have that effect.' Another psychiatric nurse claimed, 'Punishment is the only thing that makes them realize they are doing wrong. Trying to reason with them doesn't always work.' The respondents who supported the idea that the mentally ill/schizophrenic individual is not always rational and responsible, and yet would advocate some form of punishment in order to make the individual more aware that they have done something wrong, are reflecting a degree of inconsistency and confusion. The problem with this type of reasoning is that, if the mentally ill/schizophrenic individual is not rational, is experiencing disorder of thinking or believes him/herself to be rational and right and that everyone else is irrational and wrong, then is there any purpose in punishing that individual? In other words, will he/she understand and accept the reasons for punishment in the same way that the administrator of the punishment accepts and advocates it?

A number of respondents used alternative labels for what other individuals might construe as falling under the general heading of punishment (D5). As one psychiatric nurse remarked, 'I wouldn't call it punishment. We do implement Policy 20 in this hospital which is seclusion for the patient. It's not punishment because I don't think you should punish the mentally ill person.' A second psychiatric nurse commented, 'Very rarely would I advocate punishment. I would rather advocate extinction, negative reinforcement or denial.' It is evident that the meaning and use of language are central to the interpretation of the term 'punishment'.

For some respondents, punishment for the mentally ill/schizophrenic individual was seen to be dependent on whether he/she is responsible for his/her own actions (D1). As one psychiatric nurse tutor remarked, 'If a person is responsible for their behaviour then they should be punished ... If they are rational I believe they are responsible, and if they are responsible they should be punished.' The different perspectives of the appropriateness of punishment emphasize the complexity of the term, and to enhance any understanding of its application to the mentally ill/schizophrenic individual, then other complex terms and conditions need to be considered: for example, rationality and responsibility.

Interestingly, disorders of thinking (A7) were seen to be a central distinguishing feature of mental illness. According to one psychiatric nurse, 'Mental illness is some sort of malfunction of the thought processes.' A psychiatric nurse tutor remarked, 'I think rational thinking is a problem area ... they perceive life differently, understand and relate differently to the world around them.' In most cases, respondents had in mind schizophrenia when referring to thought disorder. However, to use the term 'thought disorder' only makes sense if respondents acknowledge a subjective and inferential basis, because thought is disordered it cannot be observed; nor does it follow that thought is disordered simply because speech is disordered. Further, it would have been more consistent had those respondents who supported a physical cause of mental illness/ schizophrenia spoken of neutral disorder rather than thought disorder, which would then match a descriptive and causal perspective of mental illness. For Szasz (1993) the only evidence that mental illness, in particular schizophrenia, is a genuine illness is that fact that people 'talk crazy'. Szasz prefers this expression in favour of thought disorder because the latter implies the observer or listener can know how or what the other individual is thinking. He points out that if an alteration of speech is to be interpreted as an alteration in thought, then we might as well conclude that individuals who 'hear things' suffer from some kind of auditory disorder, and that those individuals who 'see things' suffer from some kind of visual disorder.

The idea that the degree of rationality is dependent on the severity of the illness (B2) was strongly supported by the respondents. For example, a psychiatric nurse tutor commented, 'It depends on the type of the mental illness; for instance, with a neurotic type of illness such as acute anxiety the person will be rational, but if schizophrenia or a depressive illness is the problem then that person may not be as rational.' A psychiatric nurse remarked, 'With depression, the person is absolutely rational but totally lacking in emotion. With schizophrenics, they are very emotional and at times very irrational.' Two important points emerge from these kinds of claims about rationality. First, it could be argued that the type and severity of the mental illness may be dependent on or influenced by the degree of rationality. In other words, the question arises, does diminished rationality cause mental illness or does mental illness cause diminished rationality? Second, the idea that rationality and the emotions are separate appears to be implicit within many of the respondents' comments; few respondents actually acknowledged category B3.1, emotional thought disorder. It is important that the interrelationship between thought and emotion is recognized in order to enhance the understanding of mental illness. As Schacter (1971) suggests, the quality of the emotions depends on how the external world and the internal state of the person are cognitively interpreted. Similarly, Mandler (1975) supports the notion that emotions are influenced by the cognitive evaluation or 'meaning analysis' of the current state of affairs.

The suggestion that emotional problems (A8) are a distinguishing feature of mental illness was strongly supported by the respondents. Further, many respondents were more specific and referred to extreme, exaggerated and inappropriate emotions (B3) as being a feature of mental illness. Indeed, one psychiatric nurse believed that mental illness should really be referred to as 'emotional illness'. The strong support for this category and the lack of support for emotional thought disorder (B3.1) re-emphasize the necessity for psychiatric health professionals to become more familiar with the relationship between thought and emotion, and to recognize that the individual must have thought about or been cognitively aware of the circumstances or events that stimulated an emotional reaction.

There seems to be a complex interplay between rationality, the type and severity of the mental illness and responsibility. A large number of respondents held that the degree of responsibility was dependent on either the severity of the mental illness (B4) or the degree of rationality (B4.1). For example, a psychiatric nurse tutor thought, 'Schizophrenics are probably not responsible most of the time, whereas with a neurotic illness the person would be responsible for quite a lot of the time.' A second psychiatric nurse tutor remarked, 'If people are thinking logically they are responsible really.' This complex interplay of terms and their meanings is further complicated by the emotions; consequently, what becomes difficult to discern is to what extent each of these factors influences the other. In other words, to what extent do the severity of the mental illness, the degree of rationality and the emotional state interact with each other and, in turn, influence decisions about responsibility and punishment? The terms 'free will' and 'determinism' are often used to enhance the understanding of responsibility. For example, if a person is determined or influenced by external factors to behave in particular ways then they are not usually held responsible. Conversely, if a person is behaving on the basis of free will and is exercising choice and making decisions, then he/she is usually held to be more responsible. The question arises, how responsible is the person if he/she is acting freely but on the grounds of disturbed thoughts and/or emotions?

When respondents were asked about their conceptions of personality disorders, two main links were made: either a personality disorder was seen as a form of mental illness, or personality disorders conjured the idea of an 'evil' individual. it is not the intention here to discuss respondents' conceptions of evil but, when probing questions were asked of the respondents, more questions and confusion were generated. It seemed to be the case that respondents had little knowledge about personality disorders, hence their uncertainty about the meaning of the term and its relationship with other terms. It is likely that this lack of knowledge and uncertainty derive from the fact that student psychiatric nurses do not consider personality disorders to any great extent in their professional education, and from the fact that such disorders pose a number of theoretical and practical problems for the legal profession which neither moral philosophers nor psychiatrists can seemingly resolve.

The opportunity was given to respondents to reflect on their own professional education and experience, and to evaluate the curriculum for its appropriateness in understanding the term 'mental illness'. A number of opinions emerged. First, some respondents held that their professional education presented a medical perspective of mental illness with emphasis on a descriptive set of criteria, that is, the signs and symptoms. A medical perspective was thought to be too restrictive and simplistic, to the extent that social and psychological aspects were largely ignored. Such a perspective was deemed neither to match ward experience nor to enhance the relationship between theory and practice. Second, a number of respondents felt that the knowledge base was not sufficiently broad, in-depth or 'academic'. It was not seen to facilitate critical thinking, commonsense or any evaluation of complex concepts such as rationality, responsibility and personality disorders. Further, the specific subject of psychology was thought to be inadequate and to provide no foundation in different psychological approaches, and it was thought that ward experience of 'madness' did not fit with the theoretical psychology of the 'normal'. Third, some respondents perceived experience to be the most important factor in relation to conceptualizing and understanding mental illness.

Professional psychiatric education needs to place far more emphasis on the complex concepts identified as causing confusion, and needs to synthesize commonsense knowledge and experience with more formal theoretical knowledge. This ought to enhance an understanding of mental illness and related issues, and facilitate critical thinking around highly complex interdependent concepts such as rationality, the emotions, responsibility and punishment. Commonsense knowledge is taken to involve the individual's beliefs, attitudes and values, the influence of the social context, the meaning and use of everyday language and experience in a social world. It is evident that the psychiatric health professionals involved in the research utilized commonsense knowledge in order to conceptualize mental illness. One wonders what kind of knowledge these same psychiatric health professionals would have employed to understand the behaviour of the two boys held to be the perpetrators of the killing of James Bulger. For example, would they have deemed the boys to be intelligent, rational, responsible and appropriate for punishment? Or not intelligent, not rational, not responsible and unworthy of treatment and/or therapy? Similarly, would their behaviour have been attributed to external and/or internal factors? How would their emotional state have been interpreted? And to what extent might reference have been made to their moral development or lack of it?

The two boys involved in the killing of James Bulger in Liverpool have been attributed with various characteristics and labels by several professionals, including teachers, journalists, health, social and legal representatives. For example, one of the boys was said to have displayed anti-social and bizarre behaviour; the other was described as a liar, a bully and a truant who demonstrated a determination to avoid guilt and shift responsibility. Both were held to have disturbed childhoods but found to have no abnormality of mind. Further, a claim was made that the release of the boys from their respective secure units will not be based on the notion of punishment served, but on the understanding they have gained, in other words, whether they have become responsible adults. Media coverage of the story described the two boys as 'freaks of nature' and 'born to murder'. Mr Justice Morland was cited as saying the event was 'an act of unparalleled evil and barbarity'. Such an emotive use of language does not enhance understanding but serves only to confuse and fuel public outcry. Indeed, Greer (1993) remarks, '*To characterize something as evil is to refuse to try to understand it.*'

There is little understanding of why the crime did occur. Much information was gleaned about outside influencing factors but nobody really investigated the inner motives, probably because no one really knows where and how to look. This raises the question, is it appropriate to bring to bear an adult understanding to interpret the child's view of the world? For Masters (1994) '*The murder of a child by a child is entirely different in nature and frequency and must be understood apart; it reflects nothing.*' Nevertheless, many opinions were formed as to the moral character of the boys. The boys were held to be operating in a moral vacuum where, perhaps, they were left to create their own rules. According to Masters (1994) '*They were incapable of reaching a reasonable solution and had only their untutored impulses to guide them.*' It has been claimed the children were in fact taught the difference between right and wrong, and that boy boys 'legally' knew what they were doing and knew it to be wrong. However, it could be argued that 'knowing' something to be wrong requires much more than simply cognitive recognition. There needs to be some kind of emotional understanding of what makes an action and its consequences wrong. As Piaget would suggest, moral thinking cannot develop in children before they have developed the ability to reason logically and, prior to arriving at a full understanding of moral principles, children merely associate right and wrong with praise and punishment.

REFERENCES

Bentall, R.P. and Pilgrim, D. (1993) Thomas Szasz, crazy talk and the myth of mental illness. *British Journal of Medical Psychology*, vol. 66, Part 1, pp. 69–76.

Berenson, F.M. (1981) *Understanding Persons*, Harvester Press, Sussex.

Concise Oxford Dictionary (1987) Oxford University Press, Oxford.

Greer, G. (1993) Love, not hate, will heal the tragedy of three small boys, *The Guardian*, 29 November.

James, J. (1977) Ethnography and social problems, in *Street Ethnography* (ed. R.S. Weppner), Sage, California.

Mandler, G. (1975) *Mind and Emotion*, John Wiley, New York.

Masters, B. (1994) Should we throw away the key? *Night & Day*, 13 February.

Rose, S. (1987) *Molecules and Minds*, Open University, Milton Keynes.

Schacter, S. (1971) *Emotion, Obesity and Crime,* Academic Press, New York.

Szasz, T. (1993) Crazy talk: thought disorder or psychiatric arrogance? *British Journal of Medical Psychology*, vol. 66, Part 1, pp. 61–6.

5

Interpersonal and communication skills: a continuous curriculum challenge

Tom Chapman and Helen Fields

THE STIMULUS OF CHANGE

Rapid change has been a constant feature in the working environment of health and social care professionals over the last decade or so. The radical restructuring of nurse education at pre/post-registration levels and its alignment and convergence within mainstream higher education has represented a relatively rapid, fundamental and deliberate effort to advance the status of nursing and create an infrastructure which facilitates the preparation of responsive and innovative practitioners. In developing curriculum opportunities beyond Project 2000 and along the continuum of post-registration education and practice (UKCC, 1994), educators have a considerable measure of autonomy for the foreseeable future. Such autonomy needs, nevertheless, to be exercised responsively and in partnership with a wide range of key stakeholders. These include students, employers and managers, fellow health professionals and educationalists, patients and clients, and validators (academic and professional), each of whom have a varying but significant impact on the nature, relevance and demand for educational programmes and the degree of 'fit' such programmes will have within the context of wider health and social care changes.

Similarly, the considerable and dramatic upheaval caused by the UK health reforms has also had a permanent effect. Return to the *status quo* is no longer an option and there are no fixed points for the future. Inevitably, the current shape of the NHS will be largely unrecognizable by the end of this decade. The Welsh Health Planning Forum (1992), for example, have envisaged a framework of services for the year 2010 which emphasizes:

- real choice to users;
- minimum resources compatible with high-quality outcome;
- decentralized services as close to home as possible with limited concentration of high dependency/tertiary services;
- continuity of care – 'seamless care';
- staff who are responsive to users and feel valued;
- meeting health and social care needs primarily through integrated services;
- using the right level of care expertise at every stage; and
- recognition that there will be significant differences in the health of the population requiring radically different professional relationships and care strategies.

Such strategies will need to take account of the critical forces driving the changes. In particular, enhanced public expectations and user empowerment, the transformed role of acute hospitals through the use of new technology, the rapid growth in day surgery and the unrelenting pressures to provide care in the community and primary-care settings, continued sophistication in the use and application of information technology, increasingly decentralized management structures and the blurring of professional boundaries consequent upon integration, collaboration and partnership in health and social care. These changes have fundamental implications for the education of health professionals. Most recently and in anticipation of the technological, organizational, economic and demographic challenges ahead, nursing leaders in the UK have attempted to stimulate the debate through a focus on strategic issues (DOH, 1994). They have stated that:

> Education and training will be a tool in support of change. Research and development must also be called in to help. The scale and timescale of change demands that every source be used to assist the shifts in care – the service will not be able to afford the luxury of gaps between theory and practice ... training approaches will have to ensure that an understanding of the two develops together, involving the whole team. A wide variety of instruments – education, training, retraining and research – must be focused on a common objective: change within continuity.

Given this backcloth and the parallel changes that are revolutionizing the higher education sector, it is essential that educators not only prepare nurses and other professionals for a more varied and responsible role but also attempt to influence the nature of the role itself, its boundaries and parameters – and hence its public perception. In their longitudinal study of the implementation of Project 2000, Jowett, Walton and Payne (1994) suggest that in the main, early data indicate that the principles of the new preparation have been translated into practice. Nevertheless, this major shift to adult-centred learning, the reframing of long-held philosophical values and the accompanying structural reorientations will take longer to embed in professional consciousness, not least because nursing has only relatively recently turned its attention to the implications for continuing professional development and the unlocking of individual potential through strategies for personal growth. It is also in this arena that the opportunities afforded by a range of flexible and responsive educational programmes, pathways and experiences within a rigorous academic atmosphere will serve to nourish and strengthen the status of nursing, address remaining deficits and alter the traditional power relationships between health professionals in order to meet the challenges of future healthcare.

Since the inception of Project 2000 and recent government acceptance, in principle, of the UKCC Post Registration Education and Practice framework (PREP), the basic infrastructure now exists to move forward and build on the range of credit-based higher-education modules and programmes becoming increasingly available. Such programmes are becoming more responsive to the needs of education purchasers and practitioners. Within these new partnerships, the socialization of nursing within higher education has opened up opportunities to transform attitudes towards shared learning and collaboration through closer integration with other disciplines. Although in its infancy, interprofessional learning can be a powerful means of enhancing teamworking, analysing and utilizing group process skills to achieve team goals, resolving conflicts, clarifying roles and working towards consensus. These processes and elements, and, in particular, those which draw on interpersonal and communication skills, are vital if the previously outlined vision of future health and social services is to be realized.

INTERPERSONAL AND COMMUNICATION SKILLS FOR NURSING AND INTERPROFESSIONAL PRACTICE

Those interpersonal skills aimed at enhancing the psychological, emotional and social well-being of clients have, until recently, been largely neglected in that aspect of nurse education which sets the tone for professional socialization – the curriculum. Until the advent of individualized care processes and theoretical nursing frameworks, the focus of professional training had largely been on task performance, with competence measured in terms of practical, psychomotor and administrative skills which are observable and relatively easy to assess. Since patients and clients, as the consumers of healthcare, carry so much 'emotional baggage' with them, it has become increasingly recognized that their problems can only be adequately conceived and managed in a holistic sense, in their physical, psychological, social and spiritual totality. The increased attention on 'theory', facilitated in higher education, is providing greater opportunities to acquire a greater depth of knowledge and understanding of the complex interactions between the various dimensions encompassed within a holistic perspective. According to De Basio (1989), such a knowledge base is essential to the practice of nursing and other caring professions because clients continually make adaptations and adjustments to their external and internal environments.

Nursing is becoming increasingly recognized as being much more than a problem-identification and solving process. Individualized care is predicated on some degree of understanding of the client's background, personality, feelings, values and beliefs. Professional nursing is essentially an interpersonal process requiring the integration of clinical and humanistic skills (see Peplau, 1988; Hase and Douglas, 1986; De Basio, 1989; Barber, 1991). It seems clear, therefore, that continued exploration and development remains a focus for how interpersonal and communication skills can be facilitated and enhanced in nurse education programmes and also within future models of interprofessional learning and education. Since these skills are fundamental to 'good practice' and are essential ingredients of a caring relationship, the corollary is that they should also be considered central to curriculum development.

This chapter reinforces the case for giving particular consideration to the various interpersonal and communication skills required by nurses and other care professionals in higher education programmes at all levels. We have in mind a distinctive type of professional socialization which sets the tone for practitioner–client interaction. Indeed, the more progressive philosophy which seems to underpin changes in pre- and post-registration nursing education and the parallel but more gradual innovations in interprofessional learning encourages the elevation of human relationships to the centre or core of the curriculum.

The ultimate success or failure of this type of 'psychological engineering' will depend on the extent to which individual students feel better equipped to cope with the demands and stresses of their chosen career and ongoing professional development. It seems self-evident that the internalization of any aspect of an education programme depends on the conviction of students that it actually 'makes a difference to' or alters, in some constructive and lasting sense, the way they see themselves and the way they wish to act (practise). Consequently, the self-knowledge necessary before any meaningful personal change can take place in the student will only be obtained through experiential learning (see Chapman, 1974).

PHILOSOPHICAL AND THEORETICAL BASES

It is useful to start from the basic premise that nursing is a 'helping' profession', which should have as its main aim the optimum personal development of clients (consumers) of nursing services. Such a stipulation constrains attention to bio-psycho-social-spiritual needs and as such directs us to consider much more than basic 'health' needs. This prompts the question, 'How, then, can we utilize knowledge drawn from the human sciences to promote more effective practice in the helping professions?'

To achieve this goal, some study of the dynamics of human behaviour drawn from selected aspects of humanistic psychology is helpful. This leads to an appreciation of the value of a humanistic frame of reference in the increasingly wider contexts of nursing.

Within humanistic psychology, the theoretical orientation known as perceptual psychology has special utility since it provides a framework for understanding clients and co-workers as people who have needs, motives and identities that are immediately applicable to the practical problems that face health professionals. So it is not surprising that 'perceptual psychology' is called the practitioners' psychology (Combs, 1989).

In a very real sense, nursing and other health professions are applied professions in which successful practitioners do something with their knowledge. Knowledge alone is no guarantee of effective helping practice unless it can be channelled into enabling practitioners to recognize and respond to the specified needs of clients. Recent health and professional education policy changes reveal a marked shift in formal stipulations relating to conceptions of client needs. These policy changes reflect an increased respect for the rights of the consumers of public services (Department of Health, 1991; Ham, 1992; Lindow, 1993; Neuberger, 1993), an increase in the responsibility and accountability of health professionals and imply, at least in principle, radical changes in practice. In short, this new ethos requires professionals to relate to clients as individuals with unique needs; to be treated with dignity, respect and consideration; to be fully consulted on all decisions which affect their health status; and to be regarded as being capable, within sensible limits, of acting with self-responsibility.

Countless research studies in the fields of teaching, medicine and psychotherapy have revealed that effective practitioners are not distinguished by the 'methods' they use. For example, it seems that the conception that there is one best method of teaching, in any absolute sense, is a mistaken one. The same probably holds true for the practices of the helping professions. Perceptual psychology provides us with a most plausible explanation. The underlying reason why successful practice is not associated with any particular method is that it is the client's perception of both the method and the professional who is applying it, in combination, which is important. In other words, it is the meaning of the intervention of the professional for the client that significantly determines the outcome. As a theoretical orientation within humanistic psychology, perceptual psychology is predicated on the fundamental importance of the concept of self in human interaction. Perceptual psychology is closely allied with counselling psychology with which it shares a common intellectual heritage.

Counselling provides an invaluable frame of reference for the acquisition of those very skills that underpin professional practice. In the context of health and social care we take 'counselling' to be more than a set of skills employed in a limited range of situations. Counselling is represented here in the sense used by Burnard (1989) as an 'often idiosyncratic mixture of personal qualities, practical skills and interpersonal aspects of the health professional's job'. Importantly, since caring for people who are psychologically distressed inevitably places carers themselves under stress, counselling-based programmes are invaluable in helping them take care of themselves. Furthermore, since one facet of good practice is to reduce the gap between the 'all-knowing, all-powerful, all-adequate professional and the uninformed, powerless student, patient or client' (Nurse, 1983), the method of person-centred counselling in particular can be profitably explored and adapted to nursing, within the context of interprofessional care.

Sensitization to counselling skills and person centredness improves interpersonal communication in all organizational and professional contexts in which care takes place and helps to nurture the relationship which develops between nurse and client and nurse and care-team members. Person-centredness as a way of relating to other people suggests a set of beliefs, attitudes and values and not merely an adherence to standardized routines.

THE CONTRIBUTION OF HUMANISTIC PSYCHOLOGY

Much can be learned from considering some of the theoretical formulations employed by the American psychotherapist, Carl Rogers. When he was faced with the need to set out the implications of psychotherapy for education, Rogers (1967) coined the expression 'significant learning' to describe a process which is more than an accumulation of facts; it is a deeply rooted social process which 'makes a difference' in a fundamental way to the actions, behaviour and personal growth of those individuals who internalize and are penetrated by such learning, with its therapeutic undertones. To paraphrase Rogers, and at the same time adapting the learning outcomes to the health professional context, we would expect this type of orientation to produce people with an improved capacity to (a) accept themselves and their feelings more fully; (b) become more confident and self-directing; (c) become more flexible and less rigid in their perceptions; (d) become more accepting of others; and (e) become more open to evidence (ibid., pp. 280–1). The ideals of changes in nurse education, the benefits of interprofessional learning and the ethos of consumerism are commensurate with the kind of education and professional socialization which is rooted in this theoretical perspective.

DESIRED CURRICULUM SKILLS AND OUTCOMES

Some of the desired outcomes which are envisaged from the adoption of the precepts and values derived from counselling psychology include:

- improved communications in an atmosphere of trust;
- a decrease in frustration, uncertainty, anxiety and other antitherapeutic states which result from poor communication;
- a reduction in the number of clients who feel they are powerless and unable to exercise choice or express their wishes;
- a general reduction in iatrogenesis (i.e. a process of dependence created by medical/professional bureaucracy);
- an elevation of the status of clients/consumers;
- an improved coping ability on the part of professionals and clients;
- the development of a more therapeutic and caring environment;
- a better understanding of health problems (in perspective);
- the adoption by clients of more positive attitudes towards themselves and their health-related problems;
- improved efficiency as a result of more effective decision-making; and
- a greater facilitation of client advocacy.

Each of these outcomes are contingent on the level and extent to which the clients of services are exposed to 'therapeutic' interventions. From the standpoint of the care professions, systematic and thorough-going attention to interpersonal skills in the curriculum can lead to an improvement in self-esteem and self-confidence both during professional preparation and beyond qualification (see Aidross, 1985; Bond, 1986). As this aspect of the curriculum is further developed and becomes embedded as a result of education changes in the health professions, there is a greater likelihood of more effective interpersonal support in these professions, where vulnerability to stress is widely recognized.

The interpersonal skills and attitudes that dynamic curricula should incorporate include the ability to:

- orientate to the client's needs;
- value and preserve confidentiality;
- listen (incorporating sensitivity to non-verbal cues);

- offer 'free attention' (noting and accepting, not judging);
- suspend preconception; offer empathy;
- feel and show acceptance, respect and warmth;
- interact from the standpoint of 'genuineness';
- help clients at all ability levels to develop programmes to adjust to and cope with their presenting circumstances and to act on behalf of those who have long- or short-term coping deficits;
- present information (accurately and without jargon);
- analyse team-functioning and contribute to changes as appropriate;
- accept leadership directed towards group process and task achievement;
- be reflective and self-directing;
- resolve conflicts through mediation, assertiveness and diplomacy;
- tolerate ambiguity and disagreement;
- share tasks with others;
- provide clear and succinct written communication;
- accept the need of all team members for recognition and self-esteem;
- operate flexibly with a willingness to allow modification of one's role to evolve within the framework of one's developing or established professional values;
- appreciate and adapt to the different cultures and language used in multidisciplinary communication and the ways in which client problems might be interpreted and resolved; and
- use group processes to achieve team goals. (Adapted from Kane, 1976.)

Such skills will assist students to recognize and experience the creativity which can ensue from effective collaboration and orientation to the client perspective. They can also lay the foundations for co-operating across professional boundaries and translating this into practice. Naturally, there are problems, since each profession has its own body of knowledge and its own culture, but we have already outlined existing and possible future health- and social-care imperatives and policy changes which are driving an agenda based on greater intersectoral and interprofessional co-operation. Indeed, Goble (1994) suggests that the idea of interdisciplinary/professional work builds on the insight that 'modern life is so complicated that no one discipline on its own is capable of analysing and resolving the problems of everyday life'.

Bines (1992) further develops the concept of interprofessionalism by suggesting that two key related processes need to be fostered. In the case of nursing, the first would involve an analysis of the nurse's professional 'self' and the values, identities, expertise and ways of working involved in nursing. The second embraces an understanding of the professional perspectives and actions of others, culminating in a synthesis of 'self' and 'other' into what can be achieved together. Bines also postulates that despite strong arguments for postponing interprofessional learning to the level of post-registration/continuing education development, the inclusion of interprofessional learning in pre-registration preparation will avoid the risk of having to 'unpack insular attitudes and practices' developed in initial training and subsequent experience. Increasingly, this is an issue which may need to be addressed more directly by statutory and regulatory bodies in the health professions if future services are to benefit from more responsive and flexible care teams.

LEARNING EXPERIENCES

Clearly, the supervision of student-learning experiences by competent teacher/facilitators is essential to the skill-gaining process, whatever the context and application. Reflection on learning needs to be inherent to this process and is fast becoming a key feature of some professional curricula. It is deeply rooted in the humanistic tradition and is a powerful tool in developing professional awareness and effective action (Gibbs, 1988; Champion, 1991; Stephenson, 1993). An example of where reflective learning and practice is becoming commonplace is within the ENB Continuing Education Framework and Higher Award programme (ENB, 1992). This may often be facilitated through action-learning sets and can also contribute to the informal self-assessment process as students encounter issues and 'critical incidents' in the practice setting. The current debate around the notion of 'clinical supervision' (Faugier and Butterworth, 1993), its links with reflective practice and its potential adoption by the nursing profession, will also have concomitant implications for the preparation of skilled, sensitive and effective supervisors who could play a significant role in enhancing care standards through the support and development of teams, peers and less-experienced practitioners.

Creative practice experiences in a wide range of health- and social-care settings are much more evident in contemporary and newly emerging curricula and, if they are well-structured and supported, they can increasingly provide rich sources of student learning in interpersonal skills and opportunities to reflect on the issues, advantages and difficulties of collaborative working. Significantly, the increasing pressures on educationalists and supervisors to both secure and facilitate suitable practice experience may mean that insufficient attention and resources are given to the ongoing learning and support needs of the student. However, the 'practicum' is a crucial component of the professional curriculum which cannot adequately be left to chance in an unmediated or unstructured way. As Zeichner (1990) points out, attention needs to be given to three aspects in particular: organizational (length and location); curricular (what is to be learned and how) and structural (support: ensuring students are briefed, can learn, reflect and evaluate in appropriate contextual conditions). Thus the pressures to enhance the role of practice experience and deploy resources effectively are unlikely to subside and will constantly demand novel and innovative ways of facilitating practice experience within course design.

Accordingly, project and assignment work needs to be equally creative and, in relation to interpersonal and communication skills, will primarily need to be geared to student ability to work productively within groups and to interact effectively with clients. Facilitation of action-learning sets and the use of learning contracts and learning 'diaries' which detail interactions with clients and co-workers are examples of strategies which can be highly conducive to the development of important interpersonal and communication skills. Communicating the purposes of the activities is also critical, as students need to see themselves developing the skills and understanding which will support them in anticipation of their future or enhanced roles. Similarly, the skills which derive from embracing humanistic philosophy are intrinsically enabling, underpinning the shift in the power relationship between teacher and student.

Increasingly, in a political climate centred around a consumer-orientated service economy, it is also important to facilitate and nurture such personal qualities in the clients themselves so as to encourage them to play a more proactive role in the promotion of their own health and that of their families.

SUMMARY

Within nursing and other care professions, changes in policy, new and anticipated ways of delivering care through increased intersectoral working and interprofessional collaboration, mean that the dynamics of interpersonal interaction assume increasing significance for the curriculum. To this end, a study of the basic tenets of humanistic psychology and certain facets of counselling psychology, embraced in person-centred approaches, is particularly valuable.

Since the nature of interpersonal exchanges fundamentally affect the quality of care the client receives and influences the effectiveness of teamwork, attention to the processes of human interaction is and will continue to be of fundamental concern in the education of health professionals. To ensure that current and future programmes are accessible and of optimum value to students at all levels, they must be based on coherent and consistent philosophical and theoretical frameworks which substantially link with and draw from the practice context. The wider adoption and development of the techniques of reflective practice, together with creative project and assignment work which supports and underpins the gaining of interpersonal and communication skills, is therefore highly consistent with such theoretical frameworks.

In summary, the continued evolution of the caring professions, combined with greater client empowerment, means that the recipients of care will increasingly expect both to manage their own health and to participate in that management alongside professionals. The authors believe that interpersonal and communication skills are essential to realizing this shift in approach and philosophy. Regardless of recent professional education changes, this chapter underlines the continuing curriculum challenge for teachers and other stakeholders with an interest in effective and responsive education.

REFERENCES

Aidross, N. (1985) Interpersonal skills, in *Recent Advances in Nursing 12*, (ed. A.T. Altschul), Churchill Livingstone, Edinburgh.

Barber, P. (1991) Caring: the nature of a therapeutic relationship, in *Nursing: a Knowledge base for Practice*, (ed. A. Parry and M. Jolly), Edward Arnold, London.

Bines, H. (1992) Interprofessionalism, in *Developing Professional Education,* H. Bines and D. Watson, SRHE and Oxford University Press, Buckingham.

Bond, M. (1986) *Stress and Self-awareness: A Guide for Nurses,* Chapman & Hall, London.

Burnard, P. (1989) *Counselling Skills for Health Professionals,* Chapman & Hall, London.

Champion, R. (1991) Educational accountability: what ho the 1990s!. *Nurse Education Today* **11**, 407–9.

Chapman, T. (1974) The humanistic tradition in psychology and its relevance for education. *Self and Society*, **2**, 4.

Combs, A.W. (1989) *A Theory of Therapy: Guidelines for Counselling Practice,* Sage, London.

De Basio, P.A. (1989) *Mental Health Nursing: A Holistic Approach*, 3rd edn, C.V. Mosby, St Louis.

Department of Health (1991) *The Patient's Charter*, HMSO, London.

Department of Health (1994) *The Challenges for Nursing and Midwifery in the 21st Century: The Heathrow Debate*, HMSO, London.

ENB (1992) *Framework for Continuing Education and the Higher Award*, ENB, London.

Ham, C. (1992) Local heroes. *The Health Service Journal*, 19 Nov. 20–1.

Faugier, J. and Butterworth, A. (1993) *Clinical Supervision: A Position Paper,* University of Manchester.

Gibbs, G. (1988) *Learning by Doing: A Guide to Teaching and Learning Methods,* FEU, Oxford.

Goble, R.E.A. (1994) Multiprofessional Education in Europe: an overview, in

Going Interprofessional, A. Leathard, Routledge, London.

Hase, S. and Douglas, A.J. (1986) *Human Dynamics and Nursing,* Churchill Livingstone, Edinburgh.

Jowett, S. Walton, I. and Payne, S. (1994) *Challenges and Change in Nurse Education: A Study of the Implementation of Project 2000*, NFER, Slough.

Kane, R. (1976) *Interprofessional Teamwork,* Syracuse University School of Social Work, New York.

Lindow, V. (1993) Buyer beware. *The Health Service Journal,* 12 August, **23**.

Neuberger, J. (1993) Why not ask the experts? *The Health Service Journal*, 30 September, **21**.

Nurse, G. (1983) Counselling, in *Community Health* (eds J. Clark and J. Henderson), Churchill Livingstone, Edinburgh.

Peplau, H.E. (1988) *Interpersonal Relations in Nursing*, 2nd edn, Macmillan, London.

Rogers, C. (1967) *On Becoming a Person*, Constable, London.

Stephenson, P.M. (1993) Content of academic essays. *Nurse Education Today*, **5**, 81–7.

United Kingdom Central Council (1994) *Standards for Post Registration Education and Practice*, UKCC, London.

Welsh Health Planning Forum (1992) *Health and Social Care 2010: A Framework for Services,* WHPF, Cardiff.

Zeichner, K. (1990) Changing directions in the practicum: looking ahead to the 1990s. *Journal of Education for Teaching*, **16**(2), 105–32.

6

Performance indicators and changing patterns of accountability in nurse education

Ruth Balogh

INTRODUCTION

In this chapter I show some of the ways in which questions of account-ability relate to discussions about how to develop performance indicators (PIs) for nurse training institutions. The evidence I draw on is derived from material gathered over a two-year period of research for the English National Board for Nursing, Midwifery and Health Visiting (ENB), who commissioned Alan Beattie to direct a project on the subject at the University of London Institute of Education. The aim of this research was to explore the feasibility of developing PIs for nurse and midwife training institutions. The account I give of this research is intended to show how the initial findings led to further work on implementation issues and finally to a series of recommendations for the ENB to consider in formulating policy. Accordingly, the views in this section of the chapter are presented as the collective views of the research team and termed as such.

The project itself took place between 1987 and 1989 – a period it would be no exaggeration to describe as one of upheaval in the arrange-ments for the delivery of nurse and midwife training. Policies and the information required for their implementation are highly interlinked, so I intend first to locate this ENB initiative within a more general back-ground of recent changes in public sector policy, then to focus more particularly on nursing and midwifery education and to present some of our research findings within this context of wide-ranging policy debates. I conclude with a discussion about some of the general issues of accountability raised by the systematic, routine collection of this type of information.

THE GROWTH OF PUBLIC SECTOR SERVICES

The idea of gathering information to assess the performance of public sector services has been, since the development of the Welfare State at least, closely linked with the public expenditure process. Pressure to examine costs arose from a general trend throughout the developed world in the 20th century towards growth in public expenditure, especially on social, environmental and economic services and there is considerable debate among economists as to why this should be so. Peacock and Wiseman (1967) suggest that periods of social upheaval (such as the Second World War) have been a critical influence through creating an 'imposition effect' whereby the public become more willing to bear a high taxation burden, and at the same time an 'inspection effect' in which additional social problems are identified.

The complexities of these debates aside, this analysis draws our attention to a central issue in any discussion about how to assess performance in the public services: namely, the complex and changing accountability structure of modern society. Individual taxpayers today must be seen as both contributors to and recipients of public services in potentially differential degrees at different points in the lifecycle. They may also be accountable as professional service-providers or as educators of the professionals of tomorrow – or indeed both. The precise nature of these accountabilities is, however, itself a shifting phenomenon for, as Peacock and Wiseman argue, they exist against a backdrop of changing ideas about how social problems should be defined, and changing social priorities in different historical circumstances. Schon, in his influential book *The Reflective Practitioner* (1983) goes so far as to describe 'a crisis of confidence in professional knowledge ... which seems to be rooted in a growing skepticism about professional effectiveness'. Accountable to whom? – and how? – are questions that may need to be posed more frequently than they can be answered.

THE PERFORMANCE OF PUBLIC SECTOR SERVICES

Although the introduction of policies requiring performance indicators for the public sector generated a considerable amount of discussion in the 1980s, the notion of monitoring activity and performance is by no means new. Indeed, the nursing profession can legitimately claim an early advocate in the shape of Florence Nightingale, who wanted regular and systematic recording and publication of hospital in-patient activity 'to enable the work of hospitals to be assessed' (Goldacre and Griffin, 1983).

The National Health Service, perhaps of all the public sector services in the post-war period, has inquired most regularly into the costs and effectiveness of its operations. Within four months of the launch of the NHS in 1948, it had become apparent that the original costs for its first year had been underestimated by £49m, and Bevan noted to his cabinet colleagues – in terms that would be entirely appropriate in the 1980s – that 'the justification of the cost will depend upon how far we get full value for money' (quoted in Klein, 1983:34).

Successive governments, both Labour and Conservative, have pursued this question of value for money in the NHS in their different ways. Labour administrations have tried to reconcile rising costs with the principles of equity and effectiveness; Conservative administrations have attempted to justify the raising of additional revenues by (for instance) the introduction of prescription charges within a general policy of non-intervention. The early questions about the costs of healthcare derived in part from the very fact that costs had not entered into the initial debates about what form the proposed NHS should take: indeed, it had been assumed that the provision of healthcare free at the point of delivery would *save* money and it was a matter of some surprise that from the very beginning annual budgets were constantly having to be revised upwards. A committee chaired by Guillebaud was set up in 1953 to investigate the problem. It found that costs had indeed risen against early estimates; but if they were taken as a proportion of gross national product, this proportion had actually fallen from 3.75% to 3.25%. The committee drew attention to the need for better information on NHS activity, but although it recommended the appointment of a statistician at the Ministry of Health, it also argued against setting up a framework to relate costs to performance on the grounds that suitable indicators of performance were difficult to identify and even more difficult to measure (Ministry of Health, 1956).

The 1960s and 1970s brought with them attempts to introduce rational planning methods into the public sector. A plethora of new techniques emerged, complete with acronyms: Programme Analysis and Review (PAR), Planning Programming and Budgeting Systems (PPBS), Zero-Based Budgeting and Cost-Benefit Analysis (CBA), all of which sought to challenge the existing principle that 'the largest determining factor of the size and content of this year's budget is last year's budget' (Wildavsky, quoted in Likierman, 1988), by determining budgets on more rational criteria. The Plowden Committee's reform of the public spending process did not go this far, but it did transform it by introducing annual surveys of departmental spending which were scrutinised by the Public

Expenditure Survey Committee (PESC), chaired by the Treasury. For the first time, a systematic attempt was being made to discover how funds had been distributed by spending departments and to use this information for future planning.

In the NHS, the 1974 reorganization made it possible to compare the funding for different health authorities on the basis of the populations for which they were responsible and wide differences were revealed on expenditure per head. The Resource Allocation Working Party was convened to remedy this in 1976 but, coinciding as it did with a period of recession, much of the redistribution of funding was implemented as cuts.

During the mid-1970s, governments gradually began to introduce a change to the basis on which budget plans were calculated from volume to cash. In the early days of PESC, departments calculated the value of the goods and services they planned to buy according to volume and any unanticipated rises in price were covered by the Treasury. Cash-planning, on the other hand, assumes a general rate of inflation through which costs will rise and resources are allocated accordingly.

This change, from volume planning to cash and later cash-limited planning, brought with it a shift in emphasis for managers from service needs (which are more readily translated into volume terms than cash terms) to 'top-down' concerns about resource-distribution priorities. But for the Conservative administration of the 1980s there was still room for change; in September 1982 the Financial Management Initiative was launched, a top-down initiative whose aim was to hold managers more accountable for the use of resources through cash-limiting budgets, setting targets and monitoring performance. It was through this initiative that the accounting concepts of *Economy, Efficiency and Effectiveness* (the 'three Es') became a statutory element in public life, initially for local government services via the 1982 Local Government Finance Act (HMSO, 1982). This empowered auditors to look beyond their traditional concerns of accuracy and propriety to 'satisfy themselves that authorities have made appropriate overall arrangements to secure economy, efficiency and effectiveness' (Audit Commission, 1983).

Thus the trend throughout the public sector in the 1980s to gather information on performance in order to argue more closely on resource-allocation priorities was clearly associated with tighter, top-down mechanisms of accountability. In the NHS, PIs were introduced along with new mechanisms of ministerial review in early 1982, 'as a measure to improve accountability'. Similarly, in the universities new, more streamlined management structures were recommended to accompany the development of PIs in the Jarratt Report (1985) on efficiency in universities.

THE CASE OF NURSING AND MIDWIFERY EDUCATION

Until recently, nurse and midwife education has occupied a position in the public sector which can best be described as not entirely within the NHS yet only tenuously linked with higher and further education. One of the key items of evidence which has dominated discussions about policy in this area – student wastage rates – would today be called a performance indicator. As far back as 1947, the Wood Report (Ministry of Health, 1947) recommended full student status for nurses, so that 'the dissociation of training from staffing needs ... will place the student under the control of the training authority ... and not under that of the hospital'. It was high wastage rates among student nurses (nationally running at 54% at the time) which in the committee's view indicated the need for such a radical review of training programmes. To further encourage independence from the hospitals, the committee also recommended that training should be funded separately.

Though the Wood Report met with hostility from many senior members of the nursing profession, these policy issues – of where nurse education should be located, how it should be funded and what should be the contractual status of the student – have remained a central focus for debate in the succeeding 40 years. They were again underlined in the Briggs Report (1972) which looked more closely at wastage rates by comparing them with other types of predominantly female student and employee and culminated in the Project 2000 proposals put forward by the United Kingdom Central Council (UKCC) in 1985.

The ambiguous status of nurse training schools – partly funded by the new National Boards and partly funded by the Health Authorities and with variations in Scotland and Northern Ireland – perhaps protected them during the 1980s from the more robust features of the Financial Management Initiative which were encouraging some of their colleagues in further and general education to develop PIs for training programmes and institutions. But by 1985 the National Boards had come under the wing of the annual ministerial review process via the Department of Health and Social Security. The ENB – by far the biggest of the Boards, dispensing £90 million annually (in 1988) for teaching costs to 14 Regional Education Advisory Groups (EAGs) – agreed to develop PIs for training institutions to assist in its own annual reviews of the EAGs. The Board adopted a dual strategy, first by encouraging EAGs to start work at local level to develop PIs and second, by commissioning research from the University of London Institute of Education – the PI project reported on here.

During the course of this research, the pace of change in nursing and midwifery education accelerated rapidly. Policy dilemmas which had simmered away for years suddenly became subjects no longer for debate but for resolution. But most important for the PI project was the almost universal call in policy documents that the introduction and ongoing implementation of these new policies depended on developing more uniform and routine systems to collect information about what goes on in training institutions – in other words, PIs. The various policy initiatives are outlined below, illustrating the central and linking role which PIs were set to play in the future management of nurse and midwife education.

Project 2000

The radical proposals known as Project 2000 were agreed by the UKCC in 1985, but it took until spring 1988 for the Minister of Health to announce, at the annual RCN conference, that the government was prepared to support them. Their long-term effect will be to change the way nurse education is structured from a labour-market model in which schools supply recruits directly to hospitals, to an educational- investment model where students are supernumerary, where qualifications to register are approved within higher education, and for which training for the different branches of the profession is more flexible, with a greater contribution from placements in community settings

Throughout its discussions with the nursing and midwifery professions, the government was keen to estimate the costs of the Project 2000 proposals. Price Waterhouse, in a cost appraisal undertaken for the UKCC (UKCC and Price Waterhouse, 1987) acknowledged that the benefits of reducing the clinical responsibilities of students were difficult to quantify and therefore weigh against the more easily estimated costs of employing qualified substitutes in their places. However, the first 'demonstration districts', in submitting proposals to the Department of Health, were required to supply basic information which could be turned into ratios of the type used in routine cost-based performance assessment – for instance, proposed student-staff ratios and cost per student. This exercise, which took place in early 1989, revealed some important discrepancies, not only between the estimated costs of Project 2000 in different districts, but also differences between costing methods and, perhaps most important of all, major problems concerning the quality of financial and other information available to education managers. Such discrepancies, it was argued, clearly pointed to a need for generating performance-type information on a routine basis.

Clinical career structure

Recommended by the Pay Review Body early in 1988, this initiative sought to determine responsibilities and therefore grades through job appraisal using an information base which was similar to and, indeed, for teachers, overlapped with training institution PIs. The criteria used for allocating grades have differed between districts and regions and the process was strongly contested, with appeals against grades still, in 1990, taking up a major proportion of senior nurse and midwife managers' time.

The criteria for educational gradings established new relationships between the quantity and range of activities undertaken at training institution level and the numbers of teaching staff at particular grades needed to carry out these activities. The routine availability of PI-type information therefore became an essential prerequisite for the operation of the new grading system in training institutions.

ENB internal review

In 1988 the ENB commissioned outside consultants Deloitte Haskins and Sells to carry out a review of the 'interface between the ENB and the training institutions' which reported in early 1989 (ENB, 1989a). It recommended ways in which the Board might tighten up its arrangements to secure more direct lines of accountability in the resource allocation process, including the abolition of Education Advisory Groups and their replacement by Local Training Committees, permitted in the 1979 Act which established the Boards. The essential difference between the 14 EAGs and the LTCs would be that there would only be four LTCs based in the ENB's existing local premises; they would function as committees of the Board, but with greater executive input at local office level. Deloittes took the view that this new structure could not function effectively without extending the ENB's information system to permit the quarterly calculation of cost-based PIs to monitor resource allocation to training institutions.

Regional education and training strategies

It was through these strategies, developed at RHA level, that the amalgamation of schools of nursing into larger units was implemented during the period between 1987 and 1990. These amalgamations also required all training institutions to establish links with higher education and to provide courses normally in at least three specialisms. Across the country, strategies were still, during the research timescale, at varying stages of consultation and new arrangements in some places were still far from certain. Some regions commissioned option-appraisal studies from management consultants to help them decide the best way to organize local consortia of schools; the information gathered in these studies was very similar to local PI pilot studies. The ENB's own internal review (see above) identified these strategies, along with educational PIs, as a key element in taking forward the proposed new arrangements for resource allocation.

Departmental review of the statutory bodies

As non-governmental public bodies, the statutory bodies which regulate nursing (the ENB, the Welsh National Board, the National Board for Scotland, the National Board for Northern Ireland, and the United Kingdom Central Council) are subject to periodic reviews. The first review since this set of bodies was established under the 1979 Act was conducted during 1988 by outside consultants Peat Marwick McLintock, whose brief included the possibility of changes to statute. While the consultants sought to avoid such changes, their investigation -- made public in September 1989 – found that relationships between the statutory bodies were too cumbersome; they argued for a new framework which would require the assent of Parliament (ENB, 1989b: para 6). Central to the argument were the concepts of efficiency, effectiveness and accountability, as the first of the principal findings showed: 'We have identified a number of factors concerned with organizational arrangements which we believe inhibit the efficiency and effectiveness with which the statutory bodies are able to discharge their responsibilities.'

The review proposed that the Boards should cease to be elected bodies and become an executive with direct ownership of training institutions, thus severing their financial links with the NHS. In contrast, the UKCC's role as the professional body would be clarified: Council would be both funded and elected by the practitioners and would take responsibility for standards-setting.

This, the consultants argued, would enable education managers to use resource-based PIs which would more accurately reflect the true financial situations of training institutions than was possible under existing arrangements where funding was not only split between the Boards and the local health authorities, but where considerable local variation existed over the division of budgetary responsibilities. In particular, the use of student-staff ratios (SSRs) was recommended 'as an aid to improved resource allocation rather than as a measure of achievement'. However, this could not proceed until definitions of SSRs were not only based on some rationale, but above all harmonized; there were variations in definitions over what counted as a teacher, for instance whether unqualified teachers should be included in the calculations. Further research would be required, it was argued, to 'establish appropriate values of SSRs in different circumstances'. It was further recommended that the Boards develop a 'small set of resource-based PIs to be used in monitoring resource usage at institutional level'.

The White Paper: Working for Patients

The publication of the NHS Review on 31 January 1989 (Department of Health, 1989a), brought all these other initiatives into sharp focus. The idea of introducing 'internal markets' backed up by computerized resource management and clinical budgeting would, in particular, require the use of cost-related indicators. Project 2000 necessitated the calculation of some of the 'grey areas' of district health authority resource input into nurse education, the clinical grading structure established new relationships between labour costs and outputs and the streamlining of accountabilities proposed in the reviews of the national bodies would result in cost-based PI-type information flowing more directly to the Department of Health.

While the White Paper itself took no particular stand on the question of how training institutions should be managed, *Working Paper 10* (published in November 1989 and dealing with arrangements for England only) set out in more detail various options, including strong arguments for schools remaining, for the time being at least, within the NHS and managed through the regions. *Working Paper 10* also explored the way in which the new 'contracting culture' would work for nurse education. It was clear that some of the essential elements of contracts would clearly be linked to performance issues, for instance: 'ideally, the contract should be expressed in terms of the output of successful students' (Department of Health, 1989b: para. 7).

The restructuring of higher education and community care

The picture of policy debates in nurse and midwife education and their relationship to performance monitoring would not be complete without some reference to changes in higher education and care in the community, for Project 2000 requires both these areas to play a greater role in nurse education. Radical changes in the funding arrangements for the polytechnics and colleges were introduced in 1989 when they ceased to be administered through local education authorities (LEAs) and attained their own 'corporate status'. Later, in 1993, the Higher Education Bill gave the polytechnics university status and the power to confer their own awards. Resources are now distributed through the Higher Education Funding Council and the new contractual relationships are monitored by performance-type information.

Similarly, the White Paper on community-based care, *Caring for People* (Department of Health, 1990) set out proposals where local authorities, like district health authorities in *Working for Patients*, would become purchasers of 'packages' of care from outside providers, requiring contracts to be drawn up and agreed and for information systems to be developed to support these contracts.

GOVERNMENT RESPONSE TO THE REVIEWS

Taken together, these policy reviews described and analysed a range of possible options for the future management of nurse and midwife education, with an explicit emphasis on improving accountability. After more than a year's deliberation, in 1991 the government announced its response to the Peat Marwick McLintock Review. The decision was to support the Review's proposal for the UKCC to become the single elected body, but to reduce the role of the National Boards. Instead of 'providing and arranging for others to provide' courses of training (as specified under the 1979 Act), their duty would be to 'approve institutions to provide' these courses. This required an Act of Parliament, which was passed as the Nurses Midwives and Health Visitors' Act 1992.

Thus the Boards became executive bodies of the Department of Health, with its members directly appointed by the Secretary of State. The responsibility to provide training courses having been removed, the Boards no longer handled the training school budgets. For the ENB, the need for financial accountability to be monitored arose only in relation to operational matters. Nevertheless, the ENB remained the body which discharges to the profession the duty to ensure that training courses reach appropriate standards.

The question of who should manage nurse and midwife training institutions was temporarily resolved, for the English schools, by the *Working Paper 10* proposals which suggested the development of contractual relationships with the regional health authorities. However, now that the Functions and Manpower Review of 1993 has recommended a reconfiguration of this regional tier, the precise nature of these new contractual arrangements is, in 1995, still evolving.

For nurse and midwife education, the policy which has provoked the most immediate effects in the early 1990s has been the shift into higher education. In England, the pace of progress has been strongly influenced by the different approaches adopted in different RHAs. The emerging pattern is one where Project 2000 courses are validated conjointly by the awarding higher education institution and the ENB for diploma-level qualifications. Whatever the arrangements, however, there is a need for courses and programmes to be monitored with routinely collected performance-type information, eg 'annual reports on their "general health", for example recruitment and retention rates, pass rates and student evaluation' (Reed and Procter, 1993).

The ENB is no longer required, by virtue of its management of the budgets for training institutions, to demonstrate financial accountability through the production of training institution performance indicators, but it is clear that performance monitoring will remain an important task for educators to undertake. In the mid-1990s, the focus of performance monitoring in the NHS is increasingly defined by the split between purchasers and providers and the requirements for contractual arrangements to be monitored. The findings of the study the ENB commissioned to develop PIs therefore continue to be an important contribution to the enterprise of performance-monitoring in nurse and midwife education and to the issues of accountability accompanying that enterprise.

PIS FOR THE ENB

The project to investigate the feasibility of developing and implementing performance indicators (PIs) for nursing and midwifery training institutions was conducted in two phases over a period of two years. The first phase consisted of a study of the feasibility of developing PIs for training institutions, together with an exploration of the concept of 'qualitative indicators'.

We decided on an action-research approach for the project as the most appropriate way of exploring the problems of how best to develop PIs. This type of approach enabled us to take up the associated sensitive issues concerning evaluation and judgment directly with staff of training institutions by creating a series of discussion forums through which research material could be gathered. To accomplish this, we reviewed the literature from a wide range of sources, and devised techniques of structured consultation through developmental workshops which were held in all the English regions with the help of the Regional Education Advisory Groups. The results of these exercises and associated fieldwork were reported on in *Performance Indicators in Nursing Education: Final Report on a Feasibility Study* (Balogh and Beattie, 1988b) and some of the problems raised by the project for the conduct of action research have been examined in the author's doctoral thesis (Balogh, 1993).

TOWARDS A DEFINITION OF PIs

Our findings led us to propose a critique of some of the concepts currently used in connection with PIs and to propose some defining characteristics. In particular, we found an over-extension of the qualitative/quantitative dichotomy which had become over-identified with the related, but by no means identical, issues of quality and quantity. This over-extension found expression in notions such as 'quality cannot be quantified' and that performance indicators could take a qualitative form. While there do exist, beyond the realms of healthcare and education issues, indicators which express scales of measurement in qualitative terms (the Beaufort wind scale is perhaps the best example), we found no evidence in the literature, nor from other ongoing regional pilot PI studies, to support the idea that there are stable and common features concerning the performance of a training institution which could only be expressed in a qualitative way. Conversely, we did find evidence to suggest that quality could sometimes be described, though not encapsulated, numerically. We took PIs to refer to those aspects of a system which are basic to its functioning and we suggested three minimum properties:

They are guides rather than absolute measures

PIs can do no more than, as their name suggests, *indicate*. That they can measure is often assumed but, in practice, even though numerical values may be assigned, they generally fail to show the most basic requirements of measuring instruments – for example, that differences between scores at adjacent points on the scale are equal in weight. The fact that they are guides also points to the need for further information to be sought to elucidate their meaning.

They have numerical values which describe aspects of a system, most strictly in terms of inputs, activity and outputs

For educational institutions, this means that PIs are figures about:

- *student flow* intake sizes, wastage rates, completion rates;
- *teacher inputs and turnover* the range of teacher qualifications and experience;
- *cost inputs* the total costs of teaching, teaching resources, support staff and building maintenance; and
- *output of qualified practitioners* employment destinations of successful students.

Movement in indicators should be subject to unambiguous interpretation (Best 1986)

This third criterion is difficult to fulfil in practice. It means that there should be no debate about the meaning of, for example, high scores and that still higher scores should be consistent with what less-high scores denote. However, the student-staff ratio is an example of a commonly used performance indicator whose desirability is usually low both at very low (e.g. 1:1) and very high levels (e.g. 200:1), and which therefore lacks one of the fundamental properties of a measurement scale.

Elsewhere (Balogh and Beattie, 1988a), we proposed a further crucial consideration:

The 'three Es' should incorporate a fourth E which stands for an ethical dimension

By including this dimension, our aim was to underline the issues of values and accountability which arise every time a decision is taken. The simplest of data sets draws attention to the figures themselves in a way that obscures the fact that its form of presentation has been selected and that other ways of presenting the figures have *de facto* been rejected. This phenomenon has been called 'the diverted gaze' (Young, 1979) – that is, away from debates about the appropriateness of a given concept or variable.

We sought to analyse the conflicts that seemed to lie behind some of the confusions we encountered. This led us to propose a second phase of research to examine the benefits of implementing a common, nationally agreed data set for performance review, along with the difficulties encountered and prospects for resolving them.

We continued to use an action-research strategy, this time by examining implementation issues via a 'vertical' case-study, taking the viewpoints of all relevant levels at which planning takes place, from the Department of Health to the ENB, through to the EAG and training institutions in a single region, including the schools of midwifery and the views of health visiting and district nursing course leaders. Some of the workshop-based techniques we used for exploring these issues were further developed and tested and made available nationally in a 'resource guide' containing a sample data set for discussion, along with exercises and suggestions, all derived from the research process, for conducting internal reviews of the quality of educational provision and developing quality strategies. The guide, called *Figuring out Performance* (Balogh, Beattie and Beckerleg, 1989), was published by the ENB in July 1989 as a companion to their second management of change open learning pack (ENB,1989c). The research findings were reported separately in *Monitoring Performance and Quality in Training Institutions* (Balogh and Beattie, 1989).

THE IMPLICATIONS FOR ACCOUNTABILITY OF SOME OF THE PROJECT FINDINGS

Throughout our discussions with nurse and midwife teachers, we were impressed by some simple but key questions which were an almost universal focus for concern: where do standards and quality fit in? and how will PIs be used? We sought to analyse in more depth the issues behind these apparently simple questions and found a rather more complex picture.

Standards and quality

In the first phase of the project, we examined existing PI pilot projects which had been initiated by several regional EAGs. Most of them adopted a dual strategy of gathering 'manpower' figures on wastage and completion rates for students, supplemented by what was often called a 'qualitative review' of the training institution as a whole. Though information on costs was not collected in these exercises, EAGs would have been in a position to draw up crude cost-based PIs (excluding the contribution from local health authorities) by virtue of their own function in distributing funds from the ENB to the training institutions for initial preparation.

It was clear from the difficulties encountered by these local PI projects in subsequently trying to collate the information they had gathered from their 'qualitative reviews', that though the principle of PIs raising the need for further information was sound, further work was required on what form such information might take and what might be suitable techniques for gathering it. In *Figuring Out Performance* (1989) we advised schools on how to embark on an overall 'Quality Strategy' which could incorporate a variety of different techniques including standards-setting exercises and which could draw on existing evaluative activities such as the information assembled in the course approval process. The place of PIs in such a strategy would be one of 'core data': that is, they would provide some basic details about the scale and range of educational provision, ideally over a number of years, though in practice changes in institutional arrangements and course structures would preclude much stability in the definitions of data for some years to come, thus making comparisons over time potentially difficult.

The role of educational standards in developing PIs was much discussed at the developmental workshops and we found differing viewpoints. Some people thought that PIs themselves could be used to specify standards, while others felt that policy statements expressed as standards (e.g. 'learning materials should be easily accessible in the clinical areas') could be called PIs (see, for instance, RCN, 1990, where the idea of 'arising PIs' is proposed). The evidence from the case study-workshop activities suggested that neither of these positions was tenable because it is policies themselves which define what constitutes success in their achievement and local variations over policy are so great that no uniform set of standards could apply to all schools, let alone have any stability over time. We concluded that the guarantee of standards was indeed a basic requirement for performance assessment, but that they should be developed and agreed by parallel processes coming under the umbrella of quality strategies.

The role of PIs in planning and decision-making

We also found a range of views expressed in answer to the question 'how should PIs be used?', not just among senior nurse and midwife teachers in training institutions, but also among Board members and officers and DOH officials. Moreover, existing arrangements had apparently not been conducive to the use of PI-type information for planning and decision-making, either at local or national level. The picture of existing information-gathering at training institution level we found to be highly complex, with, for instance, half a day typically set aside for new students to fill in forms, most of which in some sense duplicated each other. Moreover, the ambiguous position occupied by nurse training schools also meant that their financial information was often restricted to those activities funded by the ENB , with precise levels of funding from DHAs frequently unknown.

The situation of EAGs was similarly complex, for though the groups' remit was restricted to initial nurse preparation, the casestudy EAG made a strong case for their having access to information about areas outside their responsibility, in particular for post-basic and continuing education, where levels of provision within different DHAs had a considerable impact on the quality of teaching inputs for student nurses.

At the higher levels of ENB and DOH we found a high level of agreement on the necessity for developing PIs, but views varied on how they might be used. These ranged from the 'robust' approach that they could be used to specify precise expected levels, for instance on wastage and completion rates, to the view that levels might be specified within a given range of values, to the principle that PIs are merely guides to be consulted in order to raise questions about possible problem areas. There was some support for the view that PIs ought to form the basis for resource allocation, some of the implications of which are discussed in the next section.

PIs and resource allocation

The question of using PIs for allocating funds was widely debated in all our workshop discussions and interviews. The chief problem can perhaps best be described as one of how to construct an equitable system of incentives, which in turn implies some system of rewards and penalties. Furthermore, any system so devised would have to be grafted on to current allocation procedures which varied between regions and whose rationale largely flowed from the principle observed by Wildavsky that 'this year's budget is largely determined by last year's budget' (quoted in Likierman, 1988). Education managers were very concerned that 'if you reward the successful then the unsuccessful have no prospects, it's counterproductive' (EAG financial agent, quoted in Balogh and Beattie, 1989).

An important argument against allocating resources on performance criteria derived from the finding that the directors of training institutions felt they had little control over the values which PIs would show. Quite apart from the many local and geographical factors affecting the recruitment and availability of qualified staff, our attention on many occasions was also drawn to the influence of local health authority policies on training provision, in particular via the quality of learning environments in practical areas. This is perhaps best illustrated when considering student-staff ratios, where the health authority specified the numbers of students through the provision of placements (the numerator in the ratio) and the school, in consultation with both the EAG and directly with the ENB through course approval, specified the number of teachers (the denominator). Thus any attempt to change the SSR would immediately confront the problem of 'split accountability' – on the one hand to the health authority and on the other to the ENB.

There were further complexities to this question because of the transitional state of nursing education, especially with regard to the implementation of Project 2000. The old methods of resource allocation, perhaps best described as a 'begging bowl' approach in which the onus fell to training institutions, along up the line to the EAG and the ENB, to present a case of need for further funds, have been questioned by central government policies, especially through the Financial Management Initiative. But though most of our respondents saw the future as being more dominated by rational criteria, it was far from clear what these criteria would be and how they would operate. The chief danger during such periods of transition comes from the difficulty in moving from one model of funding to another without penalizing institutions which have been performing well and with due regard to the need to raise standards in others. In such a climate it is essential for policies to be made explicit. For this reason we recommended the ENB to gather PIs for information only in the first year and to open the debate on the pros and cons of different methods of allocating funds.

FUTURE PATTERNS OF ACCOUNTABILITY

In this chapter I have traced the roots of the current concern for more streamlined accountability, to argue that they originated in government policies which aimed to tighten the financial accountability of public service managers and to show how these concerns have manifested in the various new policy initiatives which have taken nurse and midwife education into the 1990s. It is clear that the future management of nurse and midwife education will be planned with greater reference to the monitoring of performance and quality. What is perhaps not so clear is how the role of professional judgment will evolve in this process. With questions of funding increasingly pressing and lines of accountability more clearly defined with regard to resource allocation, there is a danger that these concerns will become the dominant ones. As Donabedian argues (1978), the differing focuses of professional and programme evaluation have 'raised serious ethical problems for the practitioner who is now caught between the two millstones of responsibility towards the individual patient and the collectivity'. There are some who would argue that financial and professional accountability are incompatible. Elliott (1984) makes this case for general education on the grounds that value-for-money theories are based on a manufacturing model where outputs can be clearly defined, where methods are quantitative rather than qualitative, where evaluation is summative rather than formative and where the 'audience' is the education authority and the parents or local community.

I would agree that all these distinctions apply. The dominant metaphor of financial management, however, is not so much industrial as blatantly commercial, for even manufacturing companies have problems in defining the appropriateness of their output. However, commercial enterprises assess their performance by crude output measures alone at their peril. They must also guarantee the quality of goods or services on offer *as part of the performance monitoring process*. Operating in a market does theoretically introduce the element of consumer choice as one means of guaranteeing quality, but in many cases product quality may also be bound by legislation or overseen by independent standards-setting bodies which usually incorporate a professional voice.

My concern would be more about the dangers of the metaphor taking over and here we might turn to the literature which derives from the sociology of knowledge for guidance. Schon (1983), for example, in his discourse on *The Reflective Practitioner* argues that such practitioners – indeed, the practitioners envisaged in Project 2000 – must be aware of different and perhaps competing ways of framing a problem:

> When a practitioner becomes aware of his frames, he also becomes aware of the possibility of alternative ways of framing the reality of his practice. He takes note of the values and norms to which he has given priority, and those he has given less importance, or left out of account altogether.

But, he adds, 'Frame awareness tends to entrain awareness of dilemmas'. The industrial metaphor certainly extends into the vocabulary of performance monitoring, especially with the notion of efficiency ratios which come directly from engineering. An ethical dimension must be incorporated within the three Es for public sector services in order to indicate the essential uncertainties about how, for example, efficiency is to be defined.

We have already taken a brief look at Elliott's second distinction between quantitative and qualitative methods and found they do not necessarily separate so neatly. Behind every statistic some choice, a 'qualitative' one, has been made about what to measure and what to exclude. Certainly an awareness of these qualitative issues is entirely consistent with the professional concerns about how to describe the nuances, details and 'exceptions to the rule' which are the everyday experience of practitioner-client interactions. But this does not mean these nuances cannot be described in a rigorous fashion which is open to debate. Nor does it necessarily exclude the more quantitative features of professional life which may provide a kind of background about the size and range of work undertaken. In the past, the principles of peer review have often been conducted using qualitative methods, through the use of independent judgment to protect against possible bias; more rigorous attention may be needed to these methods in the developing role of professional input to performance monitoring.

Elliott's third distinction between summative and formative evaluation may provide us with some important insights. The use of performance monitoring in a summative way implies a focus on a specified 'sum' or short-term end, perhaps without reference to longer-term strategic planning, thereby contradicting the ongoing 'monitoring" aspect of the evaluation. It therefore seems essential to stress this aspect for implementation purposes. For the ENB at least, we recommended that PIs be implemented 'within a framework of coherent strategic planning' and that the type of data gathered should be continually reviewed (Balogh and Beattie, 1989). Embedding PIs within a continuous review process should ensure that the focus will indeed be formative rather than summative.

Last, Elliott distinguishes the different audiences to which different kinds of evaluation are addressed. This raises the question of incorporating client satisfaction into the process of performance monitoring, also raised in *Working for Patients*, by the creation of market-like conditions which, it is claimed, allow patients greater choice. However, experience of implementing the review has shown that *Working for Patients* greatly over-simplified the notion of 'choice' and that patients may play many roles in influencing the shape, content, style and mode of delivery of health services (Balogh, Simpson and Bond, in press). The same may be said for the clients (students) of nurse and midwife education. Certainly what was proposed has proved to be far from any image we might have of an open marketplace dealing in goods and, as I have argued above, the mere existence of some kind of market does not itself guarantee quality. This must be done by other means.

One major problem for the incorporation of consumer or client satisfaction into performance monitoring arises from the fact that services to individual recipients are not delivered by members of one profession alone; the client's perspective in this regard is an multi-disciplinary one. There is therefore an need to consider issues such as what are the legitimate boundaries of interest of one profession in the activities and policy-setting agendas of another. Donabedian (1978) refers to this issue as one of the defining differences between professional and programme evaluation. Hepworth (in Levitt (ed.) 1987) argues that the Financial Management Initiative has raised the question of how far an auditor might legitimately comment on the effectiveness of policy and whether new relationships between auditors, inspectors and management might be called for.

For nurse and midwife education, the growing experience of developing new Project 2000 courses within higher education has become the chief focus for cross-disciplinary collaboration, but the future arrangements for purchasing nurse and midwife training, when the English RHAs are abolished in 1996, remain as yet unsettled. If the NHS continues to have a purchasing role, then it is likely that performance monitoring will take place as part of the tendering and contract monitoring process. In this case, there is a possibility that quality assurance and performance monitoring may operate as completely separate mechanisms, the former through higher education systems and the latter through contract monitoring. Nurse and midwife educators would therefore need to debate the relative merits of maintaining such a separation (as Elliott's arguments favour), or for developing a more integrated approach (as we suggested in the PI project). Either way, the discussion must hinge on analysis of how accountability to different stakeholders would be delivered.

CONCLUSION

I have given a brief overview of some of the issues of professional accountability raised by the introduction of new approaches to monitoring performance and quality in nursing and midwifery education. While it is clear that the future management of education will rely more heavily on these processes, it is also clear that the profession will need to engage in much further work and debate about how the professional voice ought to be expressed within new structures. Taking this debate forward will require, at the very least, an appreciation of the complex and multiple nature of accountability, where teachers are accountable in many respects:

- to individual patients and to populations of potential patients;
- to students in particular and to the students of the future;
- to professional peers, whether clinical practitioners or teachers;
- to line managers and superiors;
- to professional statutory bodies;
- to government; and
- to the concerns of other professionals with whom they work.

This version of accountability is by no means simple and, as Schon argues, the entertaining of multiple perspectives brings dilemmas in its wake. But unless these dilemmas are recognized, there is a real danger of falling into the trap of the 'diverted gaze', and failing to give proper attention to the rich, complex and indeed frequently contested nature of professional practice and management which lies behind the sets of numerical data that new technology allows us to generate and use.

ACKNOWLEDGMENT

The author would like to acknowledge financial support from the ENB for the research on which this chapter is based and academic support from Alan Beattie, the project director, whose ideas helped in developing many of the lines of argument.

REFERENCES

Audit Commission (1983) *Code of Local Government Audit Practice for England and Wales*, London Audit Commission.

Balogh, R. (1993) *Performance monitoring for nurse and midwife training institutions: some problems for the conduct of action research*, unpublished PhD thesis. Institute of Education, University of London.

Balogh, R. and Beattie, A. (1988a) Performance Review. *Nursing Times*, 4 May, **84**, no. 18.

Balogh, R. and Beattie, A. (1988b) *Performance Indicators in Nursing Education: Final Report on a Feasibility Study*, Institute of Education, University of London.

Balogh, R. and Beattie, A. (1989) *Monitoring Performance and Quality in Training Institutions,* Institute of Education, University of London.

Balogh, R., Beattie, A. and Beckerleg, S. (1989) *Figuring Out Performance*, ENB, Sheffield.

Balogh, R., Simpson, A. and Bond, S. Involving Clients in Clinical Audits of Mental Health Services *International Journal of Quality in Health Care*, (in press).

Best, G.A. (1986) Performance indicators: a precautionary tale for unit managers, in *Effective Unit General Management* (ed. H.I. Wickings), Kings Fund, London.

Briggs, A. (1972) *Report of the Committee on Nursing*, HMSO, London.

Department of Health (1989a) *Working for Patients*, Cmnd 555, HMSO, London.

Department of Health (1989b) *Working for Patients: Education and Training Working Paper 10*, HMSO, London.

Department of Health (1990) *Caring for People*, HMSO, London.

Donabedian, A. (1978) *Needed Research in the Assessment and Monitoring of the Quality of Medical Care* US Department of Health Education and Welfare National Centre for Health Service Research.

Elliott, J. (1984) The Case for School Self-Evaluation. *Forum*, Vol. 1, Autumn.

ENB (1989a) *Study of the Interface between the ENB and Approved Training Institutions* (Deloitte's Report), ENB, London.

ENB (1989b) *Review of the United Kingdom Central Council and the Four National Boards for Nursing Midwifery and Health Visiting* (Peat Marwick McLintock Report), ENB, London.

ENB (1989c) *Managing Change in Nursing Education*, ENB, Sheffield.

Goldacre, M. and Griffin, K. (1983) *Performance Indicators: a Commentary on the Literature*, Unit of Clinical Epidemiology, Oxford University.

HMSO (1982) *Local Government Finance Act*, London.

Jarratt Report (1985) *Report of the Steering Committee for Efficiency Studies in Universities*, Committee of Vice-Chancellors and Principals, London.

Klein, R. (1983) *The Politics of the National Health Service*, Longman Group, London and New York.

Levitt, M.S. (ed.) (1987) *New Priorities in Public Spending*, Gower House, London.

Likierman, A. (1988) *Public Expenditure*, Penguin Books, Harmondsworth.

Ministry of Health (1947) *Report of the Working Party on Recruitment and Training of Nurses* (Wood Report), HMSO, London.

Ministry of Health (1956) *Report of the Committee of Enquiry into the Cost of the National Health Service* (Guillebaud Report), Cmnd 663, HMSO, London.

Peacock, A. and Wiseman, J. (1967) *The Growth of Public Expenditure in the United Kingdom*, revised edn, Allen & Unwin, London.

Reed, J. and Procter, S. (1993) *Nurse Education: a Reflective Approach*, Edward Arnold, London.

Royal College of Nursing Association of Nursing Education (1990) *Performance Indicators for the Clinical Learning Environment*, RCN, London.

Schon, D. (1983) *The Reflective Practitioner: How Professionals Think in Action*, Basic Books, New York.

Secretary of State for Scotand (1991) *Statement by Secretary of State for Scotland on Policy Review of the Statutory Nursing Bodies and the Future Funding and Management of Nursing Midwifery and Health Visiting Education, Scottish Home and Health Department*, Scotland.

United Kingdom Central Council (1985) *Project 2000 – A New Preparation for Practice*, UKCC, London.

United Kingdom Central Council and Price Waterhouse (1987) *Project 2000 – Report on Costs, Benefits and Manpower Implications*, UKCC, London.

Young, R. (1979) Why are figures so significant? The role and critique of quantification, in *Demystifying Social Statistics* (eds J. Irvine, I. Miles and J. Evans), Pluto Press, London.

PART II

Applied Ethics in Nursing Practice

It is being increasingly recognized that a major theme that underpins healthcare is *ethics*. In fact, it becomes even more urgent to explore the ethical issues in times of radical change, particularly in healthcare organizations. The healthcare practitioner's role, and specifically nurses' and doctors' experience, is changing with the new emerging ideology of care that is continually being influenced by economic and social reorganization. Each chapter takes a particular issue of change and addresses the ethical terrain that confronts both the client/patient and healthcare practitioner's domain.

Norma Fryer (Chapter 7) and Martin Johnston (Chapter 8) explore differing ethical perspectives of the legal status of both client and professional. Stuart Horner (Chapter 9) and Barbara Shailer (Chapter 10) explore the ethical issues that arise from developing and applying ethical codes, while George Butler (Chapter 11) and Kevin Kendrick (Chapter 12) discuss the importance of ethical analysis and understanding within the research process. Glenys Pashley (Chapter 13), Christine Henry (Chapter 14) and Ruth Chadwick (Chapter 15) examine ethical issues by management organizations and advertising, all of which need addressing in times of significant reorganization and change. In contrast, Jane Pritchard (Chapter 16) and Mairi Levitt (Chapter 17) discuss and debate ethical issues that arise for nurses themselves. Kevin Kendrick and Pauline Weir (Chapter 18) take the particularly important ethical issue of truth-telling within the area of palliative care and, finally, Jeanne Siddiqui (Chapter 19) concludes this section with an examination of values inherent within the health field with specific reference to midwifery.

Ethics and the law: a right to die

7

Norma Fryer

> We do not see the law as a finely tuned instrument with which
> difficult and demanding operations can be successfully and reliably
> performed. Rather it is itself a piece of technology; a resource to be
> tapped and consumed for particular purposes and outcomes, none
> or few of which can be predicted.
>
> *(Lee and Morgan, 1990: 6)*

INTRODUCTION

It has become difficult to escape from the escalating number of
healthcare issues that are the subject of major debate and deliberation
among healthcare professionals, lawyers and, with the proliferation of
media attention and exposure, the general public. Few issues create
more ethical and legal dilemmas for doctors, nurses and midwives than
those surrounding situations of life and death. As developments in
technology provide the opportunity to preserve a life that ten or twenty
years ago would have 'naturally' perished through injury, disease or
ageing, such matters now pose questions that neither health professional, relative nor lawyer are able to answer. Meanwhile, the person at
the centre of the dilemma often remains either incapable or unable to
determine their own fate, or is restricted in some way by a system of
healthcare so strongly persuaded by either a moral, professional or
legal duty to save life.

In seeking to address any issue where attention is focused on
the 'rights' of the individual, the specific moral question of whether a
person has or should have a right to die has become one that the courts

are finding increasingly difficult to defend or oppose when, as Brazier (1992: 9) points out: 'there is no longer any general consensus on the sanctity of life, when life begins, or when it ends, or when it should end'.

For the purposes of this chapter I examine the extent to which a right to die exists within English law by seeking to examine the treatment of 'human species', from the beginning of a process where 'life' is little more than a cluster of cells, to a time where either death is imminent or where life has become of questionable purpose or quality. Issues relating to the appropriateness of any legal sanctioning will also be addressed.

It is difficult to examine questions that focus on the right to die without acknowledging the distinction, if any, between that, and any legal and/or ethical issues that encompass a right to life itself. In nursing and midwifery practice, the context of these issues may be presented from many different perspectives, particularly when clients and/or relatives are faced with decisions that require unbiased and considered options from the professionals involved. The legal implications on practice have in many ways become confused and contradictory, demonstrated in the growing dilemmas faced by the courts to provide any specific judicial solution. As Jenkins (1995: xi) remarks: 'Sometimes the law upholds the moral obligation and sometimes it appears not to be able to provide the answers.'

The present position within English law may, at first glance, seem clear. Euthanasia, i.e. any act that involves counselling or assisting a person to 'take' their own life, has no legal sanction and constitutes murder (Mason and McCall Smith, 1991). In the words of Judge Devlin, in what was one of the earliest cases in health law: 'If the act done intended to kill and did, in fact, kill, it did not matter if a life were cut short by weeks or months, it was just as much murder as if it were cut short by years' (*Rv Adams* [1957] cited in both Mason and McCall Smith, 1991: 321 and Brazier, 1992: 446–7).

In short, English law does not permit healthcare workers to 'kill' their patients. Mason and McCall Smith (1991: 178–9) suggest that while there may be seen to be no ambiguity in attitude towards the positive act of euthanasia, there is evidence that the law does permit witholding life-saving treatments in certain circumstances and acknowledges the administration of pain-relieving treatment, even in the knowledge that to do so is likely to shorten the patient's life. The implications of omitting to provide 'treatment' or its withdrawal, which may include nutrients as well as drugs, remains morally contentious and legally unclear. However, such omissions, often revered as more acceptable for the healthcare worker, reflect the view that 'passive' euthanasia is morally somehow different from that of an act of 'doing' something to procure the same end.

In contrast, it can be clearly seen through such Acts of Parliament as The Abortion Act (1967) and, more recently, the Human Fertilization and Embryology Act (1990), that the same legal protection is not afforded where life exists before birth. The Suicide Act (1961) also saw the 'right' of a person to take their life in that it is now no longer a criminal offence to commit, or attempt to commit, suicide (Dimond, 1990). The contradiction and disparity within existing law only serves to expose the legal and moral question of whether a person has, or should have, the right to die and who (if anyone) has or should have the right to make the decision.

LIFE AT THE BEGINNING – THE EMBRYO/FETUS

The point at which a human life begins has been the subject of many philosophical, scientific and theological debates, posing little concern for the lawyer until relatively recently. After many years of moral and legal deliberation, the Abortion Act 1967 undoubtedly revolutionized reproduction and childbirth. For women, greater control of their reproductive and health rights led to a violation of the rights of the new developing human life.

In superseding both the Offences Against the Person Act 1861 and the Infant Life [Preservation] Act 1929, the Abortion Act had, in effect, removed the right of the unborn child to live. Until that time it was an offence to cause the death of a child being 'capable of being born alive' unless it was for the sole purpose of 'preserving the life of the mother' (Infant Life [Preservation] Act 1929, s1). With fierce opposition from 'pro life' and 'anti abortion' groups, the act has created a plethora of passive and violent responses, providing a significant fulcrum on which all other debates about life and the right to live or die have rested.

The most recent legislation effecting this issue arises from a much earlier stage in the reproductive process. While many argue that the stage of fetal development is morally irrelevant to any decision about whether the 'unborn' child has a right to live, it became clear that the impact of reproductive medicine had provoked a new medico-legal paradigm concerning the moral and legal status of the unborn child. The position of the unborn child has moved the debate towards a woman's right to control and decide on her reproductive health outcomes into a domain where the rights of the fetus with the 'potential' for life may be seen as having equal significance both in law and from a moral perspective.

The Committee of Enquiry into Human Fertilization and Embryology, set up in 1982, examined the social, ethical and legal implications of developments in the field of human assisted reproduction (Warnock, 1985). As a consequence of this enquiry the Warnock Report (1984) provided recommendations which were given legal recognition through the Human Fertilization and Embryology Act 1990. Two major areas addressed issues concerning the use of embryos for artificial reproduction and for research. The moral argument influencing much of the enquiry focused on the 'non-personhood' status of the embryo, following much the same line as that argued for the 'non-personhood' status of the fetus in the abortion debate.

In her introduction to the report Warnock highlights the difficulties of making decisions and recommendations which 'attempt a compromise between incompatible moral positions', suggesting that 'the law is not and cannot be an expression of moral feeling' (Warnock, 1985: x). Her words best sum up the legal paradigm from which the Act was born:

> the Committee was obliged to use a mixture of utilitarian considerations of judgment. We were obliged moreover to bear in mind that any law must be generally seen to be beneficial, that it must be intelligible and that it must be enforceable. The law must not outrage too many people; but it cannot reflect the feelings of them all. It must therefore be drawn with a view to the common good, however this notoriously imprecise goal is to be 'identified'.
>
> (*xvi*)

The implications of the Act provide somewhat negligible rights/duties to the unborn, rendering ambiguous legal protection to the embryo, in so far as the storage, freezing and utilization of embryos is limited to 14 days after fertilization under s3(3)a of the Act. Prior to that stage, no such protection is given. While it is beyond the remit and/or space to discuss the moral and philosophical argument relating to the potential of the human embryo at any stage of its development, it pervades most issues and caused inevitable dissent among some members of the Warnock Committee (Warnock,1985: 90–3).

What appears, on the one hand, to offer legal protection of the right to life at one stage of embryonic/fetal development, is then violated when the law permits the termination of life, through abortion, at a later stage. Until very recently, English law has protected neither the embryo nor the fetus, suggesting that to do so would violate any civil rights afforded to the pregnant woman. Attempts to make an unborn child a ward of court have, in the main, been unsuccessful as was shown in the case of *Paton v BPSA* (1978) and more recently, in *Re F (in Utero)* (1988), where the observations of the court suggested that an unborn child has no rights of his own. Evidence in the United States, where the fetus is ascribed rights, provides a clear if not complex picture of the implications for women whose rights in law seem to depend on whether or not they are pregnant.

Where the English courts have been reluctant to interfere with the rights of the woman in childbirth is seen in the recent case of a woman who refused to consent to a Caesarean section, despite the risk of death to both herself and her unborn child (*Re S* [1992]); this seems to indicate a major shift within English law. The wishes of Mrs S were overridden by the courts in an effort to protect not only the unborn child but that of the woman herself, despite her expressed wish not to undergo what was considered to be a life-saving operation for them both. What is unclear from the outcome of this case, where the mother lived and the baby did not, is whether such a decision was based primarily on saving the child's life, or that of the woman, as the survival of the child was dependent on the operation being performed on the woman and the survival of the woman had become equally dependent on the immediate delivery of the child.

Section 37[1a] of the Human Fertilization and Embryology Act 1990 saw a revision in law relating to the viability of the fetus, i.e. the point at which a fetus is considered capable of being born alive and living independently, shifting the time at which abortion becomes illegal from 28 to 24 weeks (s37[1]b). While this appears to suggest that the fetus is protected in law for an extra month, it does not apply where there is 'a substantial risk that if the child were born it would suffer from such physical or mental abnormalities as to be seriously handicapped' (s37[1]b). Hence, the law now allows the termination of such a fetus at any stage of a pregnancy. The rights of this unborn child before or after the time of viability no longer exist.

The Abortion Act 1967, while not affording any legal rights to terminate life to any one other than a medical practitioner, provides women with an opportunity to seek such an action. Although many abortions are carried out on the grounds that 'the continuance of the pregnancy would involve risk or injury to the physical or mental health of the pregnant woman greater than if the pregnancy were to be terminated' (s1[1]a) and this decision is left to the clinical judgment of two doctors, it is clear that the moral right of a woman to choose what would be in her best interest and/or that of her unborn child is given ultimate credence to the outcome. Objections on the grounds of viability either biologically, morally or in law serve only to provide academic arguments for all involved. For example, many of the claims relating to viability, as Baylis (1990) suggests, rest on certain background assumptions about the intrinsic developmental properties of the entity in question. In law, a fetus from 24 weeks has such properties, which serve to protect it from death and, given the available resources, all efforts should and may be used to ensure its survival after birth, whatever the long-term outcome.

THE RIGHT TO DIE – NEONATES AND CHILDREN

In examining the position of neonates and children, two main aspects need to be considered. The first will focus on the neonate, born with, or acquiring during the course of labour, a 'handicap', where omission or withdrawal of existing treatment is being considered in order that it may be 'allowed to die'. Guilleminn and Holstrom (1990) describe this process in the context of one of three possible 'dying trajectories'. Where there is the possibility of a *prolonged or orchestrated death* as opposed to a *sudden* or *roller-coaster trajectory* (up and down pattern of events leading to death), medical intervention/support is withdrawn 'to limit the time of suffering by allowing the disease to take its own course' (148).

While this situation may and does extend beyond the neonatal period of 28 days, presenting all the problems involved when proxy decisions have to be made, the second area of discussion will centre around the moral and legal right of the 'mature' minor to give or refuse consent to treatment. A more general comment relating to proxy decisions on behalf of 'incompetent' persons, be they children or adults, will be made in the final section.

THE NEONATE

The amended section of the Abortion Act, which allows the termination of life for fetal handicap at any gestation, seeks to provide an alternative to any possible decision to be made after its birth, where treatment may be withheld or withdrawn. While it may have eliminated possible legal retribution for parents or professionals faced with such dilemmas, it has done little to eliminate the moral implications of such decisions. However, the burden remains one of great magnitude, with the law providing little to satisfy those parents and professionals presented with the unexpected birth of a child with a congenital or acquired handicap. Birth in effect becomes, as Brazier (1992) states, 'the crucial legal watershed', as any deliberate act aimed at destroying the child after birth is murder.

Although there is no official distinction in law between the act of homicide and that of neonatacide, the decision to withdraw treatment and/or omit to carry out life-saving procedures on severely handicapped babies appears, in practice, to generate less public debate than that of adults who become victims of the same moral vacuum. The case involving Tony Bland (*Airedale NHS Trust v Bland* [1993]), left in a persistent vegetative state after the disaster at the Hillsborough Football Stadium, provided through extensive media coverage the type of moral discourse commonly associated with neonates with similarly poor long-term outcomes.

The dilemmas of whether to initiate treatment, sustain resuscitative measures to prolong life and to what extent treatment to maintain life should be given, have remained the focus of philosophical, scientific and spiritual debate. What constitutes 'ordinary' and 'extraordinary' care has for some provided answers that support the notion that to omit treatment is morally and legally justified. What remains a problem with such a doctrine is that, in practice, it is difficult to determine what constitutes 'extraordinary' treatment. The reasoned argument suggests that efforts to treat may be withheld if the treatment is unlikely to significantly prolong life, correct the patient's condition and is more likely to cause harm than good (Wells, 1990). But who, in practice, decides whether basic nutrition is extraordinary and/or whether it is likely to cause more harm than good? How, indeed, does this apply to the use of antibiotics, physiotherapy and the administration of intravenous fluids?

Despite the acknowledgment that the act of omission does not carry the same legal stance as that of direct actions that have the same outcome, a number of cases have been debated through the courts. Some have involved professionals who have refused to treat with strong opposition from the parents (Re J [1992]). Here, the parents were found to have no legal right to demand treatment where professional opinion considered it to be 'futile'.

Other examples have involved wardships taken on behalf of minors, in cases where parents have refused treatment considered to be essential. The case of Baby Alexandria (Re B [1981]) serves as an example of such a situation where, despite the request of the parents and support of the doctors not to carry out routine surgical treatment on their Downs Syndrome baby, the courts ordered that it should be done on the basis that the life of the child would not be 'demonstrably' awful (Wells, 1990: 210). Despite such a court decision, the opinion of Lord Justice Templeman identifies the difficulties such cases pose: he suggested there may be cases of 'severe proved damage where the future is so uncertain that the court may be driven to a different conclusion' (Wells, 1990).

What is clear from the many examples of cases that have been taken to the civil courts is that there remains no absolute court ruling on a baby's right to life or that, where it may be in its best interest, to be allowed to die. Much of the case law and moral argument surrounds the omission or withdrawal of treatment and while the intention in cases where treatment has been omitted has been to allow the babies involved to die, where the doctrine is moved towards the provision of 'treatment' to hasten the process of death, the situation in law becomes one of homicide.

Probably the most cited case law that found itself in the criminal courts was that of Dr Arthur (Wells, 1990). The decision taken by both parents and Dr Arthur that the baby, born with Downs Syndrome, should be given 'nursing care only', implied and involved the omission of treatment, including nutrients, while a morphine-type drug was given at regular intervals 'to alleviate the baby's distress' (Brahms and Brahms, 1983). The baby died three days later and, as a consequence, Dr Arthur was charged with murder. This was later changed to that of attempted murder, on the basis of the defence expert's subsequent findings that showed the baby had, in fact, numerous congenital abnormalities not previously identified. While the prosecution emphasized throughout the trial that although the motives were 'of the highest order', they made it clear that the law did not allow a doctor to take steps to ensure a baby does not survive on the basis that it was mentally handicapped and that the parents did not wish for its survival. In his summary Farquharson J. explained that: 'All must be alive to the danger of giving too much power to anyone, in the medical or other professions, to exert influence over the life and health of the public at large' (Brahms and Brahms, 1983: 13).

It would appear that while the emphasis in law is on the intent to kill, the motives of Dr Arthur (despite the collapse of the defence's evidence) involved steps that appeared to bring about the death, where the intention was that the baby should die. What seemed crucial to what was an unanimous acquittal is that the jury, as in the very recent case against Dr Nigel Cox (*R v Cox 18* [1992]), had to decide whether the active steps taken by Dr Arthur did in fact ensure that the baby would die, with the intention of bringing about that event. If so, did such steps amount to murder? The outcome of this case seems to have done little to clarify the legal position, as the action taken by Dr Arthur seems clearly to have been one of intent actively to end the child's life. While it seems unlikely that any general consensus would have condemned Dr Arthur to the same fate as that of a serial murderer, there appear to be major contradictions within the present legal system as a result of this case. As Brahms and Brahms (1993:14) suggest: 'the law seems out of step and either goes by default or has evolved double standards to protect a doctor, whereas a parent would in similar circumstances almost certainly be convicted of homicide.'

MINORS – THE RIGHT TO DIE

The main issue concerning a child's right to die is grounded in the contentious view that as a minor, i.e. a person under the age of 18, decisions about treatment or non-treatment should lie with the parents or guardian and the professionals involved. Minors between the age of 16 and 18 have been placed in a slightly different category since the Family Reform Act of 1969 (s26), where a minor who has attained the age of 16 can give effective consent to any surgical, medical or dental treatment without the consent of a parent. However, as with the issues surrounding the time of viability, the question posed rests with when a child is thought to be able to act autonomously in choices relating to treatment, including the refusal of treatment which may prolong life. In essence, the law is clear in that, notwithstanding suicide, there is no right for a person to die at any age. Until the case involving Victoria Gillick (*Gillick v West Norfolk and Wisbech AHA* [1985]), which saw a shift in the application of the law relating to minors, a child under16 years was not considered to be capable of making rational choices and was denied the right to make autonomous decisions without parental consent. Where children are concerned, the position in law centres primarily on age and yet there is increasing concern about the ability and rights of children to make informed choices in many issues affecting their own welfare.

The outcome of the Gillick case provided a new paradigm for determining competence in the mature minor. The agreement in the House of Lords from this case rested on the view that 'understanding was the key element of competence' and hence a child's ability to decide on treatment, which in Lord Sharman's view involved having 'sufficient maturity to understand what was involved' (Charles Edwards, 1991). While it is argued that being capable of understanding the nature, purpose and material risks of proposed treatment provides no specific test for competence, it became a standard measure giving the mature minor rights not previously enjoyed.

In applying such criteria to a child's right to refuse treatment, as in situations where a child with a terminal illness wishes to be 'allowed to die', rather than continue treatment that they believe is no longer in their best interest, the law is less clear, providing a second dimension to the rights issue. As Brazier (1992:100) points out, the issues of consent and competence 'unlocked the door to treatment' and yet there appears to be some contradiction in law relating to a child's right to refuse treatment. The wishes of the parents in the case of *Re R* [1991], a 15-year-old girl who was given treatment against her wishes, demonstrates how 'doctors faced with willing parents and unwilling children ... could lawfully elect to act on the basis of the parental consent alone' (Brazier, 1992: 100). In other words, while present English law protects children from parents who refuse treatment to save and/or maintain the life, the rights of a child to refuse treatment, whether or not that individual be considered competent, seem to rest firmly on what other persons consider to be in the best interest of that child.

Further discussion on the right of an adult to die will focus on two main areas – that of competence and the right to choose. The 'competent' and 'incompetent' adult will be dealt with separately.

A RIGHT TO DIE – THE COMPETENT ADULT

In essence the position of the competent adult is one which links closely to the criteria set within the Suicide Act 1961. A competent adult has a right to take their own life and while there are many moral and legal implications for anyone else involved in an act of suicide, successful or not, the individual concerned is not breaking the law, whatever the outcome.

In healthcare law the specific issues concerning life and death have found themselves in both the civil and criminal courts. While the civil court in healthcare law deals primarily with negligence, the criminal courts are left to deal with more 'serious' misdemeanours and retribution. Despite the implications of a criminal act for any party involved, it is realistic to recognize that many moral issues arise which focus on the 'competence' and intent of both the perpetrator and recipient of the offence. Nowhere is this more evident than in cases of murder. When a doctor, in the course of his duty, is accused of murder, a very specific dimension is revealed, especially where that doctor has, in the course of his duty and with the consent of the patient who is competent to make a rational, informed choice, carried out an action that, in complying with the patient's wishes, breaks the law.

The act of Dr Arthur involved that of an incompetent patient, while the more recent case involving the physician Dr Cox (*R v Cox* 18 [1992]), who administered a lethal dose of a drug to a patient with insufferable pain, appears to suggest some contradiction within English law relating to a 'competent' person's right to die. The main argument in law is one that aims to determine what constitutes killing, supporting the rather tenuous claim that an omission to act is morally more acceptable in law, despite any shared intent of those involved.

The action of Dr Cox (Hewson, 1992) posed many problems. The administration of a lethal drug, despite any overriding intention to alleviate suffering, was seen by the courts as an act of murder on the grounds that the actual drug given was not one whose properties were normally associated with alleviating the pain or stress associated with a chronic, 'incurable' disorder. While the main issue in the case of Dr Arthur became one that concerned itself with whether the child starved to death as a result of the administration of a lethal dose of diamorphine, it was the action, the purpose of that action and the method used that posed grave questions in *R v Cox*; questions that in fact would probably never have been asked had a similar morphine-type substance been used. The major moral issue arising from this case strongly suggests that even though Dr Cox was acquitted of both murder and manslaughter and that the wishes of the patient to die had been fulfilled, the competent patient's right to die remains a violation in law. The impact of this case was reflected through extensive media coverage and debate among professionals from within healthcare practices and the law; and yet the outcome, which saw the acquittal of Dr Cox, did little to move the complex issues surrounding euthanasia either in law or in professional practice. Reflecting on the outcome of this case, one is perhaps left wondering whether the outcome would have been any different if the relatives had administered the drug; or do the general public and/or lawyers themselves condone the motives and actions of doctors more readily than they do relatives? Where *R v Cox* raised major issues surrounding the debate on euthanasia, other recent examples of case law have opened up wider discourse on the competent patient's right to refuse treatment.

Special attention needs to be given in the case of *Re S* [1992] where, for the first time in English law, a Caesarean section, required to save the life of a woman and that of her unborn child, was legally sanctioned despite her expressed refusal to consent to such treatment. As a 'patient' whose competence to make a choice was not in question, the outcome of this case presents a somewhat confused picture for the future, where it would appear that a woman's right to refuse treatment depends on whether or not she is pregnant. The earlier case of *Re T* [1992] also involved a pregnant woman, where a commitment to an advanced request not to be given blood was questioned by the courts on the basis that when it became necessary to provide such life-saving treatment, the woman was unconscious and therefore no longer in a position to confirm her earlier request. While other factors were seen to have influenced the outcome of the case, the eventual decision was one left primarily to the clinical judgment of the doctor who was persuaded in the end by his duty to care and to save life.

Both cases provide examples of the highly complex decisions that healthcare workers are presented with when attempting to balance an option of respecting individual autonomy through a duty of beneficence, and avoidance of harm, while seeking to prevent an unnecessary death.

A RIGHT TO DIE – THE INCOMPETENT PATIENT

The position of the incompetent patient's right to die can best be discussed by examining this last group of patients in the light of the most recent court case involving Tony Bland (*Airedale NHS Trust v Bland* [1993]). Incompetence in English law 'depends on the particular transaction in issue', with no rigid criteria to determine that a person is competent or incompetent (Brazier, 1992: 100). As a result, cases that find themselves in the English court often do little to provide a clear paradigm on which those involved in the decision-making for others can use.

Cases involving the sterilization of handicapped teenagers serve to show how, in seeking justice, decisions made by the court may differ in outcome, despite apparent similarities (Tooley, 1985). The fundamental question asked is one that seeks to decide what action or non-action will be in the best interest of the person unable to make a self-determined choice.

Adults, incapacitated with either a mental handicap or illness, pose equally difficult dilemmas when their individual level of competence is being assessed. Where rights relating to death are concerned, the incompetent adults most commonly involved are those with terminal 'illnesses'. Three main categories exist: the adult who has irreparable damage to the brain whose survival depends on artificial ventilation or, in the absence of need for such ventilation, requires other external life-saving measures to survive in what is often described as a 'permanent vegetative state'; the adult whose condition, through a process of disease, has reached a stage where only palliative treatment can be offered and where they are no longer able to participate in any decision-making; and a third category involving the elderly patient where a chronic illness provides a similar situation to that of the handicapped new-born, in that the right to die may depend on whether a decision has been made to carry out active resuscitative measures in the event of a sudden collapse. While many adults from this last group may be 'incompetent' through the process of ageing, where mental as well as physical functions have ceased, the issues involved with resuscitating the chronically ill elderly person frequently apply to those individuals who may be quite able to make such a decision but who are not given the option.

The moral issues involved in making decisions for another are grounded in doctrines that serve to offer both the best interest and dignity of that person, even and especially when that decision may involve the death of that person. The legal issue, on the other hand, is driven not only by such moral concepts but, as with the competent patient, by the distinction between the act of killing and that of allowing a person to die. *R v Cox* [1992] clearly suggests that the degree of competence is not relevant to a patient's right to die and the issue appears primarily to be one of whether the incompetent patient, either a minor or an adult, has a right to live. The main argument, therefore, seems to be one that asks whether the law offers any protection of this right, if indeed it exists at all. Philosophical arguments such as that given by Tooley (1985) suggest that to have a right to something, one must have an interest in it and to have such an interest one must have an interest in continuing to exist. The law makes no such distinction between decisions to be made for babies and that of the incompetent adult and yet, in practice, there are many situations within neonatal units throughout the country where similar dilemmas and actions defended throughout the Tony Bland hearing have occurred without consideration of any legal repercussions.

The case of *Airedale NHS Trust v Bland* [1993] focuses on the somewhat protracted question of whether any court could suggest that discontinuation of treatment on an individual in a persistent vegetative state would constitute a criminal offence. It would appear that the decision made in the House of Lords to allow such an event to occur was based on the moral premise that it was in his best interest not to prolong life and yet, in doing so, the law violated any right he had to live.

Comments made by the judges involved in the case best illustrate the justification for the decision made in the House of Lords. Lord Goff declared that the issue was not one of whether it was in his best interest to die but that it was whether it was in his best interest to prolong life by continuing treatment; Lord Browne-Wilkinson urged that the treatment was not in his best interest in that it was an invasion of bodily integrity to continue with treatment of no affirmative benefit. Perhaps the most pertinent remark came from Lord Mustill who pointed out that: 'the distressing truth which must not be shirked is that the proposed conduct is not in the best interests of Anthony Bland, for he has no best interests of any kind' (Brazier, 1993). Such a point readily moves the argument towards one that focuses on the rights of other interested parties, as it is clear that in many cases moral issues affecting the relatives, friends and professionals involved are often undermined and left unresolved once the person has died.

Lord Mustill's position reflects the existing law relating to a patient's right to die. It serves to provide rules to protect the human rights of everyone and yet cannot escape from the moral dimension associated with determining laws that will best serve such rights. What forms the basis of much healthcare law, for both the competent and incompetent patient, has revealed itself to be full of contradiction. The legal position on euthanasia contravenes a person's right to die if the assistance of another person is required. However, particularly where the incompetent patient is involved, the evidence both morally and in law appears to support an omission to act, despite the motives and/or consequences, as being more acceptable.

If we are to address the question of whether the law *should* support the right of a patient to die, the same confusion and ambiguity would exist, simply shifting the power to decide from one professional group to another. The moral issues would be exactly the same and, while it appears that there are many existing laws which confuse rather than help the decision-making process, there are others where the focus remains with that of protecting the autonomy of the patient. The reproductive rights of women until the case of *Re S.* seemed fairly clear and yet now serve as an example of how individual rights can and have been violated.

While the moral and legal position of the fetus remains contentious, it would seem that in order to protect the rights of the pregnant woman, the issue of fetal rights should never in law take precedence over that of the woman. The embryo poses a different dimension and while the Abortion Act 1967 and the Human Fertilization and Embryology Act 1990 provide many contradictions as to the rights of the unborn, it seems somewhat paradoxical that arguments against research on spare embryos has been given the legal consideration not yet afforded to animals, whose rights continue to be thwarted in the name of scientific development. If such research can be carried out on a collection of cells, albeit those of a potential human, whose destiny is destruction, there seems little justification to object, provided such controls laid down within the new Act are honoured.

The position of the handicapped baby begins to illustrate further ambiguity in law in relation to the protection of a child's right to live and yet it would seem that the issue of whose interest is best being served does, and should, be recognized further in law, especially where there is evidence that the baby involved is unlikely to ever appreciate what is in their best interest. In reality, to legalize any action that would end in the termination of life through whatever means suggests that the law as it stands does to some extent prevent what could lead to the destruction of many babies with the potential for a reasonable life. Parents, whose initial reaction to anything other than what they consider 'normal' , may subsequently find themselves in conflict with what they consider would be in their own interest, rather than that of the child. This was clearly illustrated in the case of Tony Bland, although for the adult who has enjoyed a fruitful life, the measure of potential may be more readily established both from a medical perspective and from those who believe they knew or know what the individual person would have wanted. In law the question always centres on what would the person have wished had they been able to decide for themselves. Yet it is important to consider that if Tony Bland had been consulted, would the same course of action been permitted in law or would the consultant involved have found himself in the same position as Dr Cox or Dr Arthur?

The notion of an advanced directive or 'living will', where a person decides and plans for the possibility of the type of event that befell Tony Bland, perhaps lends itself to a more acceptable perspective from which the law should operate. Kennedy and Grubb (1989: 117) examine the central moral feature surrounding what may at first glance provide some answers, suggesting that:

> Although self determination is involved when a patient establishes a
> way to protect his or her wishes into a time of anticipated incapacity,
> it is a sense of self-determination lacking in one important attribute:
> active, contemporaneous personal choice.

A written advanced instruction by Jehovah's Witness requesting not to have blood transfusions provides an obvious example of how the existing position fails to support the autonomy of an individual if 'active contemporaneous personal choice' cannot be obtained to ratify the original request (Hutchesson, 1992).

For the competent adult it would seem that the 'living will' would or should automatically provide a right for the person who is capable of deciding that they no longer wish to live. However, while the sanctioning of non-selective treatment already upheld for the competent patient could be carried out at the patient's request, it would be of little value to those where the only way to quicken the dying process would be through the assistance of another.

Perhaps the most confusing moral issue of all rests within the suffering experienced by someone where treatment has ceased to be effective, where pain and anguish is all that remains and where the only option available is suicide. The justification for the law to remain unyielding in its efforts to prevent the sanctioning of 'active' euthanasia does nothing to respect the moral rights of the person desperate for some help in the process of dying and yet provides some protection from the possible abuse of such authority.

It is clear that 'human rights' within the parameters of healthcare practice have both a legal and moral dimension, where it is no longer acceptable for practitioners to remain ignorant of the ethical reasoning that underpins the life-and-death issues that confront their daily practice. Practitioners should also be reminded that *ignorantia juris neminem excusat* (ignorance of the law does not excuse) (Curzon, 1992).

We have seen how a moral maze influencing the legal boundaries associated with rights and the termination of life begins at or, for some, begins before conception. The unborn child, at various stages of development is afforded little in the way of protection both with the advancement of reproductive technology and the wider parameters of choice given to women who wish to terminate a pregnancy. Conversely, it is becoming clear that the boundary between maternal and fetal rights is now clouded by events that suggest an alternative moral argument surrounding individual respect for autonomy, when a woman is pregnant. The journey through life and the possibility of its premature termination after birth has been presented within the context of individual autonomy and the capacity or not to use it. At what age a child should be able to make an autonomous choice to live or die, and how the best interests of an incompetent patient may be served, provide the reader with more questions than answers, demanding further exploration and deliberation at the moral-legal interface. What remains clear is that neither the lawyer nor the healthcare professional is able to address the moral complexities arising from scientific discovery which now heralds the possibility of life at almost any cost, while denying that same maxim for death.

REFERENCES

Baylis, F.E. (1990) The ethics of ex-utero research on spare non-viable IVF human embryos. *Bioethics*, Vol. 4, No. 4.

Brahms, D. and Brahms, M. (1983) The Arthur Case – A proposal for legislation. *Journal of Medical Ethics*. **9**, 12–15.

Brazier, M. (1992) *Medicine Patients and the Law*, Penguin Books, Harmondsworth.

Brazier, M. (1993) Death, dying and the law, M.A. Health Care Ethics Medico-Legal Problems Course Handout (Manchester University).

Charles Edwards, I. (1991) Who decides? *Paediatric Nursing*. Dec, pp. 6–7.

Curzon, L.B. (1992) *Dictionary of Law*, Pitman Publishing, London.

Dimond, B. (1990) *Legal Aspects of Nursing*, Prentice Hall, Herts.

Guilleminn, J.H. and Holstrom L.L. (1990) *Mixed Blessings: Intensive Care for New-borns*, Oxford University Press, Oxford.

Hewson, B. (1992) When 'no' means 'yes'. *The Law Society's Gazette*, No. 45, 9 Dec.

Hutchesson, P. (1992) Medical treatment – refusal of medical treatment – adult – refusal on religious grounds. *The New Law Journal*, Vol. 142 August 7, pp. 1125–7.

Jenkins, R. (1995) *The Law and the Midwife*, Blackwell Science, Oxford.

Kennedy, I. and Grubb, A. (1989) *Medical Law: Text and Materials*, Butterworth, London.

Lee , R. and Morgan, D. (1990) *Birthrights: Law and Ethics at the Beginnings of Life*, Routledge, London.

Mason, J.K. and McCall Smith, R.A. (1991) *Law and Medical Ethics*, Butterworth, London.

Tooley, M. (1985) Handicapped babies: a right to life? *Nursing Mirror* Feb 20, Vol. 160, No. 8.

Warnock Committee (1984) *Report of the Committee of Inquiry into Human Fertilisation and Embryology*, HMSO, London, Cm 9314.

Warnock, M. (1985) *A Question of Life*, Basil Blackwell, Oxford.

Wells, C. (1990) 'Otherwise kill me': marginal children and ethics at the edges of existence, Ch. 11, in *Birthrights – Law and Ethics at the Beginnings of Life* (R. Lee and D. Morgan), Routledge, London.

CASE LAW

Airedale NHS Trust v Bland [1993] 2 ALL ER 316 HL.

Gillick v West Norfolk and Wisbech AHA [1985] 3 ALL ER.

Paton v BPSA [1978] 2 All ER 987; [1979] QB 276.

R v Adams [1957] Crim. LR 365.

R v Cox 18 [1992] The Times, 21 September, (leader).

Re B [1981] 1WLR 1421

Re F (in Utero) [1988] 2 ALL ER 193.

Re J [1992] 4 ALL ER 614 CA.

Re R [1991] 4 ALL ER 177 CA (cited in Brazier 1993: 100).

Re S (1992) 2 ALL ER 671.

Re T [1992] 4 ALL ER 649 CA.

ACTS OF PARLIAMENT

Abortion Act 1967
Family Reform Act 1969
Human Fertilization and Embryology Act 1990
Infant Life (Preservation) Act 1929
Offences Against the Person Act 1861
Suicide Act 1961

8

Advocacy, law and the psychiatric nurse

Martin Johnston

INTRODUCTION

Over recent years, nursing commentators have given considerable attention to the themes surrounding patient advocacy (Kohnke, 1980; Jones, 1982; Wagg and Yurick, 1983; Copp, 1986; Witts, 1992; Stein, 1993). Alongside this, it is possible to identify an increasing interest in ethical and legal issues in nursing (Young, 1981; Dimond, 1984; Jameton, 1984; Burnard and Chapman, 1988; Raatikainen, 1989; UKCC 1984, 1992). Consequently, the relationship between advocacy, ethics and the law is one which merits further exploration; just such an exploration will be the primary purpose of this paper. It would be ambitious in the extreme, if not downright presumptuous, to suppose that all aspects of such an exploration could be treated adequately in a paper of this size, or indeed by a single author. I propose, therefore, to restrict discussion to selected issues which I believe to be particularly useful in elucidating some of the key themes. With this general aim in mind, the area of psychiatric nursing would appear to offer an especially fruitful basis for discussion, since it is here that conflicts between legal duties, professional codes of conduct and ethics are likely to be most apparent. Few other areas of nursing require, or indeed even permit, the type of radical interventions, such as physical restraint, enforced medication and the use of seclusion, which can often be associated with psychiatric nursing practice.

In what follows, I consider the relationship between the law and ethics in general with a view to establishing a basis for discussion. I then review the extent and nature of the psychiatric nurse's legal powers and obligations and examine the ethical rationales for their existence. From this it should be possible to explore the concept of advocacy and examine the suggestion that psychiatric nurses should serve as patient advocates.

ETHICS AND THE LAW

In the most general terms there are some features that appear common to both ethics and the law. Both can be viewed as essentially concerned with the regulation of human conduct in a variety of respects and both can be applied in judgments of behaviour which result in that behaviour being classified as right or wrong. Here, the difference between the two will prove of most interest. At the heart of this difference is the fact that what is legally permissible is not necessarily morally valid. To put this another way, the ethical merit of an action, for example, can be assessed independently of questions concerning its legality. In referring to this feature as 'moral neutrality' Lyons (1989: 104) makes the following point:

> the existence and content of law is determined by facts that make law subject to moral appraisal but do not guarantee it any moral value. The connections between law and sound moral principles (if there are any) are not necessary but contingent. Law is, in this sense, morally neutral.

It follows from this that laws, as extant social facts, may themselves be the subject of ethical evaluation. Consequently, it makes sense to talk of actual laws in terms of their being right or wrong, ethical or unethical; indeed, one need only consider the former apartheid laws of South Africa or the racial purity laws of the Nazis to identify examples of laws which were clearly unethical.

The importance of this issue lies in the relatively straightforward fact that an act being legal does not of itself also make it ethical. That the two ascriptions may on a number of occasions be appropriate to a given number of acts, and that such a coincidence of ascriptions may well be desirable, does not allow us to assume that there is any necessary relationship between the two. The psychiatric nurse, then, acting in accordance with appropriate legislation, can still find their actions to be the subject of ethical scrutiny, either by themselves or by others. This brief discussion in no way represents all that can be said about the relationship between ethics and the law. However, the ethical-legal difference identified provides us with a basis to discuss the nature of the psychiatric nurse's legal powers and obligations with a view to subsequently considering their ethical merit and influence on the idea of the nurse as patient advocate.

POWER AND THE PSYCHIATRIC NURSE

The concept of power is not easily defined in a precise manner. However, we can still offer useful descriptions and distinctions which will serve at least some illustrative purposes. Initially we can distinguish between formal and informal power. Formal power is based primarily on the law; consequently there exist a range of institutions concerned with its distribution and application. Informal power is a much broader concept and consequently harder to define, but it may be viewed in terms of the perception of particular social roles – there being some roles perceived as more important than others which in turn leads to a perceived authority being associated with those who occupy them. Clearly, this initial distinction is overly simple, but I shall elaborate upon it as I proceed. What is important for the moment is the recognition that we are essentially dealing with two poles of one continuum.

Formal powers

In the terms outlined above, the psychiatric nurse's formal powers are closely associated with their legal powers. The psychiatric nurse is subject to the same general legislation appropriate to all nurses, but here we are concerned primarily with the legal powers specific to psychiatric nurses. The nature of these legal powers is twofold.

First, the nurse is required to act in accordance with the instructions and support of other professionals such as social workers, hospital managers, general practitioners and psychiatrists in applying the statutory powers detailed in the Mental Health Act 1983, and in Scotland the Mental Health (Scotland) Act 1984. Although such legislation covers a vast array of issues, of prime importance are those sections dealing with compulsory admission to and detention and treatment in hospital. In the most general terms, the two Acts provide a sliding scale of levels of intervention, ranging from short-term detention without treatment, to long-term detention with compulsory treatment, based on the identification of specific criteria in the particular circumstances. In most cases, however, the key elements are that the individual is suffering from a mental disorder, and that it is necessary for their own health or safety, and/or for the protection of others, that those powers be applied. Again in general terms, as the level of intervention increases, so too do the extent of the controls on the application of such powers. Second, the nurse can exercise their own powers of detention under s5, ss 2 of the Mental Health Act 1983; similar powers for the nurse in Scotland are detailed at s25, ss 2 of the Mental Health (Scotland) Act 1984.

With respect to the first of these, it is apparent that the nurse's role is essentially subservient. Primarily this is a result of the nature of the nurse's conditions of employment and the duties inherent in such conditions. For example, an application for emergency admission to hospital is made to the hospital managers. Once accepted, the hospital staff then assume the responsibility for ensuring that appropriate compulsory powers are applied. In the course of this there is no requirement to take into account the views of nurses on the ward. Similarly, it is well-established (Brazier, 1992) that nurses should act in accordance with the instructions of doctors in hospital settings. Brazier (1992: 136) describes this thus: 'Within hospitals nurses may find themselves liable for negligence if they fail to take careful note of instructions given to them, or if they fail to provide adequate nursing care or attention'. Such liability is not solely applicable to psychiatric nurses, but when coupled with the requirement to act in accordance with the compulsory powers of the Mental Health Acts it becomes evident that such nurses are more dependent on the instructions of others.

In practice it may well be the case that nurses are directly involved in the decision-making process concerning compulsory admission to, and/or treatment in hospital. However, that such a democratic state of affairs pertains is largely dependent on the discretion of those directly responsible for the enforcement of statutory powers. The important point to consider here is the essentially secondary nature of the nurse's role in the proceedings. Ultimately, in most circumstances, on issues of compulsory treatment and detention the nurse is not the decision-maker, nor is there any legal requirement that they should be directly involved in the decision-making process. The bottom line is that the nurse may be required to become involved in the involuntary detention and treatment of clients. Such a situation may involve the use of physical restraint, seclusion and the enforced injection of medication.

With regard to the second aspect the situation is quite different. The employment of 'nurses' holding power', as these powers have come to be known, is a decision which is entirely in the hands of the nurse themselves. Such powers are by no means extensive. However, they do permit appropriately trained nurses (i.e. a first level registered mental nurse or registered nurse for the mentally handicapped) to directly interfere in the liberty of others. The precise wording of the appropriate sections of the two Acts is as follows:

If, in the case of a patient who is receiving treatment for mental disorder as an inpatient in a hospital, it appears to a nurse of the prescribed class –

(a) that the patient is suffering from mental disorder to such a degree that it is necessary for his health and safety or for the protection of others for him to be immediately restrained from leaving the hospital; and

(b) that it is not practicable to secure the immediate attendance of a practitioner for the purpose of furnishing a report under subsection (2) above,

the nurse may record that fact in writing; and in that event the patient may be detained in the hospital for a period of six hours from the time when the fact is so recorded or until the earlier arrival at the place where the patient is detained of a practitioner having power to furnish a report under that subsection.

(Mental Health Act, 1983, s 5, ss 4)

and

If, in the case of a patient who is already in a hospital receiving treatment for mental disorder and who is not liable to be detained therein under this Part of this Act, it appears to a nurse of the prescribed class –

(a) that the patient is suffering from mental disorder to such a degree that it is necessary for his health and safety or for the protection of other persons for him to be immediately restrained from leaving the hospital; and

(b) that it is not practicable to secure the immediate attendance of a medical practitioner for the purpose of making an emergency recommendation.

the patient may be detained in the hospital for a period of 2 hours from the time when he was first so detained or until the earlier arrival at the place where the patient is detained of a medical practitioner having power to make an emergency recommendation.

(Mental Health (Scotland) Act 1984, s 25, ss 2)

It is clear from the wording of these sections that the nurse's role is recognized as being secondary to other professionals. Nevertheless, in both Acts it is equally clear that the nurse is able, and indeed expected, to exercise their professional judgment in appropriate circumstances leading to the involuntary detention of particular individuals. In one sense the nature of these circumstances is very strictly defined in both Acts. However, this fails to take account of the inherent difficulties associated with assessing the degree of risk which a particular individual presents either to themselves or to others. (We shall not here consider the further difficulties associated with identifying what exactly 'suffering from a mental disorder' entails, nor indeed, how we are able to identify such individuals.) However, it is apparent that we are dealing here with what is primarily an emergency power of limited application, which does not necessarily have dramatic consequences for the individual so detained in the long term. But by themselves these considerations should not lead us to ignore the issues which the possession of such powers raise. The essential point concerning the provision outlined above is that, even if only for limited periods of time, appropriately trained nurses are recognized as having the requisite skills and knowledge base to allow them to act independently on the basis of their own professional judgments.

So, whether working independently or in collaboration with others, the psychiatric nurse is in possession of a broad array of legally enforceable powers over a range of individuals whose behaviour causes them to be drawn to the attention of the mental health professions. Such powers permit varying degrees of interference in the lives of others distinct from most other branches of nursing. Further, it is clear that the psychiatric nurse is obliged to apply such powers in appropriate circumstances.

Informal powers

The informal powers of the psychiatric nurse are not easily detailed. However, it is possible to identify some general features which go some way to explaining their nature and function. We are essentially dealing with perceptions associated with particular roles. Consequently, any powers will be as variable as those associated perceptions. As a result, it should not surprise us to come across contradictory views of the nature of such powers. Here we shall consider only two possible perceptions of the psychiatric nurse.

First, the psychiatric nurse may be viewed as an independent practitioner, in possession of a range of specialized skills and a sound knowledge base which enable them to exert a degree of authority in the area of mental health. When viewed in this way, the nurse is likely to command respect from others, and is in a position to wield influence over them. Second, the nurse may be viewed as essentially subservient to other more qualified professionals, such as psychiatrists. Consequently, any perceived authority is authority by association. The point here is that, given this variation in possible perceptions, it is extremely difficult to see how psychiatric nurses can influence the exercise of such informal power in any direct way, except in the most obvious sense such as general appearance and demeanour. Similarly, it is difficult to see how such power can be controlled in any remotely analogous way to that in which legal powers can be controlled. Here we can only note the possibility of the influence of informal powers in the nurse-patient relationship in a psychiatric setting.

We have now identified some features of the psychiatric nurse's powers and in the case of formal powers this has been quite explicit. We can now turn to a consideration of some of the ethical rationales given for the existence of such powers.

ETHICS AND THE POWERS OF THE PSYCHIATRIC NURSE

The starting point for the ethical rationales which seek to justify the compulsory powers of treatment and detention is entailed in the wording of the Acts themselves; we have already encountered one form of it in the two quotations above. Interventions, in general terms, under the Acts are based on a twofold concern. First, there is the concern for the welfare of the victim of mental disorder (mental disorder is not a particularly palatable term; however, since it is the term employed in the Mental Health Acts, I propose to use it in what follows), in the sense that it is recognized as being a valuable aim to prevent such individuals from harming themselves, either as a result of deliberate acts of self-injury or as a consequence of self-neglect or incapacity. The second concern stems from the potential danger which some individuals suffering from mental disorder may present to others. As with the first concern, the primary issue is a desire to prevent harm befalling others. In fact in both the United Kingdom and the United States, courts have effectively ruled that mental health professionals have a responsibility to protect others from coming to grief at the hands of their clients (*Tarasoff v Regents of the University of California* [1976]; *W v Egdell* [1990]. It may well be the case that an individual presents a danger to both themselves and others, but in such cases it would appear that our concerns simply double and our actions can be based on one or other or both of our primary concerns. It is one thing to cite general concerns but quite another to explain why we ought to act on them. The justification of our actions therefore will require far greater scrutiny if we are to consider them ethical.

The concerns identified give rise to two – although it should not be presumed that these are mutually exclusive – main types of ethical defence: paternalism and utilitarianism. I do not wish to suggest that these approaches exhaust all possibilities; rather, I identify them in particular since they are in part inherent within the wording of the Acts themselves. It will prove useful therefore to engage in further elucidation of such defences.

Paternalism

The essence of paternalism is that a given individual can be in a better position to ascertain the best interests of another person than they themselves are and should consequently act in accordance with those interests even in spite of that person's protestations. This view is fairly well captured in the old adage that 'doctor knows best'. In certain instances there is near universal acceptance of the appropriateness of some form of paternalism. Consider the cases of babies and young children and the means adults adopt to safeguard their welfare. In certain respects, the very idea of compulsory education draws on paternalism. There are limitations on the application of paternalism in such cases; nevertheless, there is a very real sense in which its value is accepted in particular circumstances and in fact those who fail to act within its terms are called to account. Clearly there is something of at least *prima facie* value in this general concern for the welfare of others and the desire to assist. The desire to prevent individuals identified as suffering from mental disorder from harming themselves, therefore, is seen in itself as a valuable goal and morally required. If this point is accepted, the remaining questions concern how we delimit the circumstances under which it is appropriate to make such interventions and what sorts of interventions will be warranted. We shall leave such questions aside and go on to consider the second type of ethical defence identified above.

Utilitarianism

For the utilitarian the consequences of an action are all-important, since it is from and to these that ethical evaluations are derived and correctly applied. The true goal of any activity, in so far as it is to be considered ethical, is the pursuit of the 'greatest happiness of the greatest number'. Accepting this at face value for the moment, it is clear that we have a case to justify the involuntary detention and treatment of individuals considered to present a threat to others, since such interventions in the long term will be justified by the general overall increase in happiness obtained. (In these types of cases it may be more accurate to talk of minimizing pain than maximizing happiness; the principle, however, remains the same.) The interests of the individual identified as suffering from mental disorder are also included in our evaluation of the consequent distribution of gains and losses, pleasures and pains. The essential point in this is the view that we are entitled to interfere in the activities of individuals where those activities present a threat to others (Mill, 1990) and, further, that if by compulsory treatment we can restore the individual identified as suffering from mental disorder to 'normality', then once again our actions are morally acceptable, given the overall positive outcome we have obtained.

These do not exhaust the entire range of possible defences. However, they do appear to be the major principles incorporated into the Acts. Our next task is to consider the adequacy of such defences, particularly in relation to the requirements placed on psychiatric nurses acting in accordance with the Acts. Of primary importance will be a consideration of respect for autonomy.

The principle of respect for autonomy

The primary difficulty with paternalistic and utilitarian defences stems from their violation of the principle of respect for autonomy: a principle which has come to take centre stage in discussions within nursing and medical ethics (Beauchamp and Childress, 1989). The concept of autonomy itself is not straightforward, but here we shall take it to involve a capacity for self-government. Self-government itself can be further described in terms of two other capacities: the capacity to determine and reflect upon one's desires and goals and an evaluative capacity whereby one can judge one's desires and goals in terms of broad categories such as right or wrong and good or bad. Where such capacities are present, it is argued (Mill, 1990), we have no grounds for interfering in the actions of another. Indeed, any such interference is seen as pernicious and detrimental to the general welfare of humanity. The most notable exceptions to this are situations where an individual's actions are likely to cause harm to others. However, such a state of affairs may lead us to presume the absence of the evaluative capacity in the individual concerned and, by association, the absence of the capacity to act autonomously. Where the capacity to act autonomously is absent, it may be argued, the principle of respect for autonomy cannot apply. This type of argument is often employed in defences of the compulsory treatment and detention of the mentally disordered.

The initial plausibility of this type of defence soon fades when subjected to more detailed scrutiny; there are two main points to make here. The first concerns the difficulty in determining the presence or absence of either of the two capacities involved in self-government. The second arises from deciding what our response ought to be to those found to lack the capacity for self-government. It is all too easy to assume that *de facto* those who are identified as suffering from mental disorder lack the capacity for self-government and consequently to allow those who are mentally well to dispose of them as they see fit. Determining a capacity for self-government is not an easy task. In our everyday lives, not all our actions are subjected to rigorous appraisal and reflection and in so far as this is the case, we cannot be said to act completely autonomously all the time. In many ways it makes more sense to view autonomy not as an absolute feature of actions which is either present or not, but rather as a variable quality of actions, present to a greater or lesser extent. This variability among those considered to be mentally well leads us to question the validity of the assumption that the mentally disordered lack any capacity for self-government. One could argue that this variability means we ought to intervene in the actions of others more frequently, irrespective of the presence of any identifiable mental disorder. However, presumably this is not a view which would enjoy widespread support. We shall not consider the issue concerning the extent of interference warranted in the actions of those found to lack a capacity for self-government other than to note that given that we are dealing with a variable quality, so too our interventions must admit of a variety of degrees.

It is beyond the scope of this paper and indeed this author to offer a definitive resolution of the conflicts between competing ethical principles identified above. However, we should note that it is possible to produce ethical rationales for the use of compulsory powers of treatment and detention, albeit incomplete and conflicting ones. Both the conflict between competing ethical principles and the conflict between legal powers and ethical principles represent potential sources of moral tension for the psychiatric nurse. It would be too pessimistic to assume that an effective resolution is unattainable. Equally, it would be over-optimistic to assume that such a resolution will be forthcoming in the immediate future. However unsatisfactory it may be, the situation is as it is. It is against this backdrop that the suggestion that nurses should act as patient advocates has arisen.

ADVOCACY AND THE PSYCHIATRIC NURSE

In recent years much has been said of the role of the nurse as patient advocate and, indeed, this can partly be viewed as a response to the demands of respecting autonomy. Given the nurse's experience and knowledge base, they are in an ideal position to offer the kind of support and information required of an advocate. In the psychiatric setting the nurse advocate is part of a process which aims at the restoration or maximization of patient autonomy. It will be helpful then to consider the concept of advocacy further and to elucidate some of the issues that arise when we take into account the legal obligations of the psychiatric nurse.

Defining advocacy

As with numerous contemporary issues in nursing, one of the major difficulties lies in attempting to provide an adequate definition of the concept under discussion. The concept of advocacy is no exception. However, for present purposes, let us consider the following: 'the role of the advocate is to inform the client and support him in whatever decisions he makes' (Gadow, 1980).

In many respects, such a definition captures the essential features of the nature of advocacy within a nursing context. If we add to this the idea of pleading the case of another, a view primarily associated with the legal origins of the concept, we have a base for discussion. We must consider how this basic definition of advocacy squares with the duties of the psychiatric nurse and the ethical rationales that underpin those duties identified above.

Advocacy and the compulsory powers

The most immediate conflict arises when we consider whether compulsory detention can ever be said to equate with our general conception of advocacy. Clearly one cannot in any usual sense be said to be supporting a decision to leave hospital by forcibly preventing an individual from doing so. Nor, indeed, can physically restraining a patient while an injection is given against their will be seen as offering support to a decision to refuse medication. Although neither of these activities represent a substantial part of the psychiatric nurse's daily activities, they are, under appropriate circumstances, required of them. The overall effect of this state of affairs is clear: the distribution of power in the nurse-patient relationship is, more so than usual, skewed very definitely in the direction of the nurse. The result of this is to make us question the possibility of the psychiatric nurse ever acting as patient advocate. Allmark (1992) puts this succinctly:

> To suggest that a patient has an advocate when it is that very person who may be involved in the treatment that the patient is resisting is analogous to suggesting that the police can act as advocates for those in custody.

Allmark's remarks are directed towards the viability of nurse advocacy in any setting and as such they apply to psychiatric nursing. But the whole viability issue becomes even more contentious when we consider the psychiatric nurse's legal requirement to act contrary to the wishes of patients in particular circumstances. It is precisely these legal requirements that render the psychiatric nurse's pursuit of the role of patient advocate inherently unrealizable, unless we substantially alter our definition of advocacy.

Such alterations are possible and perhaps even desirable. Burnard and Chapman (1988: 17), for example, describe one aspect of advocacy as follows:

> The nurse who has truly cultivated the skill of empathy and who is in frequent personal interaction with the patient may be able to interpret the patient's needs to others and to act as a go-between when other health care professionals appear, to the patient, to be unapproachable.

The move from advocate to 'go-between' or needs-interpreter may well be advisable but it takes us quite a distance from a relationship primarily concerned with the transfer of power back into the hands of the patient (Brown, 1985). But not even this type of alteration resolves the difficulties encountered by the psychiatric nurse. How can a patient be expected to identify the exercise of the skill of empathy on the part of a nurse who with their colleagues is restraining that patient in order that medication may be given by injection without consent?

Such modifications also offer little in the way of comfort or guidance to nurses who, having interpreted a patient's needs, find the rest of the team less than sympathetic to those needs. In such circumstances, what should the nurse's response be? Clearly, anything short of compliance with the decision of the senior member of staff responsible can lead to severe consequences for the nurse. In a similar vein, Bailey (1983) describes the case of two student nurses whose refusal to participate in electro-convulsive therapy led to their dismissal. It is one thing to have one's views listened to, quite another to have them acted on.

At this point, then, we have identified the nature of the problem. The possession by the psychiatric nurse of compulsory powers of detention and, by association with other professionals, of treatment essentially renders the possibility of the psychiatric nurse ever genuinely acting as patient advocate inherently implausible. One may say that these powers are only applicable to patients detained under the Mental Health Act, but the characteristic feature of a nurse's holding power is that it enables the nurse to do precisely that: to detain a patient under the Act.

CONCLUSIONS

Given the existence of and requirement to use, under appropriate circumstances, compulsory powers of treatment and detention, the psychiatric nurse is placed in a potentially difficult position. They have no right to overrule the decisions of senior colleagues irrespective of the basis for their objections. We have demonstrated that the existence and use of such powers can give rise to major conflicts between ethical principles, leaving the nurse exposed to marked moral tensions. To add to this the unrealizable suggestion that psychiatric nurses should act as patient advocates serves only to exacerbate this tension. We can dilute our conception of advocacy to the extent that such tensions are minimized. However, this move has the potential to minimize the value of advocacy in psychiatric settings. That psychiatric patients should have advocates is in principle an important suggestion which seems inherently valuable, but they do not need advocates whose activities are seriously curtailed by their other responsibilities. In fact, the provision of nurse advocates, whose activities are limited by their other legal responsibilities, would allow the more cynical elements in the mental health professions to pay lip service to the principles of advocacy and reduce the concept to empty rhetoric.

None of this suggests that psychiatric nurses can never act as patient advocates, only that the role of advocate is incompatible with the extant powers of compulsory treatment and detention. To propose that the role of advocate is central to the practice of psychiatric nursing is to implicitly call for a major overhaul of mental health legislation. This may well be a perfectly legitimate aim, but it should be made explicit.

REFERENCES

Allmark, P. (1992) The case against nurse advocacy. *British Journal of Nursing*, **2**(1) 33–6.

Bailey, J. (1983) ECT or not ECT: that is the question. *Nursing Times*, **79**(9), 12–14.

Beauchamp, T.L. and Childress, J.F. (1989) *Principles of Biomedical Ethics*, 3rd edn, Oxford University Press, Oxford.

Brazier, M. (1992) *Medicine, Patients and the Law*, 2nd edn, Penguin Books, Harmondsworth.

Brown, M. (1985) Matter of commitment. *Nursing Times*, **81**(18), 26–7.

Burnard, P. and Chapman, C.M. (1988) *Professional and Ethical Issues in Nursing: The Code of Professional Conduct*. John Wiley, Chichester.

Copp, L.A. (1986) The nurse as advocate for vulnerable persons. *Journal of Advanced Nursing*, **11**, 225–63.

Dimond, B. (1984) *Legal Aspects of Nursing*, Prentice Hall, Herts.

Gadow, S. (1980) Existential advocacy, in *Nursing Practice: The Ethical Issues*, (A. Jameton), Prentice Hall, Englewood Cliffs, N.J.

Jones, E.W. (1982) Advocacy: a tool for radical nursing curriculum planners. *Journal of Nurse Education*, **21**(1), 40–5.

Kohnke, M. (1980) The nurse as advocate. *American Journal of Nursing*, Nov, 2038–40.

Lyons, D. (1989) *Ethics and the Rule of Law*, Cambridge University Press, Cambridge.

Mental Health Act 1983, HMSO, London.

Mental Health (Scotland) Act 1984, HMSO, London.

Mill, J.S. (1990) On Liberty, in *Utilitarianism* (ed. M. Warnock), Fontana Press, Glasgow.

Raatikainen, R. (1989) Values and ethical principles in nursing. *Journal of Advanced Nursing*, **14**, 92–6.

Stein, T. (1993) A voice in the wilderness. *Health Service Journal*, 4 March, 30–1.

United Kingdom Central Council (1984) *Code of Professional Conduct*, UKCC, London.

United Kingdom Central Council (1992) *Code of Professional Conduct*, UKCC, London.

Wagg, B. and Yurick, A. (1983) Care enough to hear. *Journal of Gerontological Nursing*, **9**(9).

Witts, P. (1992) Patient advocacy in nursing, in *Themes and Perspectives in Nursing* (ed. K. Soothill, K. Kendrick and C. Henry) Chapman & Hall, London.

Young, A.P. (1981) *Legal Problems in Nursing Practice*, Harper & Row, Cambridge.

CASE LAW

Tarasoff v Regents of the University of California [1976].

W v Egdell [1990] All England Law Reports, 2, p. 835.

9

An historical and ethical perspective on a code for medical research: First do no harm

J. Stuart Horner

The modern nurse is inevitably involved in research. The increasing emphasis within the National Health Service on 'evidence-based medicine' can only result in a greater investment in research projects to obtain such evidence. Some of this research will involve nursing techniques and the use of nursing skills. In planning such projects nurses will need to consider the ethical implications and to seek the approval of the local research ethical committee. They need to know why such committees exist and why they have absolute discretion to reject an apparently desirable project. Nurses will also be involved in medical research. Almost every project doctors undertake has a direct or indirect impact on the nursing staff. Nurses may find themselves explaining such projects to patients or seeking their informed consent. They may become aware of practices which are not in accordance with the protocol approved by the ethical committee, or the patient may reveal to them concerns about the research which they have not raised with the doctors. For all these reasons nurses need to be aware of the need for ethical control over all research involving patients.

This chapter is written from a medical and an historical perspective. A broad view has been taken of research, since the modern controlled trial is a recent development. Traditionally, doctors have applied tried and trusted remedies which appear to have worked in the past irrespective of whether their effectiveness has been proved. When these remedies failed, doctors have used their theoretical knowledge to apply new remedies and have then carefully recorded their observations for their own use and that of the wider profession. Such activities are encompassed in this broader use of the term 'research'.

HIPPOCRATES AND RESEARCH

Hippocrates was born on the island of Kos around 460 BC and is alleged to have lived for 90 years. After training in medicine he eventually returned to his native island where he founded a school of medicine. At that time Greece was unusual in having no form of control over medical practice. This 'fostered opportunities for charlatanism, medical chicanery and higher than acceptable risks of abuse or permanent injury to patients' (Carrick, 1985: 169). As Hippocrates himself pointed out:

> Although the art of healing is the most noble of all the arts, yet, because of the ignorance both of its profession and of their rash critics, it has at this time fallen into the least repute of them all. The chief cause for this seems to be that it is the science for which States have laid down no penalties for malpractice. Ill-repute is the only punishment and this does little harm to the quacks who are compounded of nothing else. Such men resemble dumb characters on the stage who, bearing the dress and appearance of actors, yet are not so. It is the same with the physicians; there are many in name, few in fact.
>
> *(Chadwick and Mann, 1978: 168)*

Hippocrates represents not only a direct descent from the Asklepion tradition of magic based on a snake cult but the first major departure from it. Along with Galen in AD 200 he established a scientific basis for medical practice which was to continue in Western Europe for more than 1000 years. The Hippocratic school concentrated on detailed observation and careful recording (Chadwick and Mann, 1978: 31) and grounded their theories firmly in practical experience. McIlrath (1959: 1557) states 'in Hippocrates we find the first genuine scientific student of disease and the first doctor to insist that the physician's great duty is to do no harm'. He vigorously opposed medicine based on hypotheses or the principles of disease. He preferred observation and deduction. This has rightly become the standard of practice for modern medicine. Careful clinical observation is accompanied by rigorous scientific enquiry into the associations which those observations seem to suggest, followed by rigorous testing of proposed interventions. Hippocrates would have considered a specific intervention to be beneficial if it was associated with clinical improvement. Today this association itself is tested by using a randomized control trial so that even the clinician does not know (until the trial is ended) whether the clinical improvement he observes is due to the intervention itself or some 'placebo effect'.

Hippocrates, however, was no dreamy idealist and warmly commended the physician who made small mistakes:

> Infallibility is rarely to be seen. Most doctors seem to me to be in the position of poor navigators. In calm weather they can conceal their mistakes,

but when overtaken by a mighty storm or a violent gale it is evident to all that it is their ignorance and error which is the ruin of the ship.

(ibid: 75)

Then, as now, medicine had its critics and in a passage strangely resonant with the modern debate about whether smokers have any responsibility to assist the doctor in their own treatment he writes:

What trusty reason leads them [medicine's critics] to absolve a patient's weakness of character and impute instead a lack of intelligence on the part of his physician? As if doctors can prescribe the wrong remedies but patients can never disobey their orders.

(ibid: 142)

THE HIPPOCRATIC OATH

I swear by Apollo the healer, by Asklepios, by Health and all the powers of healing, and call to witness all the gods and goddesses that I may keep this Oath and Promise to the best of my ability and judgment. I will pay the same respect to my master in the Science as to my parents and share my life with him and pay all my debts to him. I will regard his sons as my brothers and teach them the Science, if they desire to learn it, without fee or contract. I will hand on precepts, lectures and all other learning to my sons, to those of my master and to those pupils duly apprenticed and sworn and to no other.

I will use my power to help the sick to the best of my ability and judgment; I will abstain from harming or wronging any man by it.

I will not give a fatal draught to anyone if I am asked, nor will I suggest any such thing. Neither will I give a woman means to procure an abortion.

I will be chaste and religious in my life and in my practice.

I will not cut, even for the stone, but I will leave such procedures to the practitioners of that craft.

Whenever I go into a house, I will go to help the sick and never with the intention of doing harm or injury. I will not abuse my position to indulge in sexual contacts with the bodies of women or of men, whether they be free men or slaves. Whatever I see or hear, professionally or privately, which ought not to be divulged, I will keep secret and tell no one. If, therefore, I observe this Oath and do not violate it, may I prosper both in my life and in my profession earning good repute among men for all time. If I transgress and forswear this Oath, may my lot be otherwise.

(Chadwick and Mann, 1978: 67)

The Hippocratic Oath represents the first-known attempt of a group of doctors to bind themselves to their own specific set of ethical values in their conduct towards patients. Unlike modern equivalents it was administered *before* any of the skills were taught rather than at the conclusion of initial training. It formed a unique contract between doctor and patient (Cameron, 1991) of which the essential feature was that the doctor would at all costs make the patient no worse as a result of the ministrations. Only those prepared to make that commitment could be allowed to learn techniques which had such potential for harm. Such a commitment seems fundamental for all those who wish to engage in research involving patients.

Nurses have preferred to apply a more regulated code of conduct agreed by the profession as a whole. There are benefits and disadvantages of each. A broad commitment to principles provides greater flexibility, while a detailed code of conduct makes it easier to take remedial action against those who transgress it.

Although the Oath is ascribed to Hippocrates it could not possibly have carried his approval. First, it would have been ridiculous for a man who so clearly and specifically rejected the Asklepion magic cult (although he was by no means opposed to religion and encouraged patients to maintain their faith) to swear an oath to the founder of the very arts he despised. Second, as Carrick (1985) points out, the original oath is written in the wrong dialect and the ethical values proposed were not those of contemporary practice. Respect for the sanctity of life was not the dominant ethical philosophy in Greece at the time. As in our own day, a variety of different ethical and moral perspectives were held alongside one another. Only the Pythagoreans were committed to the sanctity of life. Carrick believes that this does not necessarily make the Oath Pythagorean although it incorporates some of their ideas. He concludes that it may be the product of a very small medical reform movement. Nevertheless, the Oath is unique to Greek medicine and unique within Greek medicine in its emphasis on:

- a duty to others – to protect the patient from harm and rid him from disease;
- a duty to oneself – to preserve and promote the reputation of the craft by adopting practices to ensure the integrity and competence of its members.

The Christianized version of the Oath was probably written some time before the third century AD. As Christianity became the dominant moral philosophy in Western Europe, so an approach based on the rejection of euthanasia and abortion became the dominant ethical philosophy throughout medicine.

The Oath helps to perpetuate what Cherkasky (1973) describes as 'the Hippocrates myth'. He writes:

> In envisioning the doctor as a superhuman who would possess all virtues, Hippocrates created a myth that both physicians and their patients have willingly perpetuated. The myth is that, at the core, doctors are somehow different from other men; even now the myth continues to flourish, although all around us there is evidence that the most noble purpose and noble commitment to medicine are commonly violated; study after study shows that, for all too many doctors, the temptation to equate cash with care is too strong to resist.

Cherkasky writes from an American perspective where the tendency towards excessive surgical intervention is well known. Caesarian section, cholecystectomy and hysterectomy are all more common in the United States and many observers have imputed a cash motive for this excess, although litigious patients may be a more recent explanation. In the National Health Service the majority of doctors believe that requiring individual general practitioners to assume both financial and clinical responsibility for their patients has the potential to create similar ethical dilemmas for doctors. Reports that certain types of patient are excluded from general practitioner lists and that some patients are denied care available to others give credence to Cherkasky's rather sweeping generalization.

Yet the Oath is still as relevant today as when it was first formulated. It has something to say on key issues of modern medicine such as: patient confidentiality; abortion; euthanasia; truth-telling; and justice in the distribution of health services. It also represents a professional commitment to engage in high standards of practice and in particular to avoid intellectual dishonesty and economic and moral abuse. Carrick (1985) concludes that 'the covenant expresses the personal desire and resolve to make oneself and one's profession the very best that both can be'. These qualities surely form the basis of any sensible ethical code for medical and health service research.

STATE CONTROL OF MEDICINE AND MEDICAL RESEARCH

Self-regulation by healthcare professions is not the only way to regulate medicine or the practice of research. The Greeks were unusual in the ancient world. In central America, religion provided a powerful control on medicine, although 'ethics did not depend on religion and the law demanded cruel punishments for the use of black magic by specialists in medical sorcery' (McIlrath, 1959: 254). The Incas passed laws 'demanding that medical practitioners should be properly qualified as both surgeons and physicians' (ibid: 310). In ancient China, medical confidentiality did not exist since Chinese physicians were required to report cases to the state. In early and medieval India, 'the Indian surgeons were very observant, competent and highly skilled men'. As far as medical ethics are concerned we find that the Indians had a high code. The physician was expected to consider his patient above everything and to refrain from discussing the patient's home, relationships or condition with outsiders (McIlrath: 662).

In the Middle East, religion and the State were closely linked. In Mesopotamia, medicine was under the control of the priests but the state code of Hammurabi dating from about 1727 BC is the first attempt by any culture to protect patients from incompetent doctors. The code is largely concerned with surgical procedures and deals with them in a detailed way. This control was not limited to doctors. The code included veterinary surgeons and barbers. Even wet nurses were strictly supervised. Abortion was a particularly serious matter and was prohibited in Assyria in the 15th century BC. Research was not permitted on free men but it was acceptable to test new treatments on slaves (McIlrath, 1959: 438). Little more than 50 years ago in Germany, horrific experiments were carried out among at least 300 prisoners in the Dachau concentration camp (Berger, 1990). In 1956 mentally handicapped children in Willowbrook, New York, were deliberately infected with viral hepatitis (Phillips and Dawson, 1985) and in 1968 Chamberlain reported research on a fetus which was still alive and indeed which today would be considered capable of survival (Chamberlain, 1968). Having failed to convince the British medical establishment to take action to submit all experimental research on patients to ethical control, Pappworth (1967) published a book about current practices in medical research in the UK. Although he attracted considerable criticism, his action almost certainly led to the present [not entirely effective (Neuberger, 1992)] controls on local medical research.

The founder of medicine in ancient Egypt was Imhotep who was chancellor to the Pharaoh Djoser about 2650 BC (Aldred, 1978). The Greeks identified him with their own god Asklepios (Watterson, 1984). Egyptian medicine was characterized at this time by careful observation and recording, together with dispassionate and scientific curiosity. Egyptian physicians fully understood the key importance of the heart and came close to discovering the circulation of the blood. They were respected for their anatomical and surgical knowledge (Wilson, 1956).

There appear to have been specialists within medicine and Egyptian doctors worked by ancient rules. 'If they failed to do so and the patient died, the doctors would be tried by law with death as the penalty' (McIlrath, 1959: 370). State regulation continued well into the Christian era. The Germanic law codes of the Visigoths in Spain in the fifth century insist on women being chaperoned during medical treatment (MacKinney, 1952). A century later there are references to similar government regulations in the Ostrogothic kingdom of Italy.

A high code of professional behaviour was demanded of physicians in ancient Persia by the priests, although the Zoroastrian religion tied the conception of disease so closely to sin that it was impossible to look elsewhere for the causes and cures of disease. McIlrath concludes that this inhibited both medical research and the development of medical ethics in Persia (op. cit.).

Clearly, where professional codes of conduct are laid down either by the State or by the priesthood, considerable sanctions exist to enforce them. Paradoxically, however, such codes may inhibit the development of medical ethics and scientific research, since they cannot take account of new knowledge or new cultural attitudes. While principles such as honesty remain unchanged, the interpretation of confidentiality, for example, may change over time even though the principle remains the same. Formal codes rarely make this distinction while priests may have difficulty in determining which principles are capable of variable application and which are not.

THE HIPPOCRATIC CODE IN MEDIEVAL WESTERN EUROPE

The introduction of Christianity created some new tensions. When miraculous healing seemed to be occurring among the new believers, resort to traditional medicine could easily be seek as a lack of faith (Temkin, 1991). Gradually, however, Hippocrates was separated from the demonized Greek pantheon and the Hippocratic method was accepted by Christians as an appropriate approach to healing.

Saint Jerome, for example, late in the fourth century, writing to a priest in northern Italy, refers to Hippocrates and commends some aspects of the Oath as a suitable code of conduct for the priestly office (MacKinney, 1952). Many of the Hippocratic writings were stored and transcribed in the medieval monasteries:

> The early medieval writers seem to have combined Hippocratic and Christian ideals without any apparent feeling of conflict or inconsistency. They repeated much of the ideology of the Hippocratic Oath, notably the moral injunctions against giving poisons or abortives and against violating the patient's confidence or the virtue of his womenfolk.
>
> (*MacKinney, 1952*)

Pearl Kibre (1945) concludes:

> The medieval Hippocratic writings revered by physician and layman alike, preserved in frequent manuscripts and printed before 1500 by the incunabula presses, though comprizing only a fraction of the works now included in the Hippocratic corpus, had exercised an almost continuous influence on medical theory and practice for nearly a thousand years.
>
> (*ibid: 412*)

Nevertheless, the close involvement of the church during this period undoubtedly inhibited the experimental method and medical research.

The Hippocratic Oath was also held in high esteem throughout this period. The high ideals were held not by a few of these early doctors but were the code of the profession. Often, but not always, they held no legal sanction but were passed on by teaching or by guilds (Welborn, 1977: 204–5). Fourteenth-century medical ideals can best be summed up in the words of one of their own doctors, Guy de Chauliac,

> The doctor should be well-mannered, bold in many ways, fearful of dangers, that he should abhor false cures or practices. He should be affable to the sick, kind-hearted to his colleagues, wise in his prognostication. He should be chaste, sober, compassionate and merciful; he should not be grasping in money matters and then he will receive a salary commensurate with his labours, the financial ability of his patients, the success of the treatment and his own dignity.
>
> (*ibid: 127*)

In 1231 Emperor Frederick II required the medical students at Salerno to attend lectures on Galen and Hippocrates (Kibre, 1945: 375). After this date there was an increased interest in Hippocrates and as Galen's theories began to be dismissed so the reputation of the former began to grow. Thomas Sydenham, a famous English physician born in 1624, described Hippocrates as the 'unrivalled historian of disease' who had 'founded the Art of Medicine on a solid and unshakeable basis', namely the principle that 'our natures are the physicians of diseases' and the method of 'the exact description of nature' (Greenhill, 1844). Yet as Lloyd (1978: 59) observes:

> What these men admired in Hippocrates was not the anatomy and the physiology of the treatises, so much as two things particularly; firstly the detailed and meticulous clinical observations, and secondly the example he set of the doctor's devotion and concern for his patients and of his uprightness and discretion in his dealings with them.

The recent restatement of the core values of British Medicine (BMA, 1995) incorporates these two key features of professional competence in the practice of particular skills combined with personal attributes of care and concern for those who have entrusted themselves to the doctor's care. Neither competence nor compassion by itself is adequate.

THE RENAISSANCE AND THE ENLIGHTENMENT

Thomas Sydenham followed the Hippocratic method of exact clinical description; he also accepted his broader ideas of health and disease (Richards, 1973: 24). Western medicine finally emerged from the repression of the church in the 17th century through early reformers who were pious, God-fearing men, eager to learn more of His glorious creation. This development was part of the new learning generally known as the Renaissance in which research and investigation were actively encouraged. This approach to the natural world began to change in the 18th century in the period known as the Enlightenment. 'The Hippocratic idea of medicine assisting nature in the restoration of health began to give way to the experimental approach and its consequences' (Richards, 1973: 25). Each discovery was seen as a battle won in a relentless fight against nature and, by implication, against 'the Lord of Creation'. Hippocrates would emphasize that man must be the servant of nature and can never be its master; man must be nature's protector, not its despoiler (ibid: 28). In the Hippocratic tradition, experimental observation and what would now be called research went hand-in-hand with a particular code of behaviour by the practitioner of that research. There was an essential unity and with the advent of the Christian era that unity was seen in a common God-given origin. The Enlightenment brought an end to this unity. Experiment was not now seen as learning more about God's creation but rather about wresting knowledge from a potentially hostile environment. Moreover, with the certainty of God now under open challenge, moral and ethical values were themselves subject to evolutionary change. This perceived need for constant change is emphasized by Huxley (1940) when he writes 'man's need is for an adaptive and dynamic system of ethics rather than the conventional static system which has been accepted until today'.

Such philosophical changes do not, however, occur in isolation. Just as the end of the Hippocratic era had been accompanied by a preoccupation with relatively minor aspects of the practitioner's behaviour and etiquette, so medical ethics at the end of the medieval era had also become preoccupied with matters of etiquette and good manners. As Geyer-Kordesh (1993: 136) notes 'regulations and codes are produced in more decadent phases precisely when an inner consensus no longer holds'. Fissell (1993: 24) notes that there was no specific ethical code for doctors by the beginning of the 18th century and behaviour was based on the general conduct of a professional man, including dress and deportment. By the late 18th century there was a renewed interest in medical ethics largely from external factors such as:

- rapid commercialization which was destabilizing the traditional professional hierarchy;
- new medical institutions [the hospital] which were posing fresh problems regarding professional power, collective responsibility and the division of labour;
- gentlemanly codes of honour were proving insufficient for doctors;
- the State, the administration and the law courts offered few leads and little guidance. (See Baker, Porter, and Porter, 1993: 9)

The parallels with our own day are striking. All four factors are features of the new-style National Health Service of the 1990s.

Thomas Beddoes (1760–1808), working in Bristol, believed that doctors had become infected with the morals of the market place, encouraging consumption of their services and pursuing wealth at the expense of their patients. He was particularly critical of 'the sick person always knows best philosophy and demand-led medicine'. In a remarkable comparison with the present day he believed that a true market in healthcare did not exist because 'informed choice is a myth'. As Roberts (1993) notes: 'Managing provider markets is difficult and the training and experience is lacking in the NHS. There appears to be no one ... overseeing market competence.' Beddoes argued that 'medicine could be moved by money or it could be animated and organized by science, by the imperatives of the search for truth' (Porter, 1993: 87). In doing so he articulated one of the most fundamental issues of medical ethics and medical research.

The apparent decay in the ways that doctors behaved towards their patients and towards one another in the 18th century, which contemporary accounts seem to imply, were accompanied by changes in medical practice and a perceived inadequacy of general behavioural codes to resolve the dilemmas which such changes were presenting. Fundamental philosophical and theological precepts were being challenged by the process generally referred to as 'The Enlightenment'. It was time for doctors to re-examine their ancient values in the light of current developments. It was time for the reaffirmation of a distinctively medical ethic. (In the mid-1990s the profession seems to have begun a similar process for apparently similar reasons (BMA, 1995)).

THE DEVELOPMENT OF MODERN MEDICAL ETHICS

John Gregory is 'the first modern thinker in Anglo-American medical ethics' (McCullough, 1993: 145). Born in 1724 in Aberdeen he was much influenced by the philosopher, David Hume. He was briefly a professor of philosophy at Aberdeen between 1747 and 1749 and lectured regularly to medical students. He published his *Lectures on the Duties and Qualifications of a Physician in 1772*, a year before he died. In it he considers confidentiality; he believes that patient's suggestions should be taken seriously; he emphasizes truthfulness especially if the prognosis is doubtful; he urges doctors not to abandon dying/hopeless cases, to put patients first during consultation and to dress and behave as a physician. He emphasized the need for 'sympathy' with the patient. By this sympathy the carer shares the patient's desire to be relieved of their suffering. Similarly today in research we are enjoined to base our ethical practice on the principle of what we would expect to happen to us if we [the practitioner] were the research subject. 'Gregory wrote to defend what he took to be the traditional values of Scottish medicine (and its commonsense philosophy) against the scepticism of the Scottish Enlightenment' (Pickstone, 1993: 163).

Thomas Percival (1740–1804) also published his book *Medical Ethics* the year before he died although he had worked on the content for most of the last quarter of the 18th century. He wrote in the tradition of 'virtue ethics' and considered how the virtuous physician should behave in private practice and in public politics. Percival sensed that the previous consensus was breaking down and he drew richly on Thomas Gisbourne's idea of a social contract (Baker, 1993: 200). This gives certain privileges as a quasi-public servant. He was therefore opposed to doctors attending duels on the grounds that they were illegal and, similarly, he emphasizes the medical duty positively to help the court and without thought of remuneration. Because criticism of patient care was thought to imply criticism of the caregiver, disputes between practitioners became inevitable. If treatment was changed, the previous caregiver had effectively been slandered for giving 'the wrong treatment'. Such problems became more common as doctors became more closely involved with one another in hospitals and similar institutions. Percival's response was to submit the dispute to collective decision-making in what would now be called medical audit. 'By using the highest moral sentiments of the age in dealing with the practical problems of hospital practice, Percival cleverly adapted guild regulations to the hospital setting' (Burns, 1977: 301). He is often accused of confusing ethics and etiquette but he carefully distinguished between the two and explicitly stated that ethical duties override the etiquette of co-operation between doctors (Baker, 1993: 185).

Thomas Percival specifically acknowledged the work of John Gregory and these two doctors were largely responsible for establishing medical ethics as a separate discipline, controlled by doctors, with concepts firmly based in Christian and Hippocratic ideals.

CHANGING CONCEPTS OF MEDICAL ETHICS

The British Medical Association, established in 1832, was initially concerned primarily with distinguishing between qualified and non-qualified practitioners. Heavy penalties were inflicted on members who used any system other than allopathic medicine. In 1847 the American Medical Association was set up and adopted large sections of Percival's work on the relationships between qualified doctors to form its own code of ethics which was adopted at its inaugural meeting. A similar attempt two years later in the British Medical Association failed. Unlike their American colleagues and the nursing profession, doctors in the United Kingdom have steadfastly resisted the adoption of an ethical code (*Report of the Committee of Inquiry into the Regulation of the Medical Profession*, 1975). However, as the General Medical Council (established 1858) began to develop effective control of non-qualified practitioners in 1886, the Association felt able to take an interest in other ethical matters. A section of the annual meeting in 1895 was specifically concerned with ethical matters, but it was not until 1902 that a central ethical committee was established. For the first 30 years of its work it was mainly concerned with establishing and operating a system to adjudicate in disputes between doctors. These were largely concerned with commercial aspects of medical practice, including detailed regulations on advertising and other matters. As the State became progressively more involved in healthcare after the establishment of the Ministry of Health in 1919, the Central Ethical Committee became much preoccupied with relationships with the State and particularly with the local committees responsible for adjudication under the National Insurance Act 1911.

It was also during this period that the profession began to clearly delineate the different branches of medical practice (now usually called specialties) and the relationships that should exist between the various doctors involved. In 1937 a Matrimonial Causes Act presented doctors with the dilemma that creating benefit for one patient could often only be done at the expense of another. Such dilemmas were repeated in the 1960s with the recognition of child abuse and have formed the content of an increasing number of moral dilemmas facing doctors. A major factor in such dilemmas is, however, the relentless and increasingly rapid advance in medical innovation.

In Seattle on 9 March 1960, Dr Belding Scribner began to dialyse a patient, Clyde Shields, and in doing so started a technological revolution. Albert Jonsen (1990: 17) considers that 'this event marks a suitable inauguration of the era of bioethics'. This technological revolution has led many to conclude that research now requires close ethical control, not only in its practical arrangements but even in defining the areas in which research may legitimately be conducted. It is, for example, increasingly possible to keep babies alive at ever earlier stages of gestation. Yet the available evidence suggests that the younger the child, the more likely that it will carry major handicaps into adult life. Moreover the care involved is extremely expensive. It is not immediately obvious for whose benefit such therapeutic advances are being pursued and some have suggested that the National Health Service should not buy neonatal care earlier than a certain level of gestation. In some countries, certain forms of infertility research have been outlawed. The Association did not respond to the challenge of technological change immediately, but progressively over the last 15 years its agenda has begun to be dominated by such dilemmas almost to the exclusion of all other ethical issues.

NEW ATTITUDES TO RESEARCH

The horrors of human experimentation in Nazi Germany (Lifton, 1986) led to the Declaration of Geneva by the World Medical Association in 1948. This development, actively encouraged by the British Medical Association, is, in effect, the modern version of the Hippocratic Oath and has been used in some medical schools to gain commitment by newly qualified medical graduates to a set of ethical ideals. The Nazi experiments were not only morally wrong in so far as the need for consent was totally ignored. Deliberate harm was in many cases a key feature of the 'experiment' and there was no respect whatsoever for the dignity of the patient. The experiments were also very poor science (Angell, 1990). They revealed virtually nothing of long-term medical interest, nor did they advance the science of medicine in any significant way. Ethical review of modern research is therefore based on two quite distinct principles, both of which must be satisfied if the research experiment is to proceed. First, there must be a full recognition of the dangers, actual or potential, to the research subject. These must be fully discussed with them and attempts made to secure fully informed consent. If there is any risk, however remote, adequate arrangements through insurance and other means must be made to compensate the research subject, should such a tragedy occur.

Second, the experiment itself must be scientifically sound. An experiment which is actually or potentially flawed so that its results cannot be relied on is unethical. Some would argue that the experiment should produce a significant contribution to knowledge whether or not 'positive' or 'negative' findings result from it. Such a test would invalidate many of the experiments conducted in schools and higher-education establishments where the principal objective appears to be to provide the student with some experience of 'research'. If, however, such experiments involve potential harm to patients, compromise confidentiality or are unreasonably intrusive of personal privacy, for example by asking questions about intimate aspects of behaviour, they are perhaps best avoided. The protection of the research subject from harm must be the principal consideration in any experiment conducted with people and, some would claim, on animals too.

In recent years concern has been expressed at the number of experiments which are approved and carried out but which never reach publication. This is usually, but not invariably, because the results are not considered interesting or are at variance with conventional wisdom in the field so that editors and peer reviewers may be excessively critical. Here again there is an ethical dimension. If research subjects have been placed potentially at risk, or rules of confidentiality have been breached to allow the research to proceed, it is on the assumption that the experiment will add to the corpus of knowledge. It will not do so in the researcher's filing cabinets. Ethical committees have a responsibility not only to ensure that the research is well-constructed but that it addresses a worthwhile question and will deliver an answer capable of being published in the relevant journals. There is also some responsibility to investigate the outcome of all projects approved by the committee.

Sadly, all experimental research is at risk of the fraudulent recording of observations or the manipulation of data to support the experimental hypothesis. Some classical studies have been shown to be fraudulent in these ways. While obviously unethical, regulating authorities have been slow to take decisive action (Lock and Wells, 1993). Nurses particularly need to be aware of the need to report observations accurately, whatever the short-term consequences. They are in a very real sense the eyes, ears and conscience of medical research, as indeed of many other healthcare practices involving patients.

Local research ethics committees

The revelations of Pappworth (1967) concerning medical experimentation in the United Kingdom led to proposals by the Royal College of Physicians in London for a system of local research ethics committees. These were to be established in each health authority (DHSS, 1975). Neuberger (1992) reviewed the work of these committees. Although they are often composed of devoted members, she found they were poorly resourced and generally undertrained for the responsibilities placed on them. The Department of Health (1991) has issued revised guidelines but these are widely considered to be unhelpful. Moodie and Marshall (1992) point out that the guidelines still support the concept that committees should meet in secret; they provide no means of ensuring that consent is fully informed and fail to ensure the adequate monitoring of the committee's work or adequate compensation for those harmed by the research. Despite its wider membership, ethnic minorities are still likely to be under-represented among the lay membership (Neuberger, 1992).

National research ethics committee

Local committees were primarily designed to meet the needs of local practitioners who wish to undertake research in their own employment setting.
In order to increase statistical power there is an increasing emphasis on
collaborative research involving a large number of different centres working to a common protocol. Some studies extend beyond the responsibility
of a single local committee and some studies are conceived at the outset
on a national basis. It is time-consuming, expensive and impractical to
expect a research worker to obtain the consent of all local ethical committees before a collaborative study can be undertaken. Local committees
vary in their procedures and some meet on a long time cycle. Moreover, if
one committee insists on any amendment in the protocol it must then be
discussed and probably re-discussed with every other centre. Often
national collaborative studies are supervised by leading experts in the field,
but this has not always prevented some local committees claiming more
superior knowledge about the scientific issues involved. Over ten years ago
the British Medical Association recommended the establishment of a
national research ethics committee to overcome these and other problems.
So far its establishment has foundered on the autonomy of the local committees. Important research is currently being imperilled by this impasse
although a consensus that such a body is now needed is beginning to
emerge. Indeed, as this book went to press, the Department of Health was
preparing a consultation paper recommending suitable arrangements.

AN ETHICAL CODE FOR RESEARCH

While some principles of ethical conduct in research trials are easy to
define, there are many problems with the establishment of an ethical code
for research. Criteria for decision-making in local research ethics committees have been identified (Horner, 1993) but there is no consensus
about such criteria. Neuberger (1992) found local committees desperate
for objective measures against which to assess ethical implications.
Religious criteria seemed often to be used and I have stressed their
importance and significance elsewhere (Horner, 1993). Utilitarian
philosophers would emphasize the need for medical research and the
benefits it will bring. Others stress the autonomy of the individual subject. Consent is clearly an absolute imperative but easier to state than to
practise. The unequal relationship between doctor and patient must leave
some doubts about the level of voluntariness in participation. Indeed,
glaring examples of highly dubious practices have recently come to light.
Some patients claim not even to have been informed that they were
included in a research trial and few researchers seem willing to provide
written information leaflets which the subject can take away, study and

question before consent is finally given. Even in Hippocrates' day 'some doctors were also positively secretive about their art and prepared to write about it only in veiled language that none but the initiated would understand' (Lloyd, 1978: 21). Belkin (1993) claims that the deliberate use of technical language to confuse patients is still common.

Above all, the commercial aspects of research cannot be ignored. Commerce was a factor leading to a general tightening of medical ethics and its practice in the late 18th century; and the present emphasis on market forces in the public service, including health services and the universities, must prompt similar concerns. There are regular reports of financial inducements to doctors to recruit research subjects and there is a division of view as to whether research subjects have a right to be told what financial arrangements the researcher has made with his employers. The amount of published material is a criterion for distinction awards for hospital consultants and is increasingly used in the universities to assess individual and corporate performance. These situations must create tensions and conflicts among those who find their research ideas potentially threatened by an increasingly tight ethical framework.

CONCLUSION

The increasing involvement of nurses in all aspects of research involving patients necessitates a clear understanding of the ethical factors involved. Openness and honesty, together with freely given consent and a respect for the autonomy of the research subject, must be ethical imperatives in any well-conducted scientifically based experimental study. Nurses are in a unique position to ensure that these features are understood by all those involved, not least the patients, and that they are effectively monitored during the research project. Using a medical model, this historical review has shown how ethical codes and practices have changed over the years in the light of external pressures. Throughout history, however, many of the basic principles have stood the test of time. At certain periods it has been necessary to rediscover them and sometimes to re-apply them to new environmental circumstances. It has been argued in this chapter that recent changes in the research environment require a review of current ethical practice and the rediscovery of a common system of values against which such a review can take place. The task is becoming particularly urgent if we wish to obey the injunction to which almost everyone subscribes – 'first do no harm'.

REFERENCES

Aldred, C. (1978) *Egypt to the End of the Old Kingdom*, Thames & Hudson, London.

Angell, M. (1990) The Nazi hypothermia experiments and unethical research today. *New England Journal of Medicine*, **322** 1462–4.

Baker, R. (1993) Deciphering Percival's code, in *The Codification of Medical Morality*, Vol. 1 (eds R. Baker, D. Porter and R. Porter), Kluwer Academic Publishers, Dordrecht, Holland.

Baker, R., Porter, D. and Porter, R. (1993) *The Codification of Medical Morality, Vol I: Medical Ethics and Etiquette in the 18th century*, Kluwer Academic Publishers, Dordrecht, Holland.

Belkin, L. (1993) *First Do No Harm,* Simon & Schuster, New York, p. 270.

Berger, R.L. (1990) Nazi science – The Dachau hypothermia experiments. *New England Journal of Medicine,* **322**, 1435–40.

British Medical Association (1995) *Core Values for the Medical Profession in the 21st Century,* BMA, London.

Burns, C.R. (1977) *Reciprocity in the development of Anglo-American medical ethics 1765–1865,* in *Legacies in Ethics and Medicine* (ed. C.R. Burns), Science History Publications, New York.

Cameron, N.M. de S. (1991) *The New Medicine: Life and Death after Hippocrates*, Crossway Books, Wheaton Illinois, p. 62.

Carrick, P. (1985) *Medical Ethics in Antiquity*, D. Reidel Publishing Company, Dordrecht, Holland.

Chadwick, J. and Mann, W.N. (1978) *Hippocratic Writings*. (ed. G.E.R. Lloyd), Penguin Books, Harmondsworth.

Chamberlain, G. (1968) An artificial placenta. *American Journal of Obstetrics and Gynaecology*, **100**, 624.

Cherkasky, M. (1973) The Hippocrates myth in *Hippocrates Revisited – a Search for Meaning* (ed. R.J. Bulger) Medcom Press, New York.

Department of Health (1991) *Local Research Ethics Committees,* HSG(91)5, HMSO, London.

Department of Health and Social Security (1975) *Guidelines for Research Ethics Committees,* HMSO, London.

Fissell, M.E. (1993) *Innocent and honourable bribes,* in *The Codification of Medical Morality*, Vol. I. (eds R. Baker, D. Porter and R. Porter), Kluwer Academic Publishers, Dordrecht, Holland.

Geyer-Kordesch, J. (1993) Natural law and medical ethics in the eighteenth century, in *The Codification of Medical Morality*, Vol. I. (eds R. Baker, D. Porter and R. Porter) Kluwer Academic Publications, Dordrecht, Holland.

Greenhill, G.A. (1844) Preface to the 3rd edn (1676) of *Observationes Medicae* (ed. G.A. Greenhill) London, para. 15. pp. 13ff.

Horner, J.S. (1993) Criteria for decision-making in local research (ethics) committees, *Public Health* **107**, 403–11.

Huxley, J.S. (1940) *Scientific Monthly*, **XLV**, January–June, 5–16.

Jonsen, A.R. (1990) *The New Medicine and the Old Ethics,* Harvard University Press, Cambridge, Mass.

Kibre, P. (1945) Hippocratic writings in the Middle Ages. *Bulletin of the History of Medicine*, **18**, 371–412.

Lifton, R. (1986) *The Nazi Doctors*, Macmillan, London.

Lloyd, G.E.R. (1978) *Hippocratic Writings*, Penguin Books, Harmondsworth.

Lock, S. and Wells, F. (1993) Fraud and Misconduct in Medical Research, BMJ publications, London.

MacKinney, L.C. (1952) Medical ethics and etiquette in the early Middle Ages: the persistence of Hippocratic ideals. *Bulletin of the History of Medicine* **26**, 1–31.

McCullough, L.B. (1993) John Gregory's medical ethics and Humean sympathy in *The Codification of Medical Morality*, (eds R. Baker, D. Porter and R. Porter), Vol. I, Kluwer Academic Publishers, Dordrecht, Holland.

McIlrath, M.B. (1959) *History of Medical Ethics in the Non-Christian World before the Rise of Modern Medicine,* Vol. I, MD Thesis, University of Sydney.

Moodie, P.C.E. and Marshall, T. (1992) Guidelines for local research ethics committees. *British Medical Journal* **304**, 1293–5.

Neuberger, J. (1992) *Ethics and Health Care – The Role of Research Ethics Committees in the United Kingdom*, Research Report 13, Kings Fund Institute, London.

Pappworth, M.H. (1967) *Human Guinea Pigs – Experimentation on Man*, Routledge & Kegan Paul, London.

Phillips, M. and Dawson, J. (1985) *Doctors' Dilemmas – Medical Ethics and Contemporary Science,* The Harvester Press, Brighton.

Pickstone, J.V. (1993) Thomas Percival and the production of medical ethics in *The Codification of Medical Morality*, Vol. I, (eds R. Baker, D. Porter and R. Porter), Kluwer Academic Publishers, Dordrecht, Holland.

Porter, R. (1993) Plutus or Hygeia – Thomas Beddoes and the crisis of medical ethics in Britain, in *The Codification of Medical Morality*, Vol. I. (eds R. Baker, D. Porter and R. Porter) Kluwer Academic Publishers, Dordrecht, Holland.

Report of the Committee of Inquiry into the Regulation of the Medical Profession (1975), Cmnd 6018, HMSO, London, pp. 91 and 92.

Richards, D.W. (1973) Hippocrates and history: the arrogance of humanism, in *Hippocrates revisited – a search for meaning*, (ed. R.J. Bulger), Medcom Press, New York.

Roberts, J.W. (1993) Managing markets. *Journal of Public Health Medicine*, **15**, 305–10.

Temkin, O. (1991) *Hippocrates in a World of Pagans and Christians*, The John Hopkins University Press, Baltimore, Maryland.

Watterson, B. (1984) *The Gods of Ancient Egypt*, Batsford, London.

Welborn, M.C. (1977) The long tradition: a study in fourteenth century deontology, in *Legacies in Ethics and Medicine*, (ed. C.R. Burns), Science History Publications, New York.

Wilson, J.A. (1956) *The Culture of Ancient Egypt,* University of Chicago Press, Chicago and London.

10	# Exercising or exorcizing the code?

Barbara Shailer

For the nursing profession of the United Kingdom, the importance attributed to the code of professional conduct has gained considerable momentum since the first edition was published in 1983 (UKCC, 1983). At the heart of the code is a clear message to nurses to protect and further the interests of the individual patient and client. The basic tenet of the code reviewed by Pyne (1994) involves standards of competence with the implication that the prerequisite for good care is competent nursing practice. There are three dimensions to the code. One is ethical, as it provides a statement about the profession's values. Second, a political dimension emerges where practitioners are challenged to expose risk to patients and staff where such exists. Third, the code assists in professional self-regulation by providing a yardstick against which conduct may be measured. This code declares the business of nurses and is designed to empower them in their pursuit of professional excellence in patient care.

Surrounding the introduction of the code was a growing ethos of accountability which began in earnest with the Griffiths principles of the new 'market-driven' health service management in the early 1980s. Most professional groups, (apart from health service managers themselves), published some form of declaration to inform the consumer of standards and practice involved in its service. These declarations are published under various labels such as codes of ethics, guidelines for practice, charters and, for certain individual organizations, mission statements. Newcomers to the professions, as well as consumers, can be forgiven for being just a little confused when faced with this medley of goodness, delivered in the spirit of public altruism. Sincere statements emanate from the printed page proposing the ultimate welfare of the population served. These population members are variously described as (a) patients, the vulnerable who need our care; (b) clients, those who need our care and can expect to receive it; (c) consumers, those who need our care, sample it and can seek to improve it; and (d) customers, those who need our care, have paid for it and have the right to use official channels to improve it. The definitions vary according to the market orientation of the author. This term, the market, can be viewed as the key to some of the difficulties nurses have within the current climate. The health service is led by a new management where healthcare professionals are no longer the power-brokers and nurses are attempting to reconcile the two competing philosophies: care provision based on the economics of care and professional aspirations of the best care. Professional accountability for care is one thing but the necessary prerequisite – professional autonomy – is altogether something else.

This leads us to the questions about codes. What are their purposes and functions? Can they be upheld? Can they fulfil the aspirations of professionals in the maintenance of standards and improve care? Do codes of conduct receive the practical support of the professional regulatory bodies concerned and of management? Do they receive the wholehearted commitment of professionals themselves?

OVERT PURPOSES OF CODES

In an attempt to answer those questions the functions and purposes of codes themselves, overt and covert, will be addressed with specific emphasis on nursing.

Codes quite simply guide the conduct of professions and influence organizations, the primary focus for most being overtly stated as the welfare of those they serve. They are rooted in the concept of rights for the individual, society and the professional. Codes of conduct and practice concern individual professions and are so important that they are considered to be one of the main hallmarks of a profession (Barber, 1988). A code exhibits a profession's intent in relation to good practices. In brief, codes are said to:

- provide a moral guide for conduct;
- contain principles that state agreed standards;
- function as a public statement of ethical principles agreed through a consensus of views by members of the professional group; and
- inform others what to expect through the professional service.

Codes are published by the profession's or organization's regulatory body. For nursing this is the United Kingdom Central Council for Nursing, Midwifery and Health Visiting (UKCC) and for medicine the General Medical Council (GMC). Codes are sometimes endorsed by individual statements of professional organizations, for example, the Royal College of Nursing and the British Medical Association. Although not sustaining legal status, codes and guidelines are referred to in the daily practice of healthcare professionals and are always used in professional conduct committee enquiries as the benchmark of good practice. Certainly in the nursing and medical professions, breaches of professional codes are viewed seriously. Implicit and explicit in the documentation is the concept of professional accountability. Accountability means simply that: account ability, to give account of why we do what we do, how we do it and what the outcomes are (Simsen, 1985). A nurse is liable to be struck off the professional register should they be found guilty of professional misconduct by breaching the UKCC Code of Professional Conduct (Dimond, 1990; Pyne, 1992; Rowden, 1987).

The nurses' code is not a code of ethics as such, though one must accept that its intention must be to do good, to do right by promoting good standards of care. It is a prescriptive document, with its primary focus on patients, clients, society and the profession in that order. The introductory statement provides the context:

> Each registered nurse, midwife and health visitor shall act at all times in such a manner as to:
> - safeguard and promote the interests of individual patients and clients;
> - serve the interests of society;
> - justify public trust and confidence and uphold and enhance the good standing and reputation of the professions.
>
> As a registered nurse, midwife or health visitor, you are personally accountable for your practice and, in the exercise of your professional accountability, must:
>
> *(UKCC, 1992: 1)*

Sixteen prescriptive statements follow, embracing the 'patients first' tenet, through holistic care, confidentiality, multidisciplinary team collaboration, professional development of knowledge and skills and safe working environments. The document includes by implication the principles of justice, autonomy, beneficence and non-maleficence and truth-telling. The UKCC (1989) also published a document called *Exercising Accountability* to emphasize and further explain this aspect of role outlined in the code of conduct, relating to the general subject of truth-telling and informed consent. Guidance is offered over taking action and reporting circumstances which jeopardize or militate against safe standards of practice, concerning the environment of care and workload pressures placed on colleagues, advocacy on behalf of patients, contentious treatments, conscientious objection and collaborative working with other healthcare professionals. The primary focus of the code is repeated but the document clarifies the obligations of professionals:

The primacy of interests of the public and the patient or client provide the first theme of the code and establish the point that, in determining his or her approach to professional practice, the individual nurse ... should recognize that the interests of public and patient must predominate over those of practitioner and profession.

(UKCC, 1989: 6)

There is little doubt about the overt and public declaration of the purposes of the code for nurses, but is this professional altruism for the patient the single and over-riding concern?

COVERT PURPOSES OF CODES

Considerable thought has been given by commentators to other more covert purposes of codes. It is acknowledged that their declared primary purpose is to focus on duty to the public but it can be argued that other purposes exist, such as the enhancement of professional status and to professionalize aspiring professions (nursing is said to exist in this group), to promote the interests of professionals themselves, or for the promotion of professional disciplinary functions.

The theme of professionalizing occupations is proposed by Barber (1988: 36), who talks of the emerging professions as being partly professional: 'The medical profession is more professional than the nursing profession ... professionalism is a matter of degree.'

Emergent professions are criticized for proposing a status to which few can aspire. Professional behaviour is defined in terms of four attributes: a high degree of knowledge; primary orientation to community interests; a high degree of self-control through internalized codes of ethics organized by the professionals themselves; and a system of rewards which are ends in themselves. In an attempt to strengthen the standing of their professions, regulatory bodies and professional groups plan, construct and then publish codes of ethics. These are often criticized for their value generalities and the difficulties encountered in their application to practice because the knowledge-base of the emerging profession is not highly developed. Also inferred is the inability of emerging professions to devise mechanisms for the common interpretation and implementation of these codes. In their search for status, novice professions muster support from the public by publishing information about standards and service. The 'named nurse' concept is frequently cited in the British media. Broadcasts of this nature could be viewed as publicity stunts and window-dressing, 'in an attempt to flimflam the public with half truths and deceit' (Barber, 1988: 37). Much in these campaigns may be seen as desirable but the reality may be different because of resource constraints and lack of staff development. Only if the public's experience matches the profession's claims is it likely that the status of the profession will be elevated. Professional codes may all too often function to promote or protect the interests of a profession and its members rather than the interests of those served by the profession. Indeed, Kultgen (1982), Johnson (1972) and Randall (1979) propose four myths which serve to perpetuate the ideologies of professions:

The myth of independence with associated autonomy

Professionals are constantly depicted as having independence. In reality most are employed by large organizations, such as the NHS or Social Services, where the latitude for professional judgments is comparatively limited.

The myth of altruism

Altruism of professionals can be challenged as we have no evidence that a lawyer, nurse or doctor is more altruistic than, say, an electrician. Professional identity means upwards social mobility. The financial and social benefits which professionalism confers may be more in evidence than a national altruism which is supposed to benefit the rest of society. Furthermore, when a professional focuses primarily on research and technical advances, this may not always be in the primary interests of the client but serve simply to enhance the profile of the professional or the academic department of a university.

The myth of peer review

Peer review may be seen as a myth, due to the difficulties of one professional actually being informed of the work of another in sufficient detail. These difficulties are further compounded by strictures within some codes against public criticism of colleagues: 'gratuitous and unsuitable comment which, whether directly or by implication, sets out to undermine trust in individual colleague's knowledge and skills is unethical' (GMC, 1993: 22).

A national monitoring system of professional performance review processes has not been undertaken. The legal judgments made in the *Bolam* case [1957] also open up the peer-review process but, on the other hand, also provide a vehicle for professional solidarity in the face of adversity. The *Bolam* case advocates that when delivering a standard which should have been followed, this should relate to what a body of professionals agree should have applied at the time. To be acceptable, the local standards in question cannot be lower than those of the reasonable professional in the country at the time. However, it needs to be recognized that these cases tend to be complex, involving difficult and contentious areas of practice frequently conducted in uncharted waters.

The myth of professional wisdom

To date, we have no evidence to suggest professionals are wiser than non-professionals. Are those who rise to the upper echelons of professional hierarchies better equipped to determine their profession's role in society? Kultgen (1982) alleges that the professional hallmarks of autonomy, collegiality and meritocracy are flawed. Until professionals can demonstrate that all their practices are primarily focused on the public and that codes are used in a moral sense rather than for personal advantage, we should view professionals' claims for a privileged status with an open mind.

Another view is that of Brady (1988), who is critical of the code for nurses because of what he defines as 'the carrot and stick' approach. In one sense the code for nursing can be considered a route for fostering professional accountability – or the reverse, a vehicle for professional disciplinary proceedings. It is argued that codes should, in the general world of health policy, be preventive rather than punitive. More specifically the point of the code should be 'to improve the overall professionalism of each and every nurse' (Brady, 1988: 31). It is postulated that the heavy stick approach, with its emphasis on sanctions, could well increase tension and anxiety in some nurses and achieve the opposite of what is desirable.

Another similar view is held by Pinel (1990), who infers that maintaining professional standards may have more to do with staff discipline than patient care. Puzzling decisions of the UKCC professional conduct committee panels are evident. He refers to an example where a nurse manager was convicted and served a two-year prison sentence for sexually abusing young boys and his name was not removed from the professional register of the UKCC. In contrast, shortly afterwards, an Asian nurse's name was removed from the register for sexual harassment. At the time, the actions taken by the UKCC appeared inconsistent. The question which needs to be asked is whether the focus of the code is on client care or developing a docile workforce? In practice, the code also needs to be interpreted in a fair and a consistent manner for those who are called on to account for behaviour which allegedly contravenes it. Furthermore, Kent (1990), commenting specifically on the case of child sexual abuse, also questions whether the UKCC conduct committee is truly representative of the interests of the profession and whether its all-or-nothing powers are too blunt an instrument for dealing with such complex cases.

CAN THE CODE FOR NURSES BE UPHELD? THE ISSUE OF PROFESSIONAL AUTONOMY

Autonomy is accepted to be a partially defining feature of a profession (Bayles, 1981) and this attribute is enshrined in the codes of conduct and ethical guides of most professions. However, its utility is often compromised when competing professions attempt to exercise their autonomy. In such situations the less powerful professional is much less likely to have the opportunity to exhibit their autonomy. In the case cited by Vousden (1985), the dilemma of a nurse in charge of a patient illustrates the point. The registered nurse in question was sacked and the appeal was dismissed as he had refused to participate, against the physician's orders, in electro-convulsive therapy on a patient who, in the nurse's opinion, was too ill for the treatment. This raises a number of contemporary issues: for the physician to be challenged by a nurse is still considered to be a serious breach of respect. It is not viewed in the light of a nurse as a member of a profession exercising accountability, autonomy and acting for the patient as advocate. This nurse appealed to the UKCC code of conduct but, as this consideration was overruled, it is evident that 'the code of conduct offers no legal support at all' (Vousden, 1985: 23). Such cases are not isolated. Since Tate (1977) reported similarly in the United States, cases have been reported regularly.

In today's climate of managerial control of healthcare professionals by non-professionals, the necessary understanding relating to these issues is lacking. However , the principles are important ones. Clearly cases occur where autonomy is expected of a professional belonging to a new 'semi-profession', but this cannot be practised because of constraints imposed by members of the established professions. This raises the question as to whether autonomous practice, which entails accountability with both personal and professional responsibility (Holden, 1991), should be stated in codes if such autonomy cannot be universally upheld.

COMPETING DEMANDS OF PROFESSIONALS AND ORGANIZATIONS

A further concern about codes is expressed by Muyskens (1982), who describes nursing's double-edged sword: that of moral and professional accountability for one's own actions on the one hand and accountability to the organization and other professions on the other. The increasing publicity given to whistleblowing, internal and external to organizations, illustrates the intraprofessional and interprofessional conflicts which professionals endure and the misery they suffer when faced with competing demands of accountability to clients in upholding good standards of care and accountability to the organization. One whistle-blower, Mr Pink, whose case received much publicity for upholding the UKCC code by complaining about inadequate staffing levels and who was subsequently sacked from his post as a charge nurse, considers it should be scrapped. Certainly most nurses are unlikely to support the code if they face the emotional trauma of litigation and losing their jobs.

The constant struggle of the nursing profession is reflected in the various code changes. The current UKCC code is the third edition and continually under review.

The problem is not a new one. Indeed, the Secretary of State for Health on 12 June 1992 announced an amnesty for nurse and doctor whistle-blowers. An administrative body was announced intended to deal with aggrieved healthcare professionals. This development was seen 'to have been jettisoned into action by the Graham Pink case, recent media interest and the so-called gagging clauses in nurses' and doctors' contracts of employment' (Rea, 1992: 271). Interestingly, earlier in the same year the Health Secretary had refused to outlaw 'gagging clauses' in health workers contracts (Brindle, 1992). In fact the administrative body did not materialize but, under the leadership of Sir Duncan Nichol, Chief Executive of the NHS Management Executive at that time, government guidelines were published and circulated to health authorities and trusts entitled, *Guidance for Staff on Relations with the Public and the Media* (DOH,1993). This sought to clarify the rights and responsibilities of staff when raising concern over healthcare matters and purported to complement professional codes, ethical rules and guidelines issued by the professions. It was portrayed in the media as unhelpful and as 'Gagging guidelines' (Laurent, 1992). The document emphasizes the importance of:

1 staff rights and duties to raise matters of concern, and the right to be fairly heard;
2 the manager's duty to ensure staff may easily express concerns through locally developed procedures;
3 the normal working culture of the NHS which should foster openness and staff who express their views should under no circumstances be penalized in any way;
4 organizations should devise procedures to handle expressions of concern, through line-management structures or designation of special officers;
5 the maintenance of confidentiality of clients;
6 retention of staff rights to seek advice from unions, professional organizations and regulatory bodies.

This advice is clear and sound. It frees up the debate about expressing concern and attempts to foster a spirit of openness. Unfortunately it is also peppered with statements which can only serve to fuel the anxiety of any employee who recognizes an issue which requires reporting, the more sensitive the concern the more complex the dilemma. The contentious statements within the DOH guidelines relate primarily to the confidentiality owed to the patient and the employing organization:

> All NHS staff have a duty of confidentiality to patients. Unauthorized disclosure of personal information about any patient or client will be regarded as a most serious matter which will always warrant disciplinary action. This applies even where a member of staff believes that he or she is acting in the best interests of a patient or client by disclosing personal information.
>
> *(DOH, 1993: para. 8)*

The document continues with an emphasis on the duty owed to the employer:

> Employees also have an implied duty of confidentiality and loyalty to their employers. Breach of this duty may result in disciplinary action, whether or not there is a clause in their contract of employment expressly addressing the question of confidentiality.
>
> *(DOH, 1993: para. 9)*

The document explains the circumstances where employees might disclose confidential information:

> The duty of confidentiality to an employer is not absolute … it may be claimed that the disclosure was made in the public interest. Such a justification might, in a disputed case, need to be defended and so should be soundly based … any employee who is considering making a disclosure of confidential information because they consider it to be in the public interest, should first seek specialist advice.
>
> *(DOH, 1993: para. 10)*

The message is further reinforced in the final paragraphs of the guidelines for members who have exhausted locally established procedures including the chairman of the employing body and who have taken advice. The employee:

> might wish to consult a Member of Parliament in confidence. He or she might also, as a last resort, contemplate the possibility of disclosing his or her concerns to the media. Such action if entered unjustifiably, could result in disciplinary action and might unreasonably undermine public confidence in the service … It is expected that proper mechanisms will exist to ensure that staff concerns can be addressed and dealt with without reference to the media.
>
> *(DOH, 1993: para. 28)*

In concentrating the professional mind on confidentiality, the edicts proffer professionals an instant dilemma. All issues relating to poor standards involve patients and staff, whatever the causes may be. The complainant must provide evidence and examples of the issues of their concern which automatically requires divulging information which may be defined as confidential. If the expressions of concern over care standards are not addressed by management – and their track record to date suggests they are not likely to be (Lennane, 1993; Hunt and Shailer, 1995) – in the public interest the nurse might be forced to go public, with the threat of disciplinary action and loss of job security this entails. The regulatory body for nurses states:

> The responsibility to either disclose or withold confidential information in the public interest lies with the individual practitioner, that he/she cannot delegate the decision, and that he/she cannot be required by a superior to disclose or withold information against his/her will.
>
> (*UKCC 1987: 12*)

In doing so, it is clearly not only the might of a healthcare organization's management that professionals encounter in these circumstances but the government's as well.

THE LEGAL STATUS OF THE CODE FOR NURSING

According to Pyne (1994) the code is a means of empowerment which professionals should appropriately direct to serving the interests of patients. He argues that the source of this empowerment is found in its legal background. The Nurses, Midwives and Health Visitors Act 1979, which established the UKCC as the regulatory body, states that the principal function of that body shall be to establish and improve standards of training and professional conduct and it is empowered to give advice on standards of professional conduct. In this respect it is argued that the code arises from the law and has its backing. Pyne proposes that the code should not be regarded as ineffective simply because it is not part of the law. This proposal for the advancement of the status of the code is a reasonable one but recent history and evidence suggests that, as the code is not part of the law, professionals do encounter serious obstacles in upholding its principles and are vulnerable in situations when adversaries have the backing of the law.

Ideally there should be no divergence between the standards set by the UKCC and other professional codes, the employer and the *Bolam* case [1957]. In reality this does not happen. Where interprofessional conflict occurs, Dimond (1987) warns nurses to proceed with caution if considering non-compliance with medical requests and to consider carefully criminal and civil law, the contract of employment and the professional code. Evidence of unreasonableness of orders must exist, supported where possible by witnesses who can testify to this. A further disadvantage for nurses in relation to lack of legal status of the code emerges in cases of advocacy. Nurses feel obliged through their code to act as patient's advocates. 'Advocacy on behalf of patients or clients is an essential feature of the exercise of accountability by a professional practitioner' (UKCC, 1989: 18).

Melia (1989) and Porter (1988) advise caution, as this is a difficult area for nurses. It raises issues of compatibility with what nurses do and what they are empowered to do. Also, nurses may not be conversant with all the facts or even be competent to advocate. By exercising a form of professional paternalism they may be infringing the patient's rights of autonomy. Are nurses thoroughly conversant with the principles of beneficence and non-maleficence? If nurses speak up for the patients in the interests of justice but from a position of ignorance, they may do so at considerable personal cost.

In the advocacy role, nurses also have to face opposition by doctors who fear loss of status and senior nurses whose ideas about nursing roles are slow to change (Winslow, 1982). Jennings (1991) also warns nurses about the feasibility of advocacy questioning the possibility for the nurses to be an advocate for every patient in their care, as there is a full and lasting commitment required to resolve issues whatever the consequences. Jennings stresses that advocacy is likely to bring the nurse into conflict with employers. While organizations, such as local authorities and health authorities, may publish claims of respect for the rights of consumers by stating that provision will be available to meet local needs, these stated aims are often clouded by statements such as 'wherever practicable' and 'within the limits of available resources'.

Some commentators (e.g. Copp, 1988; Pinel, 1990; Devine, 1990; Tadd, 1994) have commented on the lack of clarity regarding the legal status of the code. In more practical terms there are also problems with the UKCC. Staff who send copies of their complaints over standards of care to this body seeking guidance and advice do not even receive an acknowledgement. 'Nurses need full and practical support from their regulatory body in this fight' (Devine, 1990: 31)

Turner (1991) affirms this argument, reflecting on professionals' feelings of betrayal due to the UKCC's apparent lack of ability to support them when they voice concerns over unacceptable standards. The regulatory body's apparent impotence in supporting individual professionals is not a United Kingdom phenomenon. In Australia this is documented by Johnstone (1989a,b) in several ethics' texts and in America by Fiesta (1990a,b) in her aptly named articles, 'Whistleblowers, heroes or

stoolpidgeons?' and 'Whistleblowers, retaliation or protection?' In a leader
on the subject, 'Controversies in Care', the *American Journal of Nursing*
(1990) ran an article called: 'Four easy ways to lose a job in nursing'.

Cole (1991) conducted a survey which examined the conflicts between
the professional code of conduct and contracts of employment.
Questionnaires were sent to all health authorities, boards, trusts and
FHSAs, of which 166 (40%) responded. They were asked how feasible it
would be to combine the code and the employment contract. All but one
accepted that nurses had an obligation under the code. Two-thirds accepted
there would be conflict between code and contract and 85% signalled their
willingness to offer nurses written acknowledgment of their obligations
under the code. However, there was a considerable difference of opinion
over whether the code or the contract should take precedence. The point at
issue is the tension between professional duty to the code and loyalty to the
employer, with all the ramifications in preserving employment status.

SHOULD THE CODE BE ENFORCED IN LAW?

While Pyne (1994) asserts that the code has the backing of the law, Tadd
(1994) argues that this serves to confuse, as legal accountability is
confined to the judicial system or specific components of legal practice,
for example, breaches of contract. Where moral accountability is involved
it is much more problematical. Dimond (1989) points out that accountability requires external standards and therefore external means of
enforcement, but the accountability that the code advocates is, by nature,
moral. So should the code be externally enforced in law?

It would seem from the evidence that nurses who refer to the code to
support practice as advocates and who generally comply with professional practice which the code specifies, may well be in conflict with other
professionals, with management and with their employment contracts, all
of which have the backing of the law. They do not receive the UKCC's
support and the code they are obliged to uphold in order to maintain
status on the professional register is not sustained in law. Taking this view
it would seem that the code should have official legal backing to
encourage and protect professionals in their obligation to enforce it.
Many laws have their origins in moral values; legal support of an ethical
code should not be unacceptable.

CONCLUSION

The code of conduct for nurses, midwives and health visitors is a guide
to professional practice rooted in moral principles and primarily devised

for the welfare of patients. It is acknowledged that it may be used to enhance the status of an aspiring profession, to promote the personal interests of individual professionals or to be used punitively in threatening disciplinary action. As long as professionals are aware of this misuse, they can collectively conspire to prevent it. After all, voluntary professional codes cannot guarantee absolute ethical conduct by all nurses.

Nurses encounter obstacles when upholding the code. There are issues of questionable professional autonomy, conflicts of interest between professional practitioners, patient's rights versus organizational needs and expressions of concern over standards in patient advocacy when patients are at risk. The nebulous legal status of the code also renders it a toothless tiger. Unsurprisingly, the UKCC is unable to support individual professionals in the face of the powers of other professionals and managers who have the full weight of the law and, at times, the government behind them. There is a danger that the code will fall into disrepute; its existence will be acknowledged by nurses but it will not be upheld.

Where does this leave nurses and the code? There is no doubt that nursing needs the code as a universal statement of the guiding principles of the profession. But what of the future?

One encouraging aspect is that nursing education is shifting to a higher education base, preparing nurses for autonomy, professional assertion and research-based practice. Cowman (1989) and Rowden (1992) imply that this significant lack of professional assertion, currently endemic in nurses, stems from professional nursing education which historically was more concerned, albeit inadvertently, with socializing recruits into bureaucratic modes of behaviour rather than educating them for professional practice.

Certainly nurses must collectively question the ability of the current code to ensure ethically sound practice and fight for its own legitimate status. Local groups in each employing institution should make a firm stand on standards, the code, professional ethics and patients' rights.

Serious attention must be given to the issue of professional ethics' education. Nurses need to be taught the fundamentals of ethical theory and application and also the art of moral reasoning and decision-making in practice (Johnstone, 1989a,b). The regulatory body, the UKCC itself, must recognize that it has a moral duty to promote sound ethical practice by supporting professionals who uphold the code and campaign for legal status. A special kind of courage as defined by Schrock (1990) accompanying total commitment is required of nurses and the regulatory body to achieve these aims. Without this support and the subsequent strengthening of the code, nurses will not be exercising the code but presiding over a silent exorcism.

REFERENCES

American Journal of Nursing (1990) Controversies in care: four easy ways to lose a job in nursing. June, 27–8.

Barber, B. (1988) Professions and emerging professions, in *Ethical Issues in Professional Life* (ed. J.C. Callahan), Oxford University Press, Oxford, pp. 35–9.

Bayles, M.D. (1981) *Professional Ethics*, Wadsworth Publishing Company, Belmont, California.

Brady, P. (1988) Code of conduct, stick or carrot? *Irish Nursing Journal and Health Services*, Nov/Dec, 31–2, 41.

Brindle, D. (1992) Bottomly rejects nurses' plea to ban gagging clauses. *The Guardian*, 28.4.92.

Cole, A. (1991) Upholding the code. *Nursing Times*, **87**(27), 26–9.

Copp, G. (1988) Professional accountability the conflict. *Nursing Times*, **84**(43), 42–4.

Cowman, S. (1989) Accountability in health services. *Irish Nursing Journal and Health Services*, Sept/Oct, 24–6.

Department of Health (1993) *Guidance for Staff on Relations with the Public and the Media*, DOH, Leeds.

Devine, J. (1990) Accountability. *Nursing Times*, **86**(21), 30–1.

Dimond, B. (1987) Doing the right thing. *Nursing Times*, **83**, 61.

Dimond, B. (1989) Accountability in the legal context. *Nursing Standard*, **3**(4), 29–30.

Dimond, B. (1990) *Legal Aspects of Nursing*, Prentice Hall, London.

Fiesta, J. (1990a) Whistleblowers, heroes or stoolpidgeons? *Nursing Management*, **16**, 16–17.

Fiesta, J. (1990b) Whistleblowers, retaliation or protection? *Nursing Management*, **7**, 38.

General Medical Council (1993) *Professional Conduct and Discipline: Fitness to Practise*, GMC, London.

Holden, R.J. (1991) Responsibility and autonomous nursing practice. *Journal of Advanced Nursing*, **16**, 398–403.

Hunt, G. and Shailer, B. (1995) Whistleblowers speak, in *Whistleblowing in the NHS*, (ed. G. Hunt), Edward Arnold, London.

Jennings, K. (1991) Speaking up for patients. *Confederation of Health Services Employees Journal*, **3**(5), 12–13.

Johnson, T. (1972) *Professionalism and Power*, Macmillan, London.

Johnstone, M. (1989a) *Bioethics: a Nursing Perspective*, Saunders/Balliere Tindall, Sydney, Australia.

Johnstone, M. (1989b) Professional ethics and patients rights, past realities, future imperatives. *Nursing Forum*, **3**(4), 29–34.

Kent, A. (1990) Protecting the public. *Nursing Times*, **6**(37), 20.

Kultgen, J. (1982) The ideological use of professional codes. *Business and Professional Ethics Journal*, **1**(3), 53–9.

Laurent, C. (1992) Gagging guidelines? *Nursing Times*, **38**(4), 19.

Lennane, K.J. (1993) Whistleblowing, a health issue. *British Medical Journal*, Vol. 307, 1 September, 667–70.

Melia, K.M. (1989) *Everyday Nursing Ethics*, Macmillan, London.

Muyskens, J.L. (1982) The nurse as a member of a profession, in *Moral Problems in Nursing, a Philosophical Investigation*, (ed. N.J. Totowa), Rowman and Littlefield, New York, pp. 158–67.

Pinel, C. (1990) Patient care or repression? *Nursing*, **4**(17), 43.

Porter, S. (1988) Siding with the system. *Nursing Times*, **84**(14), 30–1.

Pyne, R. (1992) Accountability, breaking the code. *Nursing*, **5**(3), 13–26.

Pyne, R. (1994) Empowerment through the use of the code of professional conduct. *British Journal of Nursing*, **3**(12), 631–4.

Randall, C. (1979) *The Credential Society*. Academic Press, New York.

Rea, K. (1992) The whistleblowers charter. *British Journal of Nursing*, **1**(6), 271.

Rowden, R. (1987) The UKCC code of conduct. *Nursing*, **14**, 512–14.

Rowden, R. (1992) Self-imposed silence. *Nursing Times*, **88**(24), 31.

Schrock, R.A. (1990) Conscience and courage; a critical examination of professional conduct. *Nurse Education Today*, **10**, 3–9.

Simsen, B.J. (1985) Accountability and freedom in question. *Highway*, **1**(1), 13–16.

Tadd, V. (1994) Professional codes: an exercise in ethical tokenism? *Nursing Ethics*, **1**(1), 15–23.

Tate, B.L. (1977) *The Nurses' Dilemma*. International Council of Nurses, Geneva, Switzerland, pp. 47–8.

Turner, T. (1991) A paper tiger. *Nursing Times*, **87**(24), 20.

United Kingdom Central Council (1983) *Code of Professional Conduct*, UKCC, London.

United Kingdom Central Council (1987) *Confidentiality*, UKCC, London.

United Kingdom Central Council (1989) *Exercising Accountability: A Framework to Assist Nurses, Midwives and Health Visitors to Consider Ethical Aspects of Professional Practice*, UKCC, London.

United Kingdom Central Council (1992) *Code of Professional Conduct for Nurse, Midwife and Health Visitor*, UKCC, London.

Vousden, M. (1985) Swallow your pride or lose your job. *Nursing Mirror*, **160**(1), 23.

Winslow, G.R. (1982) From loyalty to advocacy, in *Contemporary Issues In Bioethics*, (ed. L.R. Walters), Wadsworth Publishing Company, Belmont, California.

CASE LAW

Bolam v Friern Barnet Hospital Management Committee [1957] 2 ALL ER 118.

Ethical issues and research methods: covert research | 11

George Butler

The behavioural researcher whose study might reduce violence or racism or sexism, but who refuses to do the study because it involves deception, has not solved an ethical problem but only traded it for another.

(Rosenthal, 1978)

INTRODUCTION

Covert methods of investigation are now widely used in social science research. Milgram's 1960s experiments into obedience brought these methods of study to the attention of the public. This chapter examines the ethical issues surrounding the use of covert research, exploring its justification in relation to the moral principles of respect for persons, beneficence and non-maleficence. It sets out to determine the ethical parameters which require consideration in the search for scientific truth, citing examples from the healthcare professions to illustrate when the use of covert research might be justified morally.

Certainly, the use of covert or deceptive methods of investigation have become more and more extensive and are now an almost standard feature of social science research. The Milgram experiments of the 1960s into obedience brought into focus the question as to whether such methods can be justified ethically and, if so, could they be applied to research within healthcare settings where patients and healthcare professionals are involved?

Nursing research has largely focused on clinical nursing issues, where deceptive methods of investigation are not required. However, nursing is not practised within a vacuum, but within highly bureaucratic institutions where healthcare workers are subject to the same authoritative controls and abuses of power as those from a social science background. Institutional racism or other unseemly organizational practices are just as likely to be present in nursing institutions and, therefore, the use of deceptive methods of research to unearth such practices may be equally justified in nursing as it is in the social sciences.

The major ethical dilemma in research is the conflict between the protection of human rights and the generation of knowledge. This is made explicit in Bulmer's (1980) statement:

> Scientists, including social scientists, have wide responsibilities in conducting research, not only to further the ideal of scientific truth but (in research involving human subjects) to pay attention to questions of informed consent, responsibility for the well-being of research subjects and the relative importance of risk and benefit arising from the research.

Little, however, is agreed about how best to deal with these conflicting values. Caven (1977) states:

> Ethics is a matter of a principled sensitivity to the rights of others. Being ethical limits the choices we can make in the pursuit of truth. Ethics say that while truth is good, respect for human dignity is better, even if, in the extreme case, the respect of human dignity leaves one ignorant of human nature.

But what if human dignity itself is in jeopardy through the violent, sexist or racist behaviours of others? Does one have an obligation to respect the dignity of others who engage in wholesale anti-social behaviour? Douglas (1976) emphasizes the prime objective of research to be the search for truth and elaborates thus: 'Social actors employ lies, fraud, deceit, deception and blackmail in dealings with each other, therefore, the social scientist is justified in using them where necessary in order to achieve the higher objective of scientific truth.'

THE MILGRAM EXPERIMENTS: A JUSTIFICATION OF METHODS OF DECEPTION

These views must be at the forefront of one's deliberations when undertaking ethical analysis of the work of Stanley Milgram (1963), the American social psychologist who conducted a study in a laboratory-controlled environment into the propensity of male American subjects to obey commands without question, regardless of the acts demanded by the authoritative figure. Milgram had become deeply interested in the events which took place in Germany throughout the 1930s and 1940s in relation to the summary persecution and execution of Jews, among others. He maintained that in order for Hitler's evil plan to produce, as it did, the holocaust of Nazi Germany, it required the compliance of thousands of others. Milgram hypothesized that Germans had a 'basic character defect', i.e. a readiness to obey without question, regardless of the acts demanded by the authority figure. His prime interest lay in the 'readiness to obey' part of the hypothesis and he decided to carry out a pilot study in New Haven before taking his experiment to Germany. The results of the pilot study meant an experiment in Germany would have been superfluous, as the 'Germans are different' hypothesis was clearly shown to be false.

Milgram's study involved a procedure which comprised ordering a naïve subject to administer electric shocks to a victim under laboratory conditions. A simulated shock generator was used with 30 clearly marked voltage levels ranging from 15 to 450 volts, with the instrument also having indicated beside these figures in writing, designations from 'slight shock' to 'danger: severe shock'. The supposed authenticity of the experiment was heightened because each of the subjects received a 45-volt shock from the generator before commencing the experiment proper. The responses of the victim, who was a confederate of the experimenter, were standardized. The subject was told that the experiment was to study the effects of punishment on memory and the experiment involved the subject asking the victim questions. When wrong responses were received, the subject had to 'shock' the victim with increasing (up by 15-volts each time) voltage levels.

Studies into the propensity to unquestioningly obey commands from an authoritative figure had not been completed before, especially in relation to nationalist tendencies. Milgram's study was, therefore, the first of its kind but was related to earlier studies of obedience and authority (Arendt, 1958; Frank, 1944; Friedrich, 1958; Weber, 1947), authoritarianism (Adorno et al., 1950; Rokeach, 1963) and social power (Cartwright, 1959). Cormack (1984) emphasizes that not all research is necessary because research activity did not always lead to an increase in knowledge. He believed that researchers, therefore, had an obligation (especially where human subjects were involved) 'not to repeat unnecessarily that which had been substantiated by others'. Milgram's initial study into obedience certainly remained within this ethical boundary, though subsequent studies into similar areas of behaviour would have to be called into question.

Many would also call into question the way in which Milgram recruited his research subjects. His study comprised 40 males between the ages of 20 and 50 years who were recruited by newspaper as well as direct-mail advertising. The adverts had asked for volunteers to participate in a study of memory and learning at Yale University for which they were paid $4.50. This was simply for attending the laboratory, regardless of what happened after they had arrived.

The advertisements seeking recruits for the experiment clearly utilized a large degree of deception in obtaining its volunteers. Proponents of the research point to the fact that no coercion was involved in securing subjects and that they attended of their own free will. This is certainly stretching the limits of the principle of free will when we consider that those responding to the advertisement would in no way suspect that anything sinister was to take place. I use the word 'sinister' quite deliberately because, even though the experiment was simulated, the participants in no way knew this which served to further increase the deception involved, producing a most harrowing time for many of the subjects.

The experiment at face value would seem to have been designed for a most worthy purpose, i.e. the advancement of our knowledge concerning learning and memory. Because the experiments were sponsored and carried out in Yale University, an institution with an unimpeachable reputation, with personnel presumed to be highly competent and reputable, volunteers may have come forward assuming the absolute integrity of the research work, who would otherwise have not, had the experiment been advertised by a different institution.

To suggest that participants attended of their own free will is a deception in itself. Free will implies that the principle of informed consent had been addressed and this does not appear to be the case. Codes of conduct, i.e. Nuremberg Code (Bulmer 1980), stress the importance of the principle of informed consent in any aspect of research. The code clearly indicates that the responsibility for consent lies with the researcher who must communicate the facts fully, with the participant then able to make a decision, without at any time having been subject to any element of force, fraud, deceit, duress, constraint or coercion. Barbour (1979) adds that the subject must be competent, informed about the purposes of the research, understanding what they are told and then giving consent voluntarily.

Clearly, in Milgram's study most of the conditions needed to satisfy what is understood by informed consent were broken. Evidence of fraud and deceit abound, in that the subjects were kept in ignorance of the real purpose of the research until debriefing. Because of this they had no opportunity to consider the purpose and content of the research and then make a reasoned decision on whether to participate or not. Smith (1975) justifies such action in research of this nature, recognizing that 'deception or concealment may be necessary for research to be done validly'. This was apparently the case in the Milgram experiment because there would have been little purpose or authenticity to the research if subjects had not believed they were actually shocking victims. Deception was practised, therefore, throughout the entire experiment, from the façade of drawing lots (contrived to ensure the collaborator of Milgram was always to be the victim), through the subject receiving a sample shock of 45-volts (as they thought from the generator), to the victim calling out in despair once shocks were being administered at 300-volts and upwards.

Because the subject thought that he and the victim had really drawn lots, they believed that it was just a chance occurrence that they were the ones to deliver the shock. The subject generally perceived, therefore, that the victim had voluntarily submitted himself to the authority system of the experimenter and believed that, because both he and the victim had entered voluntarily, they were both under an obligation to the experimenter. This obligation was invariably heightened through receiving payment and could have had a bearing on the results, with the subject less likely to withdraw physically from the experiment. Also, the fact that subjects were told that the shocks were 'painful but not dangerous', may have led the subject to assume that the victim's discomfort was merely transient, that the benefits to be gained from the experiment may be long-lasting and therefore go on 'shocking', when in a real situation they may not. The fact that the experiments were taking place in this unimpeachable institution may also have led many to act, safe in the knowledge that the personnel of such an institution would not allow harm to occur to any of its research subjects: after all, this was the United States in the 1960s and not Nazi Germany of the 1940s.

From the stress experienced by most of the subjects, it would appear that the subjects fully believed in the authenticity of the experiment, i.e. that the victim was experiencing a great deal of pain. The principle of informed consent requiring, as it does, participation based on the full knowledge of the participant (Henry and Pashley, 1990) was clearly breached, as was the fundamental ability to withdraw at any stage once they became aware of the nature of the experiment (Smith, 1975). Such an ability to withdraw at any stage should continually be re-emphasized by the researchers conducting the experiment. But this did not happen in this experiment and, in fact, there was a degree of implied force, constraint and coercion because, when the subject questioned the experimenter about continuing with the shocks, (following the victim's verbal protestations in response to 'pain'), 'prods' to make the subject continue were utilized. The principle of informed consent was deliberately ignored, therefore, in this experiment because the results of such an experiment, with participants fully informed, would have been of little value.

ETHICAL PRINCIPLES IN CONFLICT

Henry and Pashley (1990) state, 'a major rule in any kind of applied research is "respect for persons",' which, as Harris (1985) qualifies, must necessarily involve a concern for their welfare and respect for their wishes. A general rule of research involving people is that their rights relating to privacy, anonymity and confidentiality must be upheld and, as far as publication of results is concerned, it would appear that Milgram honoured these obligations. However, subjects clearly had their privacy invaded when they were observed, unbeknown to them, by additional observers who kept notes on unusual behaviour. The recording of the sessions on magnetic tape and the taking of photographs through one-way mirrors without the subject's consent further served to contaminate the private spheres of 'self'. Nowhere is it suggested that permission was given by subjects for this to take place; neither does it suggest that such confidential data was subsequently destroyed, nor permission sought after the experiments to retain such confidential data on file.

However, as Wainwright (1994) asks: has the subject who agrees to allow access to a researcher, by their action, not given consent to some loss of privacy, in the same way as a patient who consults a healthcare professional relinquishes a restricted degree of their privacy? Beauchamp and Childress (1989) confirm that rules of privacy may be justifiably over-ridden in order to protect other moral principles and rules, providing these could not be realized or expressed without an invasion of privacy, which would appear to be the case in Milgram's study. If research leads to good moral ends, can the loss of privacy which results from research observation, therefore, be considered as lesser in merit than the benefits that will accrue for others from the research?

Is it not justifiable to place researchers as pseudopatients in mental-health institutions to assess the accuracy of psychological categorization of mental illness, as Rosenhan (1973) did? Similarly, if researchers suspected abuse of elderly or mentally ill clients, would they not be justified in placing hidden cameras within an institution to monitor activity? Is creating good (beneficence) and preventing harm (non-maleficence) by exposing and thereby preventing the abuse of patients not better than preserving privacy?

Bulmer (1980) rightly asks whether an ethical violation has been committed if you watch people, record observations about them and draw inferences from what you have seen and heard, without first gaining permission. Smith (1979) believes that, providing you do not affect the lives of the participants and preserve their anonymity so that others cannot use your observations to affect them, most would accept this. It may be argued that the benefits of research far outweigh the damage which may be done by invading people's privacy. However, in Milgram's case, because the experiments are presumably still retained on tape and photographs of subjects still held, these could potentially breach all codes of conduct related to privacy, confidentiality and anonymity should the security of this information ever be transgressed.

Two of the major principles of all ethical discussion, especially in relation to research involving human subjects, is that of beneficence (to do good), and non-maleficence (to protect against harm). Certainly in Milgram's study one has to question whether concern for the welfare of the subjects was shown. One has to ask whether adequate measures were taken to protect the subjects from the undoubted stress and emotional conflict they experienced. The research data concedes that during the procedure a degree of extreme tension was reached which had rarely been seen before in sociopsychological laboratory studies, to the extent that three subjects experienced 'full-blown uncontrollable seizures'. Many subjects became highly agitated and angry and one of them, within 20 minutes, is reported to have been 'reduced to a twitching, stuttering wreck'. One has to question the nature of the research and whether Milgram could have done more to protect the individual participants from harm.

Milgram claims to have been as surprised as anyone at the results of his experiment and maintains that any criticism of his methods was only done in hindsight: something he did not have the benefit of before the study. He emphasizes that the production of stress and anxiety in subjects was not anticipated and, in fact, if his 'Germans are different' hypothesis was to be proved, he would have expected American subjects to refuse to obey the commands, certainly beyond the point where the victim protested. If, as I suspect, it is reasonable to expect that the subjects would not 'harm' the victim and thereby would have refused to continue 'shocking', then the results of the experiment could not have been anticipated. Milgram (1974) concludes that you cannot know the results of your research in advance, maintaining, 'understanding grows because we examine situations in which the end is unknown' and, because of this, 'an investigator unwilling to accept this degree of risk must give up the idea of scientific inquiry'.

It becomes apparent that none of the subjects suffered subsequent psychological harm, despite the traumas of the actual experiment. This is probably due to the effective debriefing which took place following the experiment in which the subject was reunited with his unharmed actor-victim and was assured that no shock had in fact been delivered and that his actions during the experiment had been entirely normal. One year after the experiment, an independent psychiatrist confirmed that none of the subjects showed any signs of being psychologically harmed, nor were they suffering from traumatic reactions. In fact, 84% of the subjects indicated that they were glad to have participated and supported the use of further similar research studies. It would appear, certainly retrospectively, that the principle of non-maleficence was maintained. However, no action seems to have been taken to identify potentially vulnerable subjects after one of the subjects had suffered a full-blown seizure. I would have expected such individuals to have been eliminated from the experimental programme, knowing the effects participation could have on them.

Retrospectively, it could also be assumed that beneficence was a consequence of the study, though I am not sure that this would have been a consideration before the experiment. In an experiment of this nature, one has to weigh up the good and bad consequences. This will inevitably raise issues in relation to consequences for the individual who is participating, against consequences which may be of benefit to society as a whole. Bulmer (1980) suggests that the benefits from greater social science knowledge about society far outweigh the risks that are run in collecting data using covert techniques, i.e. the harm done by using deception is outweighed by the good that will flow from the greater knowledge about society.

When one considers the discrimination that could have ensued had the Americans continued in their belief that Germans had a flawed psyche, it makes the possible harm that could have resulted for individual subjects more acceptable – or does it? In many instances of social research, or ethics in general, this issue of individual versus societal benefits arises. Differences of opinion abound, depending on whether the observer views such circumstances from a deontological (moral duties and obligations) or a teleological (purpose or end result) point of view.

For example, a young surgical house officer visits his general practitioner complaining of lethargy and feeling unwell. Following investigation, the general practitioner confirms to the surgical house officer that he is HIV positive. The house officer asks his GP to maintain confidentiality on this matter as he intends to return to his duties as a surgical house officer. The deontologist would confirm that the general practitioner had a moral duty and obligation to maintain the confidence of his client and that this be adhered to regardless of the consequences. A teleologist, however, would weigh up the consequences or end result of the action to be taken by the house officer and if these were potentially to create harm to many patients, then confidentiality would be breached in favour of the perceived more important principle of non-maleficence.

Bulmer (1980) asks, 'In any risk-benefit equation, who is to draw up the balance sheet and determine whether particular methods are justified or not? Whose causes are the right causes in social research?' Is respect for persons or respecting autonomy more important than the principle of increasing social good? Engelhart (1984) recognizes such a conflict thus: 'Respecting freedom (autonomy) sets limits to the moral authority of others to act and this conflicts with that dimension of morality that focuses on beneficence, on achieving the good for others.'

If the causes of the majority take priority over the causes of the individual, can Milgram's experiments be defended? If, following debriefing, more than 80% of the subjects were happy to have participated, does this condone the inordinate amount of stress they suffered during the experiment? If no psychological stress befell the subjects, can the research methods be justified? Like those proponents of Milgram's study, I believe that the experiments led to the development of significant knowledge of human behaviour, dispelling the myth of a disordered German psyche to obey commands unquestioningly, thereby preventing racial discrimination and persecution against the German people. Because of this, the 'ends' could be said to have justified the 'means', although it is clear that such a consequentialist approach significantly compromises the deontological principles of autonomy, beneficence and non-maleficence.

COVERT METHODS AND THEIR APPLICATION IN HEALTHCARE RESEARCH

Can these same covert or deceptive methods of enquiry be supported in healthcare research? Could the principles employed by Milgram be justified within a healthcare setting? Can comparisons be made between the relationship of experimenter and subject in Milgram's study, to that of healthcare professional and patient?

It is important here that we make the broad distinction between patient care and researching healthcare. The therapeutic relationship between healthcare professional and patient is built on trust, i.e. where the patient believes the professional to be honest and forthright. So the use of deceit, lies, fraud, deception and blackmail as advocated in social science research by Douglas (1976) should have no place in the therapeutic relationship between healthcare professional and patient. As Yarling (1978) states, 'Lying, whatever the motive, trades on trust and truth. It can succeed only where trust is the norm. Only when the person who is speaking is regarded as trustworthy can he succeed in lying. Each lie trades on and diminishes the credibility of every truth.' Many of the major interdisciplinary ethical dilemmas in healthcare arise because the principle of veracity is in fact not adhered to, often producing conflict between physician and nurse.

This is most frequently seen when patients are not told their true diagnosis or prognosis by physicians, and nurses, through the power relationships which exist in healthcare, are expected to support such information. Yarling (1978) highlights how the practice of lying to terminal patients has made even the truth suspect, to the extent that increased mistrust has made even the truth not credible. Patients are no longer reassured when told, 'everything is fine', or 'the tumour was benign' because they know the doctor or nurse could be lying. As Curtin and Flaherty (1982) emphasize, 'Health professionals no longer are thought to tell the truth.'

Harris (1985) and Henry and Pashley (1990) earlier clarified the central issue of respect for persons in any kind of applied research and again this is paramount within the therapeutic relationship. Curtin and Flaherty (1982) clearly demonstrate how deception of patients by professionals robs them of reality and serves to destroy the human relationship between patient and professional. This fact is re-emphasized by Benjamin and Curtis (1981) who state: 'Where a doctor or nurse participate in deception, this seriously compromises the integrity of the relationship between them and the patient, both diminishing her as well as the patient's personhood.'

Naïve patients, such as the naïve subjects of Milgram, are often deceived by healthcare professionals in the use of placebos, either as part of a therapeutic programme or in researching new forms of treatment. The former category is justified on the basis of beneficence and Chadwick and Tadd (1992: 82,74) highlight how this can be used to effect in particular patients. They demonstrate in casestudy presentations how the patient with chronic back pain, who was dependent on strong analgesics, was given injections of sterile water which resulted in reduced dependency and control of pain by much milder analgesics and how a manipulative patient in hospital had his back pain relieved by injections of sterile water. The patient in the former study was furious that she had been deceived and, although a healthcare professional might argue that the patient's autonomy was increased because they had relieved her drug dependence, this does not help the complete lack of trust that may result from such action. When such deception is discovered by the patient, the trust that patients invest in healthcare professionals is irretrievably lost; such a loss of trust could result in patients not seeking professional help in the event of further illness (Bok, 1978).

The use of placebos in researching new forms of treatment brings to the fore the question of whether promoting the good of society is more important than the promotion of individual good. This compares with Milgram's experimental methods, where the potential harm to the individual subject, through repeated coercion to make the subject continue shocking, can be offset by utilitarian ideas of creating the greatest good to the greatest number. Coercion is the use of force to bring about a desired result against a person's wishes or without a person's consent. It violates a person's liberty and, therefore, this violation calls for justification (Rhodes, 1986). Rhodes (1986) indicates: 'Coercive acts are justified by the good consequences that result from the coercion – the overall well-being to the client, others and society itself.' So patients may be coerced into drug trials without knowing that they may not be receiving any treatment nor the consequences of this. In medicine, such deception has been found to have a long and sometimes tragic history (Katz, 1972; Beecher, 1970). Despite Bok's (1978) reassurances that all biomedical research is now carefully regulated, with patients having to give their consent, we have to question the degree or level this informed consent takes.

Coercive acts are also utilized in many aspects of healthcare against the person where it is perceived it produces the greater good for society. Social workers, doctors and nurses often violate a client's liberty in order to achieve what they perceive as some greater good. For example, a social worker may make a compulsory involuntary foster-home placement, thereby violating a parent and often a child's freedom in order to bring about the 'greater good' of protecting the child. Doctors and nurses behave in the same way where they believe a child is at unreasonable risk, i.e. where child abuse is suspected or where a blood transfusion request is refused for a child who is said to need one. Similarly, the Mental Health Act allows professionals to violate the liberty of certain individuals who are perceived as a threat to themselves or society. If coercion promotes utility as in the above cases and the Milgram experiments, surely restriction on liberty, albeit temporarily, can be justified.

Milgram's covert, deceptive and coercive research methods can be utilized to the benefit of society in researching healthcare, providing this research relates to interprofessional and institutional relationships. Healthcare professionals, administrators and managers have power over patients and other healthcare workers, not only because of their exper-tise but because of inequalities in society based on social class, race, professional status, institutional hierarchies and access to powerful institutions.

Just as Milgram defended his covert methods to determine the propensity of male American subjects to obey commands without question, regardless of the acts demanded by authoritative figures, similar methods are justified in healthcare research to uncover abuses of power or revelations of wrong-doing by those in positions of public trust. As Galliher (1973) states, 'No right to privacy should be applied to research on subjects involved in roles accountable to the public, because a democratic society has a moral duty to hold individuals accountable in their organizational and occupational roles.'

Fox and De Marco (1990) highlight how people gain authority, either theoretical authority through being an 'expert' on questions of truth, or practical or moral authority because they occupy positions of power or leadership. These forms of authority are typical within the framework of healthcare institutions and it is clearly necessary that such authority is seen to be good and to do good.

Some people often assume that what is right or wrong in ethics depends on who has the power to enforce their opinions on others, but it does not follow that the opinion and decisions of the stronger are necessarily the right decisions. Persons and institutions often do things which are not right, morally speaking, despite their being legal and we also know that they do things which are illegal.

The author, in exposing racial discrimination within the health service (Butler 1992, 1992a,b,c, 1993), utilized covert methods in collecting some data. As Stanfield II (1993) indicates, ethnicity and (especially) race are emotion-laden issues which are difficult matters for scholars to confront honestly: there is a great reluctance to engage willingly in introspection about these topics. Van Dijk (1993) highlights: 'given the official norm against discrimination and racism, whites will not normally admit such discriminatory practices to other whites, at least not in official contexts of enquiry', and therefore the only way open to expose this is often through covert research methods. Genuine informed consent would interfere with such a study because it is hard to imagine that healthcare professionals might voluntarily reveal the character traits or actions that such studies confirm, if told the true nature of the study beforehand. If subjects are unaware of what is being evaluated, or even unaware that research is going on, then their responses will be spontaneous.

Interference of a subject's freedom of informed choice can be justified where it exposes wrong-doing or bad practice. As Stanfield II (1993) confirms: 'The pictures may not be pretty, but at least they will be telling the truth, and certainly that is what doing social science is supposed to be all about – telling the truth, even when it hurts pretty badly.' Just as Hofling *et al.* (1966) revealed how nurses often complied with medical directives that they knew fell short of minimally decent standards of practice, Milgram exposed the same compliance to authority to act in an inhumane way to fellow human beings. Surely it is good to expose the dark side of institutional care where those in power often perpetuate systems which totally fail to respect the dignity of others. How can things be made better if the dehumanizing aspects of some healthcare institutions are not revealed through covert research? Bad practices, as revealed in the many enquiries into mental-health institutions in the 1960s, the Ashworth Inquiry of 1992 (Department of Health, 1992), and recent revelations of pindown in Derbyshire Children's Homes, only existed because those in positions of power within those institutions allowed them to happen.

Rhodes (1986) highlights the perverse nature of authority in bureaucratic organizations like healthcare institutions which severely constrain the ethical autonomy of nurses, just as Milgram demonstrated how his subjects were prepared to compromise ethical standards to obey those perceived to have an influence over them. As Thompson, Melia and Boyd (1988) confirm: 'Ethics is concerned in a fundamental way with power and power-sharing' and the issues common to all healthcare professionals relate to the way power or control is exercised over people. Benjamin and Curtis (1981) confirm how nurses feel relatively powerless because doctors and administrators severely limit and complicate their decision-making role. Because of this, morality is undermined through the gradual daily erosion of a nurses' ethical stance.

The characteristics of bureaucracies as defined by Ladd (1970) result in organizational standards that by their very nature deviate from ordinary moral ones which result in an absence of moral responsibility for actions (Rhodes, 1986). She goes on: 'Bureaucratic decision-making is based on role and legal responsibility,' whereas, 'moral responsibility by contrast involves concern for the rightness or goodness of one's actions'. Employees are, therefore, expected to undertake particular tasks, regardless of their personal feelings or beliefs – any decision they make is an instrument of the organization and for its benefit (Rhodes, 1986).

Ladd (1970) highlights how working in a bureaucracy can create a kind of moral schizophrenia, where the individual's own decisions and actions become separated from themselves as persons and become the decisions and actions of another, e.g. an organization. They become social decisions and not those of the individual which leads to the individual becoming dehumanized and demoralized. He goes on to demonstrate how morality is essentially a relationship between people as individuals; in losing this relationship, we lose morality itself.

Tadd (1991) highlights the immense problem which healthcare professionals (especially nurses) encounter when they stray from the bureaucratic expectations of their role. She demonstrates how many nurses have been forced to leave the profession, having highlighted the shortcomings of the service or incidents of malpractice. Institutions which should welcome the reporting of less-than-adequate aspects of patient care, to enable them to put these right, deal unfavourably with those who report such inadequacies. Most nurses are reluctant to report poor care because there are inadequate support systems to safeguard their interests against often hostile employers. Rhodes (1986) highlights how such organizations are in some ways the most harmful because of their false promises of caring concern.

If a democratic society has a moral duty to hold individuals in public office accountable in their organizational and occupational roles and such individuals utilize methods to sustain power and control to the detriment of their clients and employees, how will this be recognized if employees live in fear of retribution should they speak out? Surely a case can be supported for a behavioural researcher to use covert or deceptive methods of research where this may reduce violence, racism, sexism, abuse of power, inadequate or inappropriate care. After all, what have institutions to fear if they are conducting their business in accordance with public morality? Clearly, the fundamental deontological principle of respect for persons should not be compromised except in the most extraordinary circumstances. One such special circumstance must be where those who work in organizations accountable to the public seek to compromise the respect, dignity and rights of others, and therefore covert research methods in such a scenario can be entirely justified. Telling the truth, even when it hurts pretty badly, must continue to be the prime object of social science and nursing research.

GLOSSARY

Autonomy Autonomy refers to a set of diverse notions including self-governance, liberty, rights, privacy, individual choice, liberty to follow one's will, causing one's own behaviour, and being one's own person.

Non-maleficence The concept of non-maleficence or not inflicting harm has been associated with the maxim *premium non nocere*: 'Above all (or first) do no harm.

Beneficence The term beneficence suggests acts of mercy, kindness and charity, but can include any form of action to benefit another. The principle of beneficence asserts an obligation to help others further their important and legitimate interests.

Deontology A general term for those forms of ethics that base morality on duty and obligation. Deontological theories hold that acts are right or wrong in and of themselves, regardless of consequences; thus they are often contrasted with teleological theories. Deontic logic formalises our understanding of the rules of permission, prohibition and obligation.

Teleology Concerning the end or purpose toward which a process or action is directed. In ethics, a theory that the moral value of an action should be determined by its purpose or results.

REFERENCES

Adorno, Frenkel-Brunswick, Levinson, D.J. and Sanford, R.N. (1950) in Behaviour study of obedience (ed. S. Milgram) *Journal of Abnormal and Social Psychology*, Vol. 67, 371–8.

Arendt, H. (1958) in Behavioural study of obedience (ed. S. Milgram) *Journal of Abnormal and Social Psychology*, Vol. 67, 371–8.

Barbour, R. (1979) The ethics of covert research. *Network*, Sep., 9.

Beauchamp, T.L. and Childress, J.F. (1989) *Principles of Biomedical Ethics*, Oxford University Press, New York.

Beecher, H.K. (1970) *Research and the Individual*, Little, Brown, Boston,

Benjamin, M. and Curtis, J. (1981) *Ethics in Nursing*, Oxford University Press, New York.

Bok, S. (1978) *Lying: Moral Choice in Public and Private Life*, Quartet Books, London.

Bulmer, M. (1980) *The impact of ethical concerns upon sociological research.* *Sociology*, vol. 14, 125–30.

Butler, G.A.McB. (1992) Racism in employment practice within the NHS (Part 1). *Journal of Advances in Health and Nursing Care*, Vol. 1, No. 5, 85–91.

Butler, G.A.McB. (1992a) Racism in employment practice within the NHS (Part 2). *Journal of Advances in Health and Nursing Care*, Vol. 1, No. 6, 57–77.

Butler, G.A.McB. (1992b) Racism in employment practice within the NHS (Part 3). *Journal of Advances in Health and Nursing Care*, Vol. 2, No. 1, 29–57.

Butler, G.A.McB. (1992c) Racism in employment practice within the NHS (Part 4). *Journal of Advances in Health and Nursing Care*, Vol. 2, No. 2, 3–18.

Butler, G.A.McB. (1993) Racial equality in nursing and midwifery education: myth or reality? Unpublished MA Thesis.

Cartwright, S. (1959) in Behavioural study of obedience (ed. S. Milgram). *Journal of Abnormal and Social Psychology*, Vol. 67, 371–8.

Caven, S. and Douglas, J.D. (1977) Investigative social research: individual and team field research. *American Journal of Sociology*, Vol. 83, 809–10.

Chadwick, R. and Tadd, W. (1992) *Ethics and Nursing Practice: A Case Study Approach*, Macmillan, Basingstoke.

Cormack, D.F.S. (1984) *The Research Process in Nursing*, Blackwell, Oxford.

Curtin, L. and Flaherty, M.J. (1982) *Nursing Ethics: Theories and Pragmatics*, Prentice Hall, Englewood Cliffs.

Department of Health (1992) *Report of the Committee of Inquiry into Complaints about Ashworth Hospital*, CM2028–1 and CM2028–11, HMSO, London.

Douglas, J. (1976) *Investigative Social Research*, Sage, London.

Engelhart, H.T. (1984) Shattuck Lecture – Allocating scarce medical resources and the availability of organ transplantation: Some moral pre-suppositions. *The New England Journal of Medicine*, Vol. 311, No. 1, 66–71.

Fox, R.M. and De Marco, J.P. (1990) *Moral Reasoning: A Philosophic Approach to Applied Ethics*, Holt, Rinehart & Winston, Fort Worth.

Frank, J.D. (1944) in Behavioural study of obedience (ed. S. Milgram). *Journal of Abnormal and Social Psychology*, Vol. 67, 371–8.

Friedrich, C.J. (1958) in Behavioural Study of Obedience (ed. S. Milgram). *Journal of Abnormal and Social Psychology*, Vol. 67, 371–8.

Galliher, J.S. (1973) The protection of human subjects: a re-examination of the professional code of ethics. *American Sociologist*, **8**, 93–100.

Harris, J. (1985) *The Value of Life*, Routledge & Kegan Paul, London.

Henry, I.C. and Pashley, G. (1990) *Health Ethics: Health and Nursing Studies for Diploma and Undergraduate Students*. Quay Publishing, Lancaster.

Hofling, C.K., Brotzman, E., Dalrymple, S., Graves, N. and Pierce, C.M. (1966) An experimental study in nurse-physician relationships. *Journal of Nervous and Mental Disease*, **143**, 171–80.

Katz, J. (1972) *Experimentation with Human Beings*, Russell Sage Foundation, New York.

Ladd, J. (1970) Morality and the ideal of rationality in formal organisations. *Monist*, Vol. 54, No. 4. Oct.

Milgram, S. (1963) Behavioural study of obedience. *Journal of Abnormal and Social Psychology*, Vol. 67, 371–8.

Milgram, S. (1974) *Obedience to Authority: An Experimental View*, Harper & Row, New York.

Rhodes, M.L. (1986) *Ethical Dilemmas in Social Work Practice,* Routledge & Kegan Paul, London.

Rokeach, M. (1963) in Behavioural study of obedience (ed. S. Milgram). *Journal of Abnormal and Social Psychology*, Vol. 67, 371–8.

Rosenhan, D.L. (1973) On being sane in insane places. *Science*, Vol. 179, 250–8.

Rosenthal, R. (1978) Unpublished working paper for a conference on deception in research, in *Lying: Moral Choice in Public and Private Life* (ed. S. Bok), Quartet Books, London.

Smith, H.W. (1975) *Strategies of Social Research: The Methodological Imagination*, Prentice Hall, Englewood Cliffs.

Smith, M.B. (1979) Some perspectives on ethical/political issues in social science research, in *Federal Regulations: Ethical Issues and Social Research* (eds M.L. Wax and J. Cassell), Westview, Boulder, Colorado.

Stanfield II, J.H. (1993) Methodological reflections: an introduction, in *Race and Ethnicity in Research Methods,* (eds J.H. Stanfield II and R.M. Dennis), Sage, Newbury Park, California, pp. 3–15.

Tadd, V. (1991) Where are the whistle-blowers? *Nursing Times*, Vol. 87, No. 1, 42–4.

Thompson, I.E., Melia, K.M. and Boyd, K.M. (1988) *Nursing Ethics*, Churchill Livingstone. Edinburgh.

Van dijk, T.A. (1993) Analyzing racism through discourse analysis: some methodological reflections in *Race and Ethnicity in Research Methods* (eds J.H. Stanfield II and R.M. Dennis), Sage, Newbury Park, California, pp. 92–134.

Wainwright, P. (1994) The observation of intimate aspects of care: privacy and dignity, in *Ethical Issues in Nursing* (ed. G. Hunt), Routledge, London, pp. 38–54.

Weber, M. (1947) in Behavioural study of obedience (ed. S. Milgram). *Journal of Abnormal and Social Psychology*, vol. 67, 371–8.

Yarling, R. (1978) Ethical analysis of a nursing problem, II. *Supervisor Nurse*, Vol. 9, No. 6, 29.

Considerations of personhood in nursing research: an ethical perspective

Kevin Kendrick

Act in such a way that you treat humanity, both in your own person and in the person of all others, never as a means but always equally as an end.

(*Immanuel Kant,*
Groundwork of the Metaphysics of Morals)

There has been a progressive increase in the amount of nursing research being carried out in Britain over the past 25 years. This is a promising trend which illustrates that nurses are becoming increasingly aware of the need to utilize research in their practice. The result of this has been that the delivery of care is now more likely to be based on insight and understanding rather than tradition alone. To a certain extent, this is a valid response to demands for nursing to become a research-based profession. If other professionals are seen to engage actively in research, then nurses must do likewise if a position of real parity is ever to be achieved.

Many different types of research methodology can be used as a tool for enquiry. To a large degree, the type of method used is often dictated by the nature of the research which is to be carried out and by the personal bias of the researcher. Although there is a choice available regarding what research method is used, the differences between them must be explored if clarity is to be achieved. In order to address the opposing perspectives that exist, consideration must be given to the philosophical differences that occur between quantitative and qualitative research.

QUANTITATIVE RESEARCH

One of the most fundamental of philosophical issues can be found in the question: is social research a science? Quantitative researchers would undoubtedly agree that it is possible to apply the laws of the natural sciences to the social arena and establish causal relationships which are consistent with scientific enquiry. This perspective is sometimes referred to as 'empirical positivism' and it has a long tradition in the historical development of quantitative research.

The person accredited with introducing the notion is Auguste Comte (1798–1857), who believed that it was possible to have a science of society based on the principles of cause and effect which are found in the natural, physical sciences. This approach makes a number of assumptions about the nature and behaviour of persons. If positivism is considered in terms of logical progression, then the behaviour of people is said to be open to the same objective measurement as matter. If scientific rationale is to be considered valid, then it is necessary to quantify this matter in terms of some acceptable measurement. This type of enquiry has been largely adopted and accepted as a positive mechanism by medical scientists. There are many example of causal relationships in the aetiology of disease processes; we are told that smoking cigarettes causes lung cancer, that atheroma causes heart disease and that viruses cause influenza. All these examples can be considered through scientific scrutiny and may be open to a certain amount of quantifiable observation. However, for the positivist it is feasible to take the methods used in this type of enquiry to establish causal links for human behaviour.

If we consider elements of nursing research which may be quantified, it seems reasonable to accept the notion that certain physiological parameters may fit the criteria for being considered as 'facts'. A person may have measurements taken of temperature, weight or blood pressure which can be taken as objective statements of physiological fact. The quantitative researcher who wishes to pursue a line of pure, positivistic enquiry would also argue that similar criteria could be devised to predict the behaviour of patients under certain circumstances. For example, the majority of people entering hospital put on their nightwear even during the day; this is in compliance with the unwritten code of the hospital ethos. This is a type of behaviour which can be observed and quantified without having to give any interpretation to the meanings that people associate with it. The end of this scenario is that nurse researchers who take this approach believe that it forms a valid foundation for reliable data.

The orientation which Comte instigated gained further support from the work of Emile Durkheim, who argued that science was concerned with the study of 'things' and that social observation should be carried out in the same way. He tried to illustrate that concepts such as religious belief or societal customs could be observed in the same way as objects in the physical world. The central theme which Durkheim tried to present was that social facts may impinge on the individual's consciousness but that they still remain external and, therefore, may be studied by using objective criteria. Human behaviour is shaped and influenced by these social facts which contribute towards a collective way of thinking or acting. Durkheim produced a famous work on the nature of suicide to try to validate his positivistic stance. This presented an argument that suicide is not merely an act of individual consciousness but is influenced and caused by external social factors. This gave Durkheim a firm conviction that social phenomena are similar to natural phenomena in respect of the laws which govern their action. Given this fact, Durkheim maintained that the only valid criterion for producing research in the social realm is to use natural science methodology.

The concept of cause and effect is very much reflected in the philosophy of biomedical science, and to a certain extent this is acceptable because it is physical phenomena which are being observed. However, if we accept the perspective of philosophers like Comte and Durkheim then the same approach may be taken in observing human behaviour. This may be expressed in the following way:

$$C \longrightarrow E$$

This is an acceptable model if 'C' represents a person sitting on a pin and 'E' represents the recoil due to pain. This simplistic representation shows that it is possible to explain human behaviour when it operates at the level of a reflex. The methods of causation become more complex when a number of factors are introduced into the equation. Let us consider the example given earlier of the person who enters hospital and puts on night attire in the middle of the day. Quantitative researchers would argue that the observation of this act is sufficient to validate it as data. The higher-order cognitions to do with why the person acted in this way and what meaning they can bring to illustrate their present state are thought to be unimportant in the search for scientific objectivity. The glaring problem with taking this approach is that the individual who is supposed to form the focal point of nursing or health research seems to have been left out of the equation.

If we leave a person out of the research process in terms of ignoring their cognitive elements then it would appear impossible to claim anything like an approximation towards understanding a given social reality. At this point we can introduce the concept of qualitative research as an alternative perspective in research methodology.

QUALITATIVE RESEARCH

In sharp contrast to the philosophy of positivism, qualitative research places a great deal of emphasis on the importance of interpreting meaning in the research process. This reflects the ethos of a philosophical theme called phenomenology.

Phenomenology is concerned with placing the person at the centre of the research process; persons are more than just a collection of atoms and molecules. Duffy (1985) continues this theme by arguing that persons cannot be viewed merely as objects. In the social arena, qualitative researchers take the stance that persons are not merely acted upon by social forces but that they react to them through a dynamic dialogue with fellow actors. If a researcher accepts that a person plays an active role in creating social reality, then research must be aimed at gaining insight and at interpreting the meaning people give to social phenomena.

It is because emphasis is placed on the importance of meaning that qualitative research believes that the notion of values cannot be divorced from an enquiry which involves people. This is in contrast to the central theme of positivism which maintains that research must be value free if a position of true scientific objectivity is to be achieved. If phenomenology is used as the underpinning philosophy, then the main focus must be placed on research which attempts to understand human behaviour from the agent's perspective.

From the perspective of phenomenology, there exists a fundamental difference between the subject matter of the natural sciences and that of persons. Physical matter does not have cognitive processes which are expressed through the conscious elements of the person. It is justified, therefore, to consider the reaction of matter when subjected to external stimuli. Matter is compelled to react in a preordained way because it cannot introduce any sense, interpretation or meaning to its behaviour. However, a person does have the facility to bring meaning to a given behaviour and to interpret and experience the construction of social reality.

Phenomenology research argues that attempting to quantify human behaviour is not possible through the use of scientific enquiry in the objective sense. If we consider the human condition in the same way as the physical sciences, then we present a threat to the unique nature of individuality and freedom. It seems difficult to conceptualize a person as being at liberty to interact if the positivistic stance of being constantly under the influence of societal laws is to be understood in terms of the definitive. Howarth (1981) considers that positivistic research imposes a view of the person which is reminiscent of the reductionistic and materialistic perspectives favoured by the natural sciences. If an individual is seen through the perspective of positivism, then they are reduced to the unconscious level of elements used in the physical sciences. The term 'materialistic' is used because the person's cognitive processes are ignored in the search for an objective equation which will explain causal links in human behaviour.

What is starting to emerge here is similar to the stance which Henry (1986) takes in arguing that the concept of personhood is central to nursing and, therefore, must also take a dominant theme in any research which is carried out. This approach may be represented in the following way:

$$C \longrightarrow P \longrightarrow E$$

The important issue here is that the person has been placed firmly at the centre of any observable phenomena. The cause does not bring about an immediate effect; the person at the centre of the dynamic interprets whatever the information is through the avenue of cognitive processes. The effectual end of this scenario will be the result of a person bringing interpretation and meaning to a given situation.

Taking either a positivist or a phenomenological approach to research will strongly influence how it is conducted. Each philosophical theme will have an effect on the way in which measures are made or interpreted in a particular research project. However, it must be emphasized once again that natural science explanations of the world are based on conceptions of things. In nursing research, it is essential to explore forms of knowledge more appropriately matched to conceptions of care. The main focus for the nurse researcher is interacting with persons within a healthcare environment. In this respect, the term 'person' is an evaluative oral term and is not used to describe an object or a thing in the world.

The process of research in nursing can strongly influence how we construe things. Because this process is concerned with two dominant elements – the concept of the person and the concept of care – then it is suitable to consider the ethical dimensions which can be introduced as a means of enhancing the relationship between the researcher and persons involved in the study. The most essential ethical principle when undertaking nursing research must be an acknowledgment of 'respect for persons'.

RESPECT FOR PERSONS

This is a central ethical doctrine which demands that any research involving people should place a great deal of emphasis upon the importance of autonomy, partnership and informed consent. If these concepts are acknowledged as playing a central role in the research process, then it suggests that the researcher accepts that persons have both an inherent worth and value. This is an excellent basis for enquiry because it means that persons are not merely being used as vehicles for substantiating the validity of a given theory. In terms of the approach which the philosopher Immanuel Kant would take, the researcher who has a respect for persons is using them not merely as a means to an end, but as valued ends in their own right. It is of the essence that nursing research should hold this principle at the centre of any project which involves persons and their care.

We have said that a respect for persons involves the acceptance of them having intrinsic worth and value. Harris (1985) argues that it also means that someone who has a respect for persons must show both a concern for their welfare and respect for their wishes. In healthcare ethics there is sometimes a degree of conflict between the wishes of the patient and concern for their welfare. For example, a person may express an intense desire to smoke following surgery of the stomach. The nurse realizes that this might result in a coughing episode which could rupture the wound. In this instance, the nurse would probably go against the patient's wishes in trying to maintain a respect for their physical welfare. This scenario is fraught with ethical issues regarding patient autonomy, paternalism and competency. There is no need to consider these concepts in detail as they were only introduced to show that conflict can occur between the expressed wishes of the patients and respect for their welfare. However, in nursing research it is unlikely that dilemmas of this nature will arise and the relationship between respect for a person's welfare and wishes should be both complementary and reciprocal.

Earlier in this chapter it was stated that the type of methodology employed will be influenced by the personal bias of the researcher and the type of data to be collected. The central theme of this chapter is concerned with presenting ethical and philosophical considerations about personhood in the research process. Because nursing research is concerned primarily with studying the delivery and effect of care, then the nature of ethical principles will be considered within a methodological framework which enables the nurse researcher to practise while formulating and collecting data; the research tool being referred to here is participant observation.

PARTICIPANT OBSERVATION: RESEARCH AS AN ADAPTIVE PARTNERSHIP

Participant observation has a long history in social science research and involves the researcher joining in the everyday routines of those who are to be studied and observed. For the nurse researcher, this would involve joining the normal, natural environment of the ward. Although participant observation may be used by researchers with either a quantitative or a qualitative background, it is particularly favoured by those who adopt a phenomenological approach. However, like all methods of research, participant observation has both positive and negative aspects associated with it.

1. Participant observation (PO) allows the nurse researcher to consider the patient's conception of objects and events by being a part of that person's activities during the hospital stay.
2. PO is sometimes criticized on the grounds that the researcher cannot gain access to the group's social reality because the presence of a stranger will inhibit normal social intercourse. This criticism is not valid in nursing research because the process is usually carried out by a nurse who is familiar with the norms, culture and values of the hospital environment.
3. Because a nurse is already a part of the world which they wish to study, there is little likelihood of them imposing a false and detached reality on the social world they are seeking to understand. If a structured methodology was introduced, for example, a structured interview with a predetermined set of questions or a questionnaire with pre-set questions, then the researcher has already decided what is important. If a nurse researcher takes a number of prepared enquiries to a patient, then a framework is being introduced which imposes personal research priorities upon those who are to be studied. When this is done, assumptions have already been made about how the patient perceives social reality within the confines of the hospital.
4. Positivistic researchers claim that the data that are obtained from participant observation are unreliable. Objective scientific research involves using the same method of investigation on the same types of material and that this should reproduce the same types of result. Very few social researchers would claim that the same degree of exactitude could be achieved in the area of social research. However, they do claim that a certain degree of reliability is possible to achieve. Criticism is levelled at participant observation because its procedures are not made explicit, that the observations do not follow a systematic pattern and that the results obtained are rarely quantified.
5. Participant observation relies greatly on interpretive skills, and their value lies in providing useful insights into the meanings which persons put on events which form social reality.

If the nurse researcher utilises participant observation as a tool, then they are attempting to come face to face with the reality of the patient's experience. It is possible only to approximate towards an understanding of socia! reality; participant observation acknowledges this problem, but still enables the researcher to make valid observations. The researcher who adopts this approach must gain the trust of those who are to be observed. This demands that certain ethical principles are adhered to. The most effective means of achieving this is by viewing the person in a research programme as an equal partner in the understanding of our social world. This last point is of the essence when applied to nursing research.

Adaptive partnership

The notions of adaptation and partnership are not new to nursing theory but basing them firmly within a framework of ethical rationale and principles certainly is. The way in which people react to being in hospital can cover every aspect of the emotional spectrum. The nurse researcher can provide an avenue through which these issues can be addressed. In this way, a vital element of participant observation is advanced, the process of sharing information which reflects the meaning which patients put upon events relating to their present state.

Another proviso for partnership is that the nurse researcher must treat the patient as a complete equal. As Seedhouse (1988: 132) states:

> The requirement to respect persons equally when working for health follows from the requirement to create and respect autonomy in all people, and from the work by philosophers establishing basic criteria for personhood. We regard people as valuable not only because of what each person can do, but essentially because of what each person is.

The requirement to treat people as equals is very important when considering the process of adaptation. A person in hospital has to adapt to a whole plethora of changing circumstances; treating the person as an equal demands that the nurse researcher complement the uniqueness of the patient by adapting knowledge to suit the patient's abilities and demands. If this approach is taken, it forms a foundation on which to base a plan of action which views the nurse researcher and the patient as equals in an adaptive partnership.

We have already discussed the rationale for utilizing participant observation in the process of nursing research. The next stage must be to consider certain ethical principles which must be recognized if the concept of the person is to remain central to the notion of research.

Ethics in nursing research

The concepts of autonomy and informed consent are of vital importance in nursing research. In certain respects the two terms are inextricable, but, in order to achieve clarity, the concepts will be considered separately before common strands and themes are drawn together.

Autonomy

In its purest form, the term 'autonomy' is used with reference to self-rule or self-government; Beauchamp and Childress (1982: 59) present the following interpretation:

> The most general idea of personal autonomy is still that of self-governance: being one's own person, without constraints either by another's action or by psychological or physical limitations. The autonomous person determines his or her course of action in accordance with a plan chosen by himself or herself. Such a person deliberates about and chooses plans and is capable of acting on the basis of such deliberations, just as truly independent government is capable of controlling its territories and policies.

The interpretation of autonomy suggests a number of things. It implies that persons have the ability to express a dynamic and subjective orientation; furthermore, it suggests that autonomy is expressed through active participation within decisions. It also leads us to the position that an autonomous person is able to think about ends and to decide what means shall be utilized to achieve those ends. However, if we apply this to healthcare ethics, it becomes evident that a person is unable to take any action in isolation because it is highly unlikely that any social factors are not involved and also that it will not affect somebody else. As an example, if a nurse researcher takes an action within their professional role, it is difficult to envisage this as not having some sort of effect on other people within the healthcare environment, be they colleagues, patients or visitors. This brings us back to an earlier position: it is difficult to separate and isolate social actions from the meanings and consequences they bring. Therefore, if all observable phenomena in the social realm are interrelated with factors such as judgments, interpretation and other subjective operations, then it is impossible to compartmentalize them in terms of a purely objective framework. The phenomenological researchers call this the relationship between the knower and the known (Henry, 1986).

Autonomy is vitally important in nursing research if the patient is to be viewed as an end in their own right. This ties in completely with the notion of 'respect for persons' because it emphasizes that any person who forms the subject of a research project should be enabled to express autonomy within that context. In practical terms, this means that the nurse researcher must give the person as much information as they require, not only regarding the nature of the research but also relating to the nursing care which is an inherent part of using participant observation in nursing research. The concept which is used to describe this process of information exchange is 'informed consent'.

Informed consent in nursing research

Herbert (1988: 1043) offers us a traditional interpretation of what is meant by the doctrine of informed consent:

> An informed consent is that consent which is obtained after the patient has been adequately instructed about the ratio of risk and benefit involved in the procedure as compared to alternative procedures or no treatment at all.

It has already been said that the principles of informed consent and autonomy are largely interwoven. In terms of nursing research, this refers to the researcher's obligation to maintain the patient's dignity and integrity while attempting to achieve a partnership which will allow access to how a person perceives reality in the hospital environment. The doctrine of informed consent is of vital and central importance to anybody involved in nursing research; a patient must be privy to the aims and objectives of how the programme will relate to them if the research is to be viewed as ethically valid. Faulder (1985: 32) comments on the importance of gaining a position of clarity over informed consent by stating:

> This is not obtuse pedantry. An important principle lies behind a deceptively simple formula; its words are burdened with shades of meaning which we must clarify in our own minds before we can use it.

If a person does not give a nurse researcher permission to take a certain form of action, then the researcher has no moral basis for instigating the action. It follows from this that it is vitally important that the patient understands, as far as is possible, the different permutations associated with the research. The nurse researcher, who is also practising, must ensure that the person is as fully aware as they wish to be regarding a given nursing action. If this position is not adhered to, then it is not possible to say with certainty that a person has given a full and informed consent. If a nurse researcher performs a given action without the permission of the patient, then they perform an act which violates the individual. The consequences of such a situation can be grave and may even constitute negligence in legal terms (Kennedy and Grubb 1989: 225).

It is important that a great deal of emphasis is placed on autonomy and informed consent during the research process in nursing. We discussed earlier the nature of qualitative and quantitative research and that it is the concept of the person which must form the focal point of whichever philosophical perspective is followed. However, if this is to be a formative endeavour, then it must be underpinned with an ethical rationale such as that suggested here with autonomy and informed consent. Adopting this perspective provides us with the fundamental ethos of the relationship which should exist between persons in the research process, as Dyer and Bloch (1987: 12) have argued:

> It is the principle of partnership endowed with the qualities of mutual trust and human sincerity which may help health professionals aspire to the pursuit of the ethical principles which underlie informed consent.

The concept of freedom also plays a fundamental role in discussions concerning consent. It is not possible to do justice to a topic as vast as freedom in the confines of this discussion owing to its immense complexity; but it does merit some mention.

For the nurse researcher, freedom should be used to mean the liberty with which the patient can do one thing rather than another. This is an integral element of enabling the person to express autonomy. This is another reason why the research process should be based on the interpretation of meaning; persons cannot be restricted by the clearly defined criteria of natural scientific enquiry, as Haring (1975: 135) informs us:

> The transfer of the natural scientific model to society is criminal in the eyes of critical theory. It represents the original sin of positivistic society.

CONCLUSION

This chapter has been concerned with the philosophical and ethical issues relating to persons in nursing research. If the people taking part in the research are fully informed of the ramifications associated with it and knowingly give their consent, then autonomy, individuality and dignity are being respected. Research in nursing can do much to enhance the care which people receive from practitioners; it can help deliver the nurse from being a dictator of practice to becoming a partner in practice with the patient. As Faulder (1985: 106) tells us:

> Their trust must not be abused, nor their altruism. These human and moral considerations are more important than any scientific advance, and it is these obligations which impose the limits to science.

REFERENCES

Beauchamp, T.L. and Childress, J.F. (1982) *Principles of Biomedical Ethics*, Oxford University Press, Oxford.

Duffy, M. (1985) Designing nursing research: the qualitative-quantitative debate. *Journal of Advanced Nursing*, **10**; 225–32.

Dyer, A.R. and Bloch, S. (1987) Informed consent and the psychiatric patient. *Journal of Medical Ethics,* **13**; 12–16.

Faulder, C. (1985) *Whose Body is It? The Troubling Issue of Informed Consent*, Virago Press, London.

Haring, B. (1975) *Manipulation: Ethical Boundaries of Medical, Behavioural and Genetic Manipulation,* St Paul's Publications, Slough.

Harris, J. (1985) *The Value of Life: An Introduction to Medical Ethics*, Routledge & Kegan Paul, London.

Henry, I.C. (1986) Conceptions of the nature of persons. Unpublished PhD thesis, Leeds University.

Herbert, V. (1988) Informed consent – a legal evaluation. *Cancer*, 46(4): 1043.

Howarth, C.F. (1981) The nature of psychological knowledge, in *The Structure of Psychology,* Allen & Unwin, London.

Kennedy, I. and Grubb, A. (1989) *Medical Law: Text and Materials*, Butterworth, London.

Seedhouse, D. (1988) *Ethics: The Heart of Health Care*, John Wiley, Chichester.

FURTHER READING

Alderson, P. (1995) Consent to research: the role of the nurse. *Nursing Standard*, **9**(36), 28–31.

Consumers for Ethics in Research (CERES) (1994) Spreading the word on research: notes on writing patient information leaflets. CERES, London.

Kendrick, K. (1995) An ethic of care in nursing research, in *Community Ethics and Health Care Research* (eds I.C. Henry and G. Pashley), Mark Allen Publishing, Dinton.

Competition or collaboration in the health and social services | 13

Glenys Pashley

The traditional bureaucracy underpinning the health and social services was seen to be too big, too wasteful and too powerful; therefore some of it was sold off and some of it was reformed by the government. Both these government strategies resulted in the services being subject to the rigours of the market place, a move which was supported by Porter (1990) who believes a government should intervene, stimulate change and innovation and promote domestic rivalry. He further maintains that a government has a role to play by functioning as a catalyst and challenger and by encouraging organizations to raise their aspirations and move towards higher levels of competitive performance. The current government, through legislation and major reforms, is presently challenging health and local authorities to improve their performance by: being accountable; providing value for money; achieving efficiency gains; being flexible; affording users and carers wider choice and improving quality at the lowest possible cost. The government has fuelled market forces in the sense of explicitly encouraging competition between providers of health and social services, thus increasing the rivalry between providers for resources and users. Being competitive therefore seems to be one of the unavoidable aims for the health and social services, affecting both purchasers and providers. So what was the rationale behind the introduction of competition and what do we understand the term 'competition' to mean? Further, is competition and gaining an advantage over competitors the best way forward, or is collaboration and co-operation a more appropriate strategy?

There can be no doubt that competition does have a place and can be of some value in organizational practice. According to Mullins (1993), competition can be productive in three principal ways. First, in the setting of standards; second, in stimulating and channelling energies and providing a common sense of purpose; and third, in distinguishing better from worse. For Solomon (1992) the purpose of competition is to produce and deliver the best and usually the least expensive products and services. For Smith (cited in Shaw and Barry, 1992), free competition is the regulator that keeps a community, activated only by self-interest, from degenerating into a mob of ruthless profiteers. When traditional restraints are removed, or when all have access to the market, then all are free to pursue self-interest. In this scenario we confront others who are also pursuing self-interest. Hence competition regulates and steers self-interest in a socially beneficial way. Indeed, competition could be described as a corrective and a constraint, 'not the carrot but, perhaps, more the stick that serves as a constant warning: nothing here is guaranteed or assured' (Solomon, 1992). If an organization fails to succeed in serving a purpose or fails to satisfy its customers and someone else can do the job better, then, 'the stick finds its mark and measures out its punishment' (Solomon, 1992).

Any organization can become lazy, incompetent, ineffective and inefficient because of a lack of competition but is the introduction of competition into the health and social market place the only solution? – unlikely! It could be argued that people within organizations are motivated by the excitement of their ideas, by the challenge of a service, by the promise of success but not particularly by competition. Indeed, competition may well be perceived as an obstacle to be overcome. Organizational practice adhering to a battlefield mentality and emphasis on competition can have some adverse effects, not only on the stability and culture of the organization but also in terms of the outcomes characterized by short-term thinking, an impoverished sense of innovation, a loss of standards of service delivery and poor employee morale (Shaw and Barry, 1992). Further, in a scenario where organizational practice is driven by competition, exploitation, rivalry, secrecy and ignorance, then nearly everyone can become a loser. For instance, two providers of care services may find themselves in a position of having to set their prices in competition with one another without knowing what the other is going to do. Each participant in the 'game' may be cautious and set a lower price than they might if they were confident the other would set a suitably higher price. In such a case, competition is mutually disadvantageous because of a lack of co-operation. It should be noted, however, that the customer (the purchaser) will benefit and tend to support the practice of price wars and laws against collusion and price-fixing. Competition needs to be healthy, fair, positive and encouraging of excellence, innovation, efficiency and productivity, and not merely focus on eliminating competitors or maintaining a competitive edge over rivals, say, through secrecy or dishonesty; although for Grant (1991) competitive advantage 'requires the existence of barriers to imitation'. But here the question arises: should health and social services agencies and organizations be secretive about examples of good practice?

The term competition is multidimensional and very dependent on its meaning and use in a particular context. As Paine (1990) remarks, 'There is healthy competition and there is sick, debilitating and depraved competition. There is fair competition and there is underhanded competition. There is constructive, positive even inspiring competition, and there is mutually destructive, negative, inhibiting competition'. Being competitive ought to involve a focus on developing core competencies, avoiding activities that do not add value, ensuring rapid response times to market trends, continuous quality improvement and by encouraging collaboration. As Solomon (1992) argues, organizational practice is fundamentally co-operative and it is only within the parameters of mutually shared interests, agreed rules of conduct, trust, the honouring of contracts, respect for the law and rules of fair play that competition is possible. Competition ought not to be understood as the means of success or as an end in itself. It makes sense only within a framework of mutual interest, co-operation and collaboration; and when healthy, positive competition can be distinguished from unhealthy, negative competition. In effect, an ethical or collaborative edge, as opposed to a competitive edge or advantage, may well be the way forward, particularly in the light of the recommendation that health and local authorities ought to produce joint and consultative plans which cover funding arrangements, reach agreement on common goals for particular client groups, key areas of operation and joint working and contractual relationships between purchasers and providers. Handy (1993), however, warns that in most organizations the conditions for fruitful competition will be difficult to realize because of limited resources and opportunities and the different cultures present in different organizations. A strong organizational culture provides structure, standards and a value system in which to operate. It is a social phenomenon which recognizes the centrality and importance of people and shared values and embraces the idea of ethics. Although ethics may be described as relying on personal beliefs, opinions, experience and values, the resulting decisions and actions impact on the culture and corporate image of the organization.

Competition can be based on any number of factors such as organizational image, price, productivity increases, differentiation or quality; and competitive advantage could be said to exist where one agency or organization has, say, a more positive image than a rival or provides a better quality of care and at a lower cost. It is important to point out that customer perception has an important role to play in the attribution of features like a more positive image. According to King (1992) 'Corporate images, consumer speak and user friendliness are the language of community care in the nineties. Disseminating information to the public, and to users of services and carers is a key component of new legislation'. One particular social service department in the UK is committed to raising its profile and promoting a positive image to both employees and the public. It aims to meet the needs of its customers 'first time every time'; it has produced a user's and carer's charter, a mission statement, a 'people first' logo, utilized the expertise of an advertising agency, reorganized and appointed four local service development and planning officers who have a remit to collect information regarding users' needs and whether these are being provided for. Other social services departments are following suit, showing initiative and creativity in their attempt to raise profiles, organizational image and to convince all of the range of impressive services available.

However, as King remarks, are such aggressive advertising and promotion strategies raising expectations unrealistically? The goal of advertising, more often than not, is to persuade people to buy/use the goods/services that are being touted. The idea of advertising, though, does not seem to sit well with the notion of a free market. One of the features of a free market is that everyone has full and complete information, but if this were the case then surely it could be argued that advertising is pointless. The suggestion could be made that advertising moves us closer to the ideal of full information, though there are sound reasons to doubt this. There can be a tendency for advertisers to exploit ambiguity, conceal facts, exaggerate and peddle psychological satisfaction. For example, it is questionable whether a health or social services organization could meet all of the user's needs 'first time every time'. A related concern is: how honest can health and social services organizations be about dealing with unmet need when there is a threat of legal action if promises are broken? This potential threat is resulting in some organizations, especially social services departments, not recording need if it cannot be met. There is an element of dishonesty in this practice and one seeking to reflect service delivery as it relates to available resources rather than reality. It seems odd that health authorities record the need for medical patients and acknowledge a waiting list, but that local authorities feel unable to pursue this same more open and honest practice. Empowering people implies giving them choice; and choices can only be made on the basis of information, including an honest assessment of need. It is important, therefore, for local authorities to acknowledge unmet need and, like the health authorities, perhaps introduce something akin to a waiting-list on the grounds of resource constraints. Perhaps a 'pending allocation list' could be introduced, but which takes account of statutory requirements. In other words, the legal differences between health and local authorities in relation to meeting identified need is an important distinguishing feature. Advertisers have a responsibility and obligation to provide clear and truthful information in order to avoid misleading people. At stake is people's money, health, social well-being, loyalties, expectations and informed choices. Further, one could argue that advertising and related practices use resources which may have been better spent on the services themselves.

The creation of a competitive environment and the introduction of market mechanisms is seen to offer a context where health and local authorities can achieve an efficient an effective use of resources by those individuals responsible for providing public services and negotiate favourable financial terms for the purchase of services from a range of providers who are great in number and can enter the market with ease. Common, Flynn and Mellon (1992) suggest market reforms have been designed to achieve changes in managerial behaviour and competition is expected to generate an impetus among providers for survival and/or growth which should result in a concern for price and quality. Supporters of the idea of free and competitive markets usually view them as promoting efficiency, improving responsiveness and accountability and expanding the range of opportunities and choices open to users.

The following features typify a free market:

- people who are in a position to choose the provider of the service they are opting to purchase;
- providers of a service who are free to attract customers by providing what people want with specific regard to price and quality;
- freely available information on price, quality and availability which is sufficient to ensure the market can operate;
- a large number of purchasers and providers such that both parties are able to make an informed choice;
- a context in which neither an individual purchaser nor provider can determine the price.

In a market place reflecting these criteria, the positive outcomes desired by supporters of market mechanisms may well be realized. But are such favourable circumstances applicable to the health and social services? Le Grand (1994) cites five key conditions which must be satisfied in order for a health and social care market to achieve their ends without adverse consequences:

- the market must be competitive on both sides;
- both sides need access to cheap and accurate information regarding costs and quality (providers need to cost services in order to price them appropriately, purchasers need to monitor quality to ensure providers do not reduce the costs by lowering quality);
- the costs of running a market must be low, since high administrative costs may offset efficiency gains;

- providers need a financial motivator and not simply be driven by a sense of public duty; the latter may well serve to lead such providers to be less proactive in response to market changes;
- neither the purchaser nor the provider should be allowed to discriminate against a potentially expensive user of services.

Most of these features and conditions of a free market, however, are rarely met. The user's degree of autonomy, power and freedom envisaged in a pure market philosophy is, in reality, debatable. The user is not free to purchase their own care; rather a GP or care manger has a major input to the decision-making process. Such professionals will be influenced by many factors, including cost and a consideration of whether health and social care is an individual 'good' and/or a social benefit, for example, the value of purchasing immunization programmes. Health professionals are more familiar with having to make such decisions. This is an area relatively new to social professionals, for example, deciding the value of block- or spot-purchasing arrangements; hence social care professionals may well benefit from the mistakes and elements of good practice and decision-making displayed by healthcare professionals. Le Grand (1994) emphasizes the lack of user autonomy by remarking that some GP practices have fund-holding budgets to purchase hospital treatment or care on behalf of their patients and some care managers hold budgets to purchase community care on behalf of their clients. For Le Grand, markets foster and maintain inequalities and therefore social injustice.

Common, Flynn and Mellon (1992) suggest, at its minimum level, the introduction of market reforms simply divides the organization into two parts which are labelled the purchaser and provider and, if nothing else changes, this is likely to have little impact. They offer the example of an area which has one district health authority and one district general hospital to illustrate the point. In this kind of scenario the district health authority functions as the purchaser and the hospital serves as the provider of services. If no other hospital is accessible and there are no GP fund-holders, there will be no significant impact on the managerial behaviour of the hospital management and staff because patients cannot choose where to go, the providers of services have no incentives to do better, no other provider is encouraged to enter the market and, in effect, there is no real competition.

The relationship between purchasers and providers is open to many dilemmas. First, purchasers would prefer a choice of providers, flexibility, lower prices, spot-purchasing arrangements implying a process of being able to buy a particular service for a particular client and to operate in a market where competition between providers is great because this context often places purchasers in a commanding position to demand flexibility, short-term contracts and more choice. It is important to point out that the issue of more choice for users is perhaps really one of increased choice for purchasers. On the other hand, providers of services would prefer financial stability over a period of time and block-purchasing arrangements to enable them to plan service delivery and reduce the risks involved. The commanding position held by purchasers in a competitive market is counteracted in a market where providers are scarce. In this situation, providers could wield sufficient power to control the price, nature, quantity and quality and then, maybe, the market would be working against the interests of users and taxpayers. Provider power of this kind might arise if markets became highly specialized and segmented with only a few providers in each. However, it does seem to be the case that providers of services tend to believe the way forward is through joint planning and co-operation, through collaboration and partnership.

Just from these few examples it becomes evident that the relationship between purchasers and providers raises a stream of important issues and dilemmas. Different health and local authorities are approaching the task in hand in individual ways: some are working together with providers to develop sound arrangements which are beneficial to all concerned, others in a less co-operative way. One suggestion is for health and local authorities to shape the new market by encouraging new providers and diversification; by avoiding standardized commissioning/purchasing arrangements if these inhibit the providers in responding to the diversity of need and by not rewarding price-cutting if this is a short-term measure to encounter competition. Health and local authority purchasers need to take a long-term perspective because if price is the main consideration, quality could well diminish. Conversely, if profit is the main criterion for providers, survival and the winning of contracts will probably not materialize. It follows that if only major providers survive then competition is reduced which, in turn, limits choice, encourages higher prices and without necessarily higher levels of quality. It may well be the case that competition should encourage providers to push service quality up and prices down, but will there be, indeed, should there be, sufficient competition to enable this pattern to develop?

An important question worth raising here is: are the health and social services operating in a freely competitive environment or are there restraints and interventions? As we have seen, there is certainly a problem with the notion of a freely competitive market and the relationship between purchasers and providers presents a range of complex dilemmas still to be resolved. There is also the issue of government intervention, for example, how can health and local authorities flourish in a system which claims to be market driven and encourage diversity and strategic planning when it is actually operating in an increasingly centralized bureaucracy where authorities are governed by national directives and have their resources controlled, for instance, the requirement of local authorities to provide evidence of their care plans? The present intensity of government intervention is, perhaps, too excessive and constraining to enable a true market philosophy.

Leat (1993) remarks consultation between the health and social services and the independent sector is now mandatory, but she asks how genuine are the attempts at joint planning and collaboration and how do these fit with the notion of competition? On the basis of a report by KPMG in 1992 (cited by Leat) it was concluded that there appears to be 'widespread and participative involvement' between social services departments and the voluntary sector, but little evidence of the private sector being consulted or participating in the planning process for service delivery. It seems to be the case that purchasers prefer to contract with voluntary organizations, perhaps believing their non-profit motivation will reduce potential exploitation, perhaps on the grounds of trust and a proven track record, perhaps due to an assumption that voluntary organizations are not familiar with the competitive scene and do not possess the resources and skills to compete on a 'level playing-field'. Purchasers seem to be more wary of the private sector because of the existing competition within the sector and because this sector is deemed to be less concerned with the earlier stage of planning (needs assessment). It is obviously important to question the assumption that voluntary organizations are not competitive and the private sector is. Further, how can a market be increased and freely entered if trust and a proven track record are prerequisites? This would certainly appear to inhibit the social services changing their culture from one of being a provider to one of enabling other agencies to become providers.

If the most recent approach to community care is to work, the key agencies of both the health and social services must work well together. This presents a challenge; the traditional roles, cultures, priorities and organizational styles within the two establishments are different. Further, if local authorities are to fund social and healthcare and health authorities are to fund health and social care, then active co-operation is essential. Mutually acceptable plans that hold authorities together and which identify each authority's responsibilities will have to be developed. The smaller the number of authorities working together, the more likely is a successful outcome. However, there is a danger of the primary emphasis on users and carers being shifted to a preoccupation with policy formation and joint working. Wistow and Robinson (1994) reviewed the research carried out in 1993 by a national focus group for the King's Fund Centre for Health Services Development and the Nuffield Institute of Health. They remark that demands on community health services appear to be intensifying and there is concern over the apparent and continuing deterioration in service provision, especially in areas that lie between health and social care. Further, there seems to be discrepancy between views held by managers, users and carers as to the issue of rights and responsibilities. This becomes a major problem when the disputes are between health and local authorities about who is to pay for particular services. Managers, though recognizing disagreements, are keen to point out how much improved the collaboration is between health and local authorities, how successful agreements have been in resolving problems and how the prospect of joint commissioning health and social care services will lead to shared responsibilities and end uncertainty. Of more concern to users and carers is the issue of diminishing entitlements, for example, as respite care crosses the boundary from healthcare to social care, what was once a free entitlement under the NHS is now a means test for local authority services or non-existent if neither agree. The conflicting concerns and priorities seem to suggest that managers have been more concerned with systems, finances and administration, whereas users and carers would be more appreciative of clarification as to their rights, the element of choice, flexibility and care services which match their individual needs.

The present emphasis on an enabling, rather than a providing, role for health and local authorities, coupled with encouraging words for the service users such as support, independence, dignity and involvement in the decision-making process, ought to result in service users feeling less like passive recipients and more in control of their own lives,. On the surface, then, one could assume that paternalism is a diminishing practice. However, with the continuing shortfall in resources and services now being targeted only on those in danger or in 'need', it becomes important to question whether a massive cultural change away from paternalism and control towards freedom, accountability and respect for individual rights is actually taking place. Indeed, one could question whether the implementation of the National Health Service and Community Care Act 1990 has served to remove the rights of people. The pressure on resources inevitably leads to attempts to find ways to legitimize the denial of care. Indeed, there is a danger of growing discrimination against whole groups of people and the possibility that certain groups will be at a disadvantage in the distribution of health and social care. The principle that people have equal worth is fundamental to health and social care and to decide to offer care to one person rather than another indicates that the principle of equality has been abandoned. Practitioners make many decisions in their working day which entail issues of right or wrong, fairness, justice and the allocation of harm or benefit. An important issue for the value basis of health and social care is justice. As Raphael (1981) remarks: 'Everyone is in favour of justice, but not the same interpretation of it.' A whole web of policies and procedures exist which reveal disregard for the principle of justice and autonomy and make it virtually impossible for certain groups within society to be able to access services. The principle of autonomy involves liberty, freedom of choice, respect for persons and the decisions persons make about themselves. Problems such as disability, illness or disease may well lessen a person's potential to be autonomous. It becomes important, therefore, to create autonomy for those who are unable to live autonomously, for whatever reason, through the use of advocates.

Advocacy is concerned with ensuring that a person is treated with dignity and that their needs and rights are met. It requires that practitioners act on behalf of their users, either by providing them with information which will enable them to make an informed decision or by pleading for their cause as they would have done themselves if able. To override a person's autonomy can only be considered morally legitimate when it is intended to promote, provide or protect the rights of that person (Seedhouse, 1986). However, one has to question the extent to which this ethical principle is being adhered to. For example, do professionals exercise power and/or paternalism in their relationships with clients and are managers more concerned with resource issues than with the empowerment of clients and perhaps professionals? For James (1994) the health and social services are created on behalf of vulnerable people. However, she acknowledges reality and comments: 'The primary task of public services is to represent, to advocate and to empower that group of people within a set of competing political, economic and social choices ... Public authorities are forced to make choices between the heard and unheard, the seen and unseen.' Similarly, Wilson (1994) is realistic about what may be happening within the health and social services. She remarks:

> Empowerment, whereby individuals and groups are enabled to take more control over their lives, is an alien concept; thus the new managerialism encourages the preservation of existing power relationships between officers and users. Where there are value judgments to be made, the public may be consulted but managers will ultimately make the decision.

Indeed, one could argue that to ensure the effectiveness of applying market principles and the idea of competition to health and social services, it becomes necessary to crush the power of the professionals in order to facilitate managerial control. The 'new right' politics are based on values such as personal freedom, individualism, inequality, features of social authoritarianism, control and the idea of a free and competitive market economy. The introduction of these values into the public sector rests on the underlying assumption that the efficiency of service provision will be improved by encouraging an enterprise culture without bureaucracy and with managers rather than professionals to control resources, pursue governmental goals and objectives and manage rather than administrate change.

With massive organizational changes in the health and social services, people need to understand how to play the new ground rules of collaboration. If an organization, through decisions made by its managers and professionals, do not reflect the values shared by other organizations and its people, then fruitful competition via co-operation and collaboration is highly unlikely and organizational conflict may well arise. Imagine the difficulties of establishing common goals and principles when several organizations may have incompatible missions and cultures. For Grant (1991) a sharp dichotomy exists between organizations intensely competing for customers and resources and organizations seeking to enhance their competitive position through collaboration and co-operation with one another. To achieve maximum benefit from collaboration, organizations need to adopt more effective management strategies for these arrangements. The key, according to Hamel, Doz and Prahalad (1989), is to recognize that: 'collaboration is competition in a different form'. Inter-organizational relationships during the 1990s, which will break up large bureaucratic and vertically structured organizations, enable flexibility, innovation and opportunity and encourage a wider repertoire of capabilities to probably flourish. According to Grant, some of the emerging trends for organizational structure and management are:

- the breakdown of structural rigidity;
- less distinct organizational boundaries;
- new models of management;
- the resolution of organizational problems of accountability and legitimacy; and
- co-operation within the organization.

Underpinning these trends is an important focus on teamwork. The importance of teamwork to the effectiveness of health and social work practice is imperative. Its absence would be bewildering to staff and service users alike. However, where competition is promoted as increasing user choice and quality, it must be remembered that competition at the expense of co-operation and collaboration between teams will probably lead to reduced quality and a breakdown of services rather than a better service.

Without doubt competition, innovation and change are commendable strategies to pursue, but their success might be questionable if the complementary resources are not forthcoming. Williams (1992) implies it is difficult to do something new without the means to fund the changes. More often than not developing and implementing change means giving up something old. For example, a recent debate concerns whether social-work values can be distinguished from and replaced by care-management values. Investment and change are difficult to operationalize if not paid for. Investment from the government in the guise of additional resources would be the obvious preference, but it is highly unlikely. Given the restraints, there is a danger that quality as well as costs will be driven down, especially since there are significant intangible aspects of quality that cannot be expressed in conventional cost-benefit terms. For example, if profit or low costs are a driving force and measure of success, then values which cannot be quantified in monetary terms such as compassion, empathy, respect and anti-discriminatory practice may well be discarded. The question must be asked: would the health and social services be deemed to be successful if they lacked these values? An important distinction here lies with the idea that the value base and power of health professionals has long been established and explicitly influenced health-service policy. Conversely, it could be argued, although social professionals clearly have a value base, their power to influence the social services is less formidable, hence a context of policy informing practice has been the dominant relationship. Perhaps the 'stick', implicit within the idea of a free and competitive market, serves to ensure policy informs practice. Hopefully, however, collaborative and co-operative, rather than competitive strategies, will be a convincing reminder of the 'carrot' and its role in enabling a compromise between an ethical value base and a concern for the new managerialism and that, equally, practice should inform policy.

REFERENCES

Common, R., Flynn, N. and Mellon, E. (1992) *Managing Public Services*, Butterworth-Heinemann, Oxford.

Grant, R.M. (1991) *Contemporary Strategy Analysis*, Blackwell, Oxford.

Handy, C. (1993) *Understanding Organisations*, Penguin Books, Harmondsworth.

Hamel, G., Doz, Y. and Prahalad, C.K. (1989) Collaborate with your competitors and win. *Harvard Business Review*, Jan./Feb., 133–9.

James, A. (1994) *Managing to Care*, Longman, Harlow.

Leat, D. (1993) *The Development of Community Care by the Independent Sector*, Policy Studies Institute, London.

Le Grand, J. (1994) Into the quasi market. *Community Care*, 27 Jan.

Mullins, L.J. (1993) *Management and Organisational Behaviour*, Pitman Publishing, London.

Porter, M.E. (1990) *The Competitive Advantage of Nations*, Harvard Business Review, March/April.

Raphael, D.D. (1981) *Moral Philosophy*, Oxford University Press, Oxford.

Seedhouse, D. (1986) *Health – the Foundation for Achievement*, Wiley, Chichester.

Shaw, W.H. and Barry, V. (1992) *Moral Issues in Business*, Wadsworth, California.

Solomon, R.C. (1992) *Ethics and Excellence*, Oxford University Press, Oxford.

Williams, G. (1992) What price market forces in the quality stakes? *Times Higher Education Supplement*, July.

Wilson, E.M. (1994) *Managerialism, management competencies and values*. Paper: British Association of Social Workers, Annual General Meeting, April.

Wistow, G. and Robinson, J. (1994) Trial and Error. *Community Care*, 27 Jan.

FURTHER READING

King, J. (1992) Raising profiles. *Community Care*, 3 Dec.

Paine, L.S. (1990) Ideals of competition and today's marketplace, in *Enriching Business Ethics* (ed. C. Walton), Plenum, New York.

<table>
<tr><td>14</td><td># Principles and values: an ethical perspective in healthcare organizations</td></tr>
</table>

14	# Principles and values: an ethical perspective in healthcare organizations

Christine Henry

THE ETHICS AND VALUES AUDIT

The aim of the audit was to ask the question: 'Do we practise what we preach?' In the foreword of the audit report it is claimed that while every organization should ask itself this question, both a healthcare organization and a higher education institution has a responsibility to do so encapsulated within the very nature and purpose of the two organizations. While the first Ethics and Values Audit (EVA) was carried out in a university it can be readily applied to a healthcare organization. Apps (1993) remarks that the EVA report is extremely useful and she draws parallels with the health service, particularly in 'relationships to mission statements and ward philosophies' (p. 47). It is commonly assumed that healthcare and higher education institutions have a caring ethic simply as a result of their inherent values of care. However, it is suggested by some that in times of dramatic change, competition may become the only value, especially if individual healthcare communities are clearly restructured to reach targets and compete with each other. There is a perception of double standards where the values that are preached are not the values that are practised. In times of change it is even more important that organizations specifically assumed 'caring' institutions ought to enhance further their professional standing by presenting a higher ethical profile. Furthermore, because of the implicit values and guiding moral principles, institutions have a duty to identify ways in which quality can be enhanced through good practice. This means caring for patients and staff.

The objectives of the EVA project were:

- to produce a profile of shared values;
- to explore and evaluate policy;
- to assess the teaching of ethics across the curriculum (in healthcare organizations the objective would be an assessment of professional practice) and to develop recommendations which would enhance organizational policy.

The EVA was a research-based audit and therefore used several methods for collecting data. These included a questionnaire, an open-ended interview, a values grid, and an 'ethics hot line', which resulted in case studies and a selective policy analysis. The findings supported staff concerns and resulted in specific recommendations. The emphasis was placed on values in all dimensions of the organization.

On the one hand there are many values that are shared; on the other hand, there are practices that do not live up to the values identified. The findings resulted in identifying the following themes:

- an informal, supportive staff network;
- peer-group integrity;
- poor information flow;
- non-participation in important decision-making processes;
- the abuse of power and role when management practices and styles are inappropriate;
- a potentially disruptive and charged working environment affecting the climate of the organization;
- the provision of staff resources;
- inappropriate provision for research and advanced study (Henry *et al.*, 1992: 6–7).

The recommendations were a set of draft resolutions intended for wide debate across the institution and addressed ways in which to improve the staff and client experience, the organizational culture and support the achievement of organizational goals. These were:

- the leadership of the organization: its management style;
- its organizational culture;
- the mission statement;
- the need for a code of professional practice;
- the establishment of a director of human resources and communications;
- a staff handbook;
- further improvements in the working environment;
- the development of a cross-university learning community;

- an ethics and values audit for students/clients;
- an audit of values in the curriculum; and
- the appointment of an ethics and values adviser/facilitator.

(*Henry et al., 1992: 32–7*)

With some modifications, most of the recommendations have been implemented. A discussion of moral principles and values may help to clarify not only the usefulness of an ethics and values audit, but support the processes of policy implementation and professional practice.

VALUES AND PRINCIPLES

Values

According to Henry *et al.*, (1992) values are much more subjective than principles and need not necessarily be moral. There is little doubt that Hitler had some very clear values that he shared with others. Values are central to a society's culture, individual experience and attitudes; they influence the way we behave. Some organizational values may conflict with professional or personal values. **Moral values** have a personal interpretation and support moral principles. There are values that may be termed instrumental, such as self-affirmation and competence; while these values have a psychological element and may not be viewed as strictly moral, they are still within the boundaries of an ethical frame-work. People will devote their time and energy working for an organization if there is a belief that they are valued members of that organization. However, if self-esteem and self-affirmation is harmed through poor communication as in the instance of bad management and low morale, levels of competence are affected. Enhancement of such **instrumental values** are essential for the fulfilment of an organization's mission.

Professional life, guided by shared values, will empower and affirm members of the organization's community. The values that are shared in both professional and organizational terms must support moral principles. It is perceived that healthcare practice, generally, ought to promote the values that are held by the organization itself. Nevertheless, there is tension between what the organizations appear to promote and the way in which patients and staff are treated, particularly in times of change.

Ethics, as a discipline, is part of theoretical enquiry within the philosophical field but it is also part of everyday commonsense in our interactions, exemplified in the ways in which we behave towards each other and the choices we have to make. Ethics, as a form of theoretical enquiry, studies the ways in which we behave and may give justification for the actions we take. Ethical theory may help to solve dilemmas and may be viewed as more than just a set of principles. While principles are necessary for ethical theory, they also act as a guide to human conduct and, therefore, underpin practice.

Principles

Central to the idea of a caring community is an understanding of important moral principles. It is necessary for moral principles to underpin a mission statement, a charter, a professional code of ethics or a general organizational code. A code, while not solving a moral dilemma, will provide guidance for human conduct. Codes will not change the way people behave but a code will raise levels of awareness and can act as a guide for the ways in which we behave towards each other. However, in order to enhance the function of a generalized or specific code or a broad charter like the Patients Charter, it is essential to educate the healthcare professionals and the managers in practical ethics, particularly those relating to the organizational culture, its processes, policies and organizational goals. Not only would an in-house staff-development programme in ethics raise levels of awareness and understanding but it would ensure the development and function of realistic codes and charters so that its implementation might improve professional practice. Henry's (1986) study shows that we are not only influenced at an early age by the experiences we have but our occupational training and education will influence the sort of ethical and philosophical conceptions we adopt.

The first major moral principle that underpins practice within a caring community is the principle of respect for persons. Keyserlingk, 1993: 390 says:

> Most Western, principle-based ethical systems have long tended to consider respect for persons a central and indispensable normative principle in moral reasoning.

Henry and Pashley (1990) support the view that the term 'person' is a moral term in the sense that it may be viewed as a value term like 'good'. If this is the case, then it follows that respect for persons is an important moral principle. The use of the term person as a moral term implies that the individual valued as a person has rights, is free and responsible, is self-determined and interactive. Persons are also capable of making choices and as the result of having a level of autonomy are capable of being moral agents. Respect and value involve other regarding principles. If respect for persons, regardless of their being male or female, black or white, young or old or handicapped, is not both the focus and guiding principle to the mission, charter or code and to healthcare communities generally, then it follows that the individual will be disadvantaged. When individuals are not treated as persons or valued as persons, unethical practices occur. It is worth remembering what may happen when a group of people have their rights, identity, freedom, choices and responsibilities taken from them. During the Second World War, groups of individuals were not valued as persons. By taking away social identity and all the commensurate rights, persons were treated as objects. This allowed for inhumane practices where individuals were perceived as dispensable items or units for disposal. Furthermore, closely allied to the value of 'respect for others' is the principle of 'care'. The principle or 'ethic of care' (Gilligan, 1977) is not only a major central concern for healthcare professionals and the organization but also involves aspects of empathy, compassion and emotional sensitivity. An ethic or principle of care emphasizes action through practice and 'caring action' is bound by the ties and relationships between professionals and clients/patients. It also involves the ties and relationships between employers or managers and employees. The principle of care will give credibility to the ideal abstract conception of 'respect for persons and encourages practising what is preached'. Gilligan's view of a mature morality involves interaction between understanding ideal, generalized principles like the Kantian principle of respect for persons and those of personal relationships and care (Blum, 1993).

Respect for persons relates closely to other moral principles considered important for a caring community. The **principle of autonomy**, while an ideal principle, means having the freedom to choose, to be able to carry out plans and policies, make decisions and be held accountable for actions and behaviour. The principle of autonomy is a distinctive mark of the person. However, in reality, one can never have absolute freedom and in some cases autonomy may be impaired by physical, social or psychological factors. Furthermore, while respect for persons, responsibility and trust are essential for autonomy, the individual in the real world cannot always and absolutely act in their self-interest. The principle of autonomy is an ideal conception and may cause tension between other principles. Once again the value must rest with respect for a person's autonomy. Respecting a person's autonomy involves other regarding values and relates to the principle of care.

The moral **principle of non-maleficence** simply means to take due care not to harm others and is not as forceful as the **principle of beneficence**. This principle means to positively help someone whenever necessary. However, beneficence may conflict with the principle of autonomy. For example, if one acts in the best interest of a patient in order to avoid harm, the action may interfere to some extent with the patient's own wishes, values or beliefs. Respect for the patient's autonomy is crucial when decisions are made by professionals in 'the patient's best interest' even though it may go against the patient's wishes or beliefs. The danger arises when only one specific group decides what is in 'the patient's best interest'. The subjective views of one professional group often based on professional judgment may be classed as paternalism. When dilemmas of this sort arise, the professionals (often the doctors) will seek legal support in the civil courts. However, in order to make the most informed decision in solving a moral dilemma, one principle may have more weight given to it than others. Beneficence clearly means to positively help and obviously relates closely to the principle of 'care', not only for healthcare organizations but also for action taken in order to prevent harm. This perhaps highlights the conflict that emerges between two principles. The principles of respect for persons, autonomy and beneficence are generalized principles and it is perhaps through the application of the principle of care that these generalized principles may be put into practice. The principle of care, taken as a moral principle of action, concerns the practical.

The moral principle of justice is closely linked to respect for persons. Furthermore, the principle is central to legal, moral and political issues. The principle of justice governs interactions with individuals and groups and concerns concepts of fairness and equity. It involves informed decisions concerning the welfare of clients/patients/staff, aspects of equal opportunities and the fair allocation of resources. Justice is supported through legislation and the judicial system. However, justice also relates to the moral principle of care because within the organization it ought to involve policies that support the welfare of both patients and staff. Action that encourages the well-being of staff may involve not just paying lip-service to a policy of equal opportunities but finding ways through action to ensure fair treatment and the just distribution of resources.

VIRTUES

May (1994) and others have claimed that if there are more evaluations (like the EVA) and monitoring of organizations, less emphasis will be placed on virtues. However, virtues for the health professional remain important and are a central concern for behaving in a professional way. Principles involve rules and guidelines and are concerned with producing good acts; values are more subjective and diverse and will either support or negate principles; while virtues are a part of the domain of professional ethics because they are concerned with being good. May remarks that those who wield power within the professional field ought to be virtuous simply because of the position they are in. According to May, being virtuous means being good when no one else is watching. Beauchamp and

Childress (1979) remark that virtues are settled habits and dispositions to do what we ought to do. Virtues are acquired human characteristics such as honesty and being virtuous means having personal or professional integrity. MacIntyre (1981) states that virtue should be valued because the virtuous person will achieve what is central for 'good' practice, for example, trust between health professional and patient or client.

While in any community of professionals, the occupational and organizational structures ought to be monitored, virtues must also be viewed as important to the moral climate of the organization. Self-discipline and professional integrity are virtuous and necessary for self-evaluation and the regulation of professional practice.

EQUAL OPPORTUNITIES VIEWED AS AN ETHICAL POLICY

Equal opportunities ought to be taken as an ethical policy and a working principle. It may also be noted that virtues such as honesty and openness are essential for successful implementation. To be treated equally means to be treated as an equal but is not necessarily the same. For example, it is not seen as unfair in giving preferential treatment to someone who has a disability. Everyone should be treated the same unless there is a morally relevant difference between them. Equal opportunities is clearly a moral issue and concerns values. The equal opportunities policy has the advantage of being recognized and supported by law. Legislation exists to prevent discrimination and to allow for positive action to correct previous injustices. Healthcare organizations, in particular, ought to have developed a framework for recognizing the importance and seriousness of equal opportunities for both patients and staff. The most plausible argument for preferential treatment for past wrongful injuries relies on the actual principle of equal opportunities (Boxill, 1991). Healthcare organizations within an NHS structure rest on every member of society having the right to healthcare treatment. Underpinning the NHS system are the principles of social justice, welfare and the principle of care. Nevertheless, in times of changes in the NHS structure where healthcare organizations are encouraged to compete with each other, the principles and values of welfare and care may be overridden by values inherent in competitive market forces. In times of scarcity of resources, access to hospital treatment and shorter operation waiting-lists may be perceived as a 'double-edged sword'. Account may not be taken of poor environmental factors, scarcity of staffing and other resources possibly resulting in lower standards of care.

Equal opportunities are seen as a means to achieving the end but are not an end in itself. However, the principle of respect for persons is central here and underpins any policy of equal opportunities in that persons are valued as ends in themselves. A member of staff or a patient may experience a sense of helplessness or loss of personal autonomy through unfair treatment if the policy of equal opportunities is not coherent or adequate. For example, if abuse of power and role occurs through the unequal relationship that exists between a patient and a healthcare professional, or between manager and professional, then positive action ought to be taken to correct previous injustices. A member of staff, for example, may experience a lack of value or respect and this may affect levels of performance (instrumental values). While some institutions have a separate harassment policy, from the present author's perspective a harassment policy comes under the umbrella of equal opportunities. Harassment is seen as a feature of discrimination which requires a sensitive approach if progress is to be made. Nevertheless, it is valued as a policy because it involves the principles of fairness and justice (Henry *et al.*, 1992).

Equal opportunities and sensitive implementation may improve the quality of the staff or clients'/patients' experience. In times of dynamic changes where the level of uncertainty increases, policies such as equal opportunities need revision and continual evaluation. Furthermore, the pursuit of fair and just treatment is necessary in relation to practising care.

REFERENCES

Apps, J. (1993) Nursing education and practice. *Journal of Advances in Health and Nursing Care*, vol. 2, No. 3, 47–54.

Beauchamp, T. and Childress, J.F. (1979) *Principles of Biomedical Ethics*, Oxford University Press, Oxford.

Boxill, B. (1991) Equality, discrimination and preferential treatment, in *A Companion to Ethics* (ed. P. Singer) Blackwell Publishers, Oxford, pp. 333–43.

Blum, L.A. (1993) Gilligan and Kohlberg: implications for moral theory, in *An Ethics of Care* (ed. M.J. Larrabee) Routledge, London, pp. 49–68.

Gilligan, C. (1977) Concepts of the self and of morality. *Harvard Educational Review*, **47**, 481–517.

Henry, C. (1986) Conceptions of the nature of persons. Unpublished PhD thesis, Leeds University.

Henry, C., Drew, J., Anwar, N., Campbell, G. and Benoit-Asselman, D. (1992) *The EVA Project: Ethics and Values Audit*, University of Central Lancashire, Preston.

Keyserlingk, E.W. (1993) Ethics codes and guidelines for health care and research: can respect for autonomy be a multi-cultural principle? in *Applied Ethics: A Reader* (ed. E.R. Winkler and J.R. Coombs) Blackwell Publishers, Oxford, pp. 309–415.

May, W. (1994) The virtues in a professional setting, in *Medicine and Moral Reasoning* (eds K.W.M. Fulford, G. Gillett and J.M. Soskice) Cambridge University Press, Cambridge, pp. 75–90.

MacIntyre, A. (1981) *After Virtue: a Study in Moral Theory*, Duckworth, London.

FURTHER READING

Henry, C. and Pashley, G. (1990) *Health Ethics*, Quay Publishers, Lancaster.

Nursing, advertising and sponsorship: some ethical issues

15

Ruth Chadwick

INTRODUCTION

Clause 16 of the third edition of the UKCC *Code of Professional Conduct for the Nurse, Midwife and Health Visitor* states that every registered nurse, midwife and health visitor must 'ensure that your registration status is not used in the promotion of commercial products or services, declare any financial or other interests in relevant organizations providing such goods or services and ensure that your professional judgment is not influenced by any commercial considerations' (UKCC, 1992). In 1985 the UKCC issued an elaboration of the advertising clause (then clause 14) of the second edition of the Code of Professional Conduct (UKCC, 1984). The trend in healthcare provision towards a market-based system has produced some problems for nurses in this area and in 1990 the UKCC circulated a further document on advertising and commercial sponsorship in response to the 'variety of innovative schemes and proposals ... being devised and considered to generate income to supplement resources allocated to health authorities and boards from Government sources' (UKCC, 1990: 1).

The purpose of this chapter is to look at the ethical issues involved in advertising by nurses, with special reference to the matters covered by UKCC statements: the wearing of logos on uniforms, advertising in the healthcare environment and commercial sponsorship. In the context of a society which has embraced publicity and in which the General Medical Council has relaxed its rules on advertising, what are the ethical arguments for the position taken by the UKCC, and how, if at all, can it be defended against objections? Is there something about healthcare in general, or about nursing in particular, which is incompatible with advertising?

First, it is necessary to be clear about what advertising is.

ADVERTISING

According to the Oxford English Dictionary, an advertisement is a public notice or announcement; a statement calling attention to anything (OED, 1971). As Don Evans (1990) notes, however, ethical questions arise when such an announcement becomes promotional. We may understand a promotional advertisement to be one that attempts to further the success of a particular organization or product by, for example, boosting sales.

Advertising – is it an ethical issue?

It has been suggested (Carroll and Humphrey, 1979) that the question of whether advertising is appropriate for nurses is a matter of etiquette rather than of ethics. In the context of nursing ethics, 'etiquette' can be interpreted in the following way: 'the unwritten code of honour by which members of certain professions (esp. the medical and legal) are prohibited from doing certain things deemed likely to ... lower the dignity of the profession' (OED, 1971).

Those who see advertising as an ethical issue for nurses, however, look beyond the notion that advertising might be considered undignified and stress its capacity for 'undue influence' on patients who are vulnerable (Miles *et al.*, 1989). The claim is that the interests of patients may be adversely affected by the promotion of the interests of particular advertisers. If this is so, we have an ethical issue. Ethics is, after all, concerned with finding principles to resolve conflicts of interests.

Truth-telling and misleading advertisements

There is a view that there is nothing wrong with advertising as such, even when it is promotional; that moral problems arise only in relation to misleading advertisements – ones that make false claims for products or organizations.

Certainly, if the advertisement is making false claims, this introduces the question of harm to those misled: the harm not only of being deceived but also of being injured by useless or even dangerous products. In the health-care setting this is particularly worrying, as the controversy over misleading advertising by pharmaceutical companies illustrates (see Melrose, 1982).

But what is misleading is a matter of degree. John Berger, who was instrumental in defining the terms in which recent debates on advertising have been conducted, argued that it is in the nature of advertising to mislead and suggested that: 'Publicity speaks in the future tense and yet the achievement of this future is endlessly deferred' (Berger, 1972: 146). In other words, advertising perpetuates itself by promising more than it can deliver. Nevertheless, even if we accept that it is in the nature of advertising to mislead, there will be differences of degree according to the amount of harm that may be brought about by a particular deception. Thus we might consider an advertisement which promotes in the Third World a drug which has been banned elsewhere, worse than an advertisement in the West for health-giving properties of some harmless but ineffective food supplement. And again, in some advertisements which draw attention to services offered, it may be difficult to find any false claims: in so far as the advertisement misleads it is because it participates in the system.

The extent to which an advertisement is misleading, however, is not the only factor to be taken into consideration. First, there is the question of the relevance of the beliefs of the person involved in advertising. This will be taken up in the discussion of the wearing of logos on nurses' uniforms.

Second, we have to address the issue of whether the appropriateness of advertising is context-dependent. In particular, is the healthcare environment one from which advertising should be excluded and if so why? This takes us to one of the three aspects of advertising considered in the UKCC circular.

The healthcare environment will be taken to include not only the physical spaces in which healthcare is provided (e.g. hospitals and GPs' surgeries), but also advertising which relates to the provision of health services generally (e.g. advertisements which might attract potential clients to those physical spaces). The issues will be approached by looking at justifications of advertising and the extent to which they apply in the healthcare context. As indicated above, we have as our focus of concern specific types of advertising that might involve nurses. It is in relation to these that we primarily need to think about moral arguments in general and possible lines of argument that might be used to support permitting its use in the healthcare setting.

ADVERTISING AND THE HEALTHCARE ENVIRONMENT

Berger (1972: 130–1) sets out the standard justification of what he calls 'publicity':

> Publicity is usually explained and justified as a competitive medium which ultimately benefits the public (the consumer) and the most efficient manufacturers – and thus the national economy. It is closely related to certain ideas about freedom: freedom of choice for the purchaser; freedom of enterprise for the manufacturer. The great hoardings and the publicity neons of the cities of capitalism are the immediate visible signs of 'the Free World'.

There are in fact two arguments here. The first is that advertising produces good results by promoting the interests of all, especially the consumer; the second is that advertising should be permitted in the name of freedom.

The interests of consumers

Let us look closely at the argument that advertising promotes the interests of consumers. The benefit is said to lie in the information they receive about competing products which enhances their power of choice. The objection to this view is that advertising is essentially not about providing information which enables consumers to choose. Berger's point remains valid that, while choices may be offered between one type of car and another, 'publicity as a system only makes a single proposal. It proposes to each of us that we transform ourselves, by buying something more' (Berger, 1972: 131). Advertising, then, is not about providing information which enables us to choose: it is about making us buy more.

It might be argued that this does not apply to all types of advertising. Don Evans (1990: 23), in discussing advertising by doctors, seems to be supporting a version of the consumer interest argument when he refers to the 'general gain in public awareness of doctors' services produced by advertising' and says that 'the relaxation of restrictions on advertising ... constitutes an important advance on what can be regarded as the provision of good health care'.

Evans seems to be assuming that the Berger point does not apply in the healthcare setting: that, where what is under consideration is advertising by doctors, it is simply a question of the public being informed about what services are offered by different practices and practitioners so that potential patients can choose which to consult. There is no suggestion that the purpose of advertising might be to boost consumption of the services offered. The picture given is of people who have particular needs but who realize that not every professional will be equally competent to meet those needs. Advertising will help them to find out who is competent.

It might be argued that in the context of healthcare these are reasonable assumptions to make. Surely, apart from one or two people who are obsessive about their health (with or without advertising), people consult medical practitioners when they are ill and so need to know where they can obtain the best care.

First, however, it seems fairly clear that the most effective advertisers are not necessarily the best providers of care. Second, the prevailing political ideology not only advocates greater consumer choice in healthcare but also the other side of the coin, which is personal responsibility for health. In such a setting, advertising by doctors may indeed lead people to perceive themselves as having a larger set of healthcare needs than they would otherwise have done. As Berger pointed out, 'all publicity works upon anxiety' (Berger, 1972: 143). An 'unworried well' person might be transformed into a 'worried well' person by the advertising of preventive medicine and screening services, for example.

It is not the purpose of this chapter to downgrade the importance of preventive medicine and screening. The value and effectiveness of such programmes must be assessed on a case-by-case basis. What *is* being argued is that it is not possible to support advertising, in the healthcare setting or in any other simply by claiming that it is in the general interest because it increases the information available to consumers and leads to an improved service by stimulating competition. The social and political context also has to be borne in mind. We have to ask, for example, whether there are incentives for practitioners to target certain groups in the population and, if so, what kind of incentives these are and which groups.

The interests of advertisers and the interests of all

Advertisers, however, have interests as well as consumers and it has to be admitted that advertising makes them a great deal of money which, they argue, ultimately benefits the economy and thus the interests of all. It is so profitable to large companies to advertise that they are willing to pay handsomely for space in which to do it, those with space available to sell.

An argument about the interests of advertisers is unlikely, however, to carry weight with the nursing profession. As the Code of Professional Conduct indicates, it is the duty of every nurse to act to safeguard and promote the well-being and interests of patients/clients (UKCC, 1992). The argument therefore needs to be extended beyond the interests of advertisers to the interests of all. In the healthcare context, it is fairly clear how this would go. More money is needed for healthcare provision; the healthcare environment has space that could be used for advertising; advertisers will pay healthcare providers money for the use of their space; everyone will benefit, including the patients who can be provided with improved facilities out of the income so generated.

This is a difficult argument to counter. If it really can be shown that it is to the ultimate benefit of patients to allow advertising in the healthcare environment, how can it be argued against? In order to answer this we need to look first at Berger's freedom argument and the related issues of autonomy and paternalism.

Freedom

In the context of debates about advertising, the role of the appeal to freedom is linked primarily, as indicated above, to freedom of choice and freedom to market. But Berger's point that publicity is related to 'certain ideas' about freedom draws our attention to the fact that there are other ideas which are being denied in this form of argument. Freedom is an 'essentially contested' concept (see Gallie, 1955–6): there are opposing, irreconcilable political philosophies in which 'freedom' takes on different meanings. The freedom to compete, which capitalism promotes, is opposed to the notion of freedom from poverty and want: conditions which are arguably, to a certain extent, effects of the implementation of the first notion of freedom.

From its beginning, the National Health Service incorporated into its aims the second notion of freedom: that of freedom from, not poverty and want, but avoidable ill-health and disease. Over the past few years there has been an attempt to replace this 'freedom from' concept by the 'freedom to' concept, linked with the (at least partial) replacement of the idea that the State has a responsibility for health by the view that individuals should take personal responsibility for their own health. As the meaning of freedom is contested, the issue remains unresolved.

Autonomy and paternalism

There has been a related long-standing conflict between two models of healthcare: the autonomy model and the beneficence model. The autonomy model, resting on the principle of autonomy, suggests that because adults of sound mind have a capacity to think, decide and act on the basis of such thought and decision (Gillon, 1985), we should respect the decisions they make and so facilitate, for example, informed consent. The beneficence model, on the other hand, adopts the view that people who are ill may not be in the best position to make decisions about their own welfare; illness diminishes the capacity for autonomy and it is thus up to healthcare professionals (primarily doctors) to make decisions about what is in the best interests of their patients.

In the context of this debate, to try to prohibit advertising in the healthcare setting on the grounds that patients are vulnerable may seem to be a paternalistic siding with the beneficence model. Don Evans (1990: 24) argues against too strict a control on advertising by doctors on these grounds: 'Too tight a control by the GMC will harm the interests of the consumer and will represent an unwelcome paternalism. We do not want to see every doctor's advertisement qualified by the GMC warning "Danger: this advertisement may damage your health".'

There does seem to be a potential problem here for anyone who wants to oppose paternalism in healthcare and yet prohibit advertising on the grounds that patients are in a vulnerable condition. If we think that, despite their vulnerability, they are perfectly capable of making autonomous decisions about their treatment, why are they not, despite their vulnerability, equally capable of responding to advertising in an autonomous way?

There are three points to be made here. The first two relate to the situation of those in the physical spaces of the healthcare environment, the third to advertising in healthcare generally.

Berger (1972: 130) has something to say about the relationship between the advertisement and the recipient:

> Usually it is we who pass the image – walking, travelling, turning a page; on the TV screen it is somewhat different but even then we are theoretically the active agent – we can look away, turn down the sound, make some coffee. Yet despite this, one has the impression that publicity images are continually passing us ... We are static; they are dynamic.

It is fairly clear that in the healthcare setting, people waiting for appointments will be 'static' in the literal sense. Thus in a letter to *The Times*, Malcolm Miles and others wrote (1989: 13):

> Most people enter a hospital in fear of a disease they or a relative may have. When they wait for an appointment they are stressed – a fact which the cunning psychology of advertising could exploit. Amidst the notices displayed, an advertisement may take on an authority, as if from the caring professions, to which it has no claim; yet its vulnerable recipients may make no such distinction.

The second point was made by the UKCC in its 1990 circular: that the physical surroundings can in themselves contribute to, or detract from, the therapeutic process. So it is suggested that the physical environment 'should be conducive to healing, recovery, care and calm' (UKCC, 1990: 2). The description given by Berger, of being continually passed by a plethora of advertising images, hardly meets this requirement.

The third and final point under this heading is the most important. It disputes the validity of the analogy between advertising and the 'informing' part of informed consent and so holds that the prohibition of advertising is not unjustifiably paternalistic.

The importance of patient autonomy has been increasingly emphasized, at least since the mid-20th century, to the extent that the autonomy model has arguably become the dominant model of healthcare, especially in the USA, but also in the United Kingdom. It implies that healthcare professionals should avoid using their authority to influence patients unduly, but should try to facilitate the expression of informed choices by them.

Advertising, on the other hand, as we have seen, is not primarily about facilitating informed choice. If it is the case that it feeds on anxiety in order to produce a particular result, it is not autonomy enhancing. So it is quite consistent for one who supports the autonomy model of health-care to oppose advertising to those who are ill.

Without being unduly paternalistic, then, these arguments suggest that a concern for patients' interests will lead to the opposing of advertising in the healthcare environment. It is still arguable, however, that patients have other interests, in improved facilities, which could outweigh these consid-erations. This will be considered further in the context of examining the arguments for and against logos on nurses' uniforms.

LOGOS ON UNIFORMS

Logos have become a pervasive feature of our culture. We buy clothing and carry bags with brand names prominently displayed. The fact that it is not only acceptable but desirable to adorn our own persons with advertising designed for the promotional benefit of others is particularly significant: it shows how deep the uncritical acceptance of publicity is. Given this back-ground, why should it be thought impermissible for this feature of our society to spread into healthcare, particularly if it is done in a discreet way?

The position of the UKCC (1990: 1) on logos in its statement was as follows:

> The use of professional uniforms, or the use of the clothing worn by professional staff who do not wear uniform, to carry advertising through the use of emblems or other embellishments used for commercial promotion is not acceptable as this implies the endorse-ment of the product or service so advertised by the individual practitioner.

Since the wearing of logos implies endorsement, then, it constitutes a violation of Clause 16, which prohibits the use of registration status to promote commercial products or services.

Means and ends

But why should this be so? What if nurses really do think that the products of a certain company are worthy of promotion, as being the best? This recalls the truth-telling argument outlined above, where the relevance of the agent's beliefs was mentioned.

There are two possible scenarios to consider. The first is where an indi-vidual nurse wishes to endorse a particular product or company and uses their professional qualifications to give it backing. The problem with this is that if they use professional qualifications to do so it can be seen as endorsement not by an individual, but by the profession, and in this sense it is a misleading advertisement.

The second type of case concerns a group of nurses in, for example, a hospital setting who are instructed by management to wear uniforms carrying logos because to do so will bring the hospital a considerable sum of money. We have talked about the selling of space in healthcare settings to advertisers but what is now being suggested is, in effect, the selling or hiring out of the nurses themselves. Now it is conceivable, though statistically unlikely, that every single nurse will agree that this product should be endorsed, but it is probable that at least some will disagree or will not have given thought to the matter. In that case they as individuals are being asked to endorse a product which they do not wholeheartedly support. And not only may they not support the product, they may also be opposed to this form of advertising. In such a case, an appropriate way of describing what is going on may be to use a Kantian argument to the effect that nurses are being illegitimately used as means to ends they do not agree with, rather than as ends in themselves.

One possible reply to this would be that in many aspects of their work nurses are used as means. In the first place, they are used as a means to the end of promoting patient welfare. This, however, is an end with which they presumably agree if they are to enter the profession in the first place. Advertising is not such an end. In several other types of situation, they may have to do things with which they personally do not agree, but they have an obligation to co-operate with other members of the healthcare team in order to promote the interests of patients.

There are limits to the extent to which nurses are expected to accept things, however. It is part of the point of the UKCC Code of Professional Conduct to encourage nurses to be people who challenge (Pyne, 1988). The ultimate test is whether or not they believe that a particular course of action is in the interests of patients. This brings us once more to the crux of the matter. Is it in the interests of patients to raise money by such methods as wearing logos on uniforms? The answer to this does not depend on a crude analysis of the amounts of money that can be made available by different methods, e.g. public-funding versus commercial sponsorship. There are wider questions about the ethos of the service, public expectations and the nature of nursing as a profession.

Nursing as a profession: two kinds of power relationship

The notion of publicly provided healthcare has its origins in the ethics of charity on the one hand and in public responsibility for welfare on the other. Of those professionals who work in healthcare, nurses in particular have been associated with notions of altruism and an ethic of care. The image (whatever the reality) of the medical profession has been associated to a greater extent with career advancement and social position than has that of nurses.

The image of nurses has changed from that of doctors' handmaidens to that of professionals in their own right. But the realities of the power relationships in the healthcare context are still of interest and particular relevance in thinking about logos for nurses' uniforms.

First, nurses still have less power than doctors because doctors have ultimate authority in determining how patients should be treated. Their power, however, does not stop at this but spreads in other directions. While doctors may perhaps be seen using pens emblazoned with the name of a pharmaceutical company, it is difficult to imagine them wearing logo-bearing uniforms, however much money it might raise for their patients. But if it were acceptable for nurses, why not for doctors? This may say something about the relative status of the two professions. (An additional point, however, is that the advertising of pharmaceutical companies to doctors is largely aimed at persuading them to prescribe certain drugs, rather than encouraging patients to buy.)

The point about the relative power of doctors and nurses is one that has frequently been made. Also significant is the difference in power between the nurse and the patient. Here the practitioner has the power. Patients who are ill are vulnerable. In this situation they want to put their trust in somebody and it is nurses in whom it is normally placed. The advertisers will be well aware of this. Not only are there more nurses than doctors, but they spend more time with patients with whom they can develop a relationship of trust. The potential for influencing patients is thus enormous.

An argument against the use of nurses for advertising through logos, then, might be that this is an illegitimate exploitation of differences in power that already exist – first, of nurses *vis-à-vis* other professional groups, and second of patients who are in a vulnerable position with regard to health professionals generally, including nurses.

The professional and the patient

Beyond this, however, there is a point about the ways in which nurses and patients are viewed. We have already said something about the way in which the image of nurses generally has changed. Reg Pyne has argued that the UKCC Code of Professional Conduct presents an image of what a nurse is (Pyne, 1988). This image, according to the UKCC, is incompatible with the nurse as advertiser. The nurse's primary duty is to act at all times to promote the welfare of patients. While it has been suggested that the strongest argument in favour of advertising is that it can contribute towards this end by raising money for new or improved facilities, the reply to this can be put in the following way: using nurses to advertise to patients alters not only the image of the nurse but also that of the patients. To see patients as customers marks a radical change in how they are regarded, a change which patients themselves might resent and which might lead to a weakening of that very trust advertisers would like to exploit.

In another context Ronald Green makes this point in relation to fee-splitting (the practice of paying a percentage to doctors who refer patients to clinics). He notes 'a fear that fee-splitting encourages a "trafficking' in sick people and a view of patients as financial resources rather than persons. A further assumption is that even the appearance of such practices might seriously undermine patients' trust' (Green, 1990: 24). The point being made here is that if patients suspect that someone has something to gain financially out of certain advice they are given, they are likely to distrust both that advice and the professionals who give it.

In addition to this argument about the possible undesirable consequences for trust in the professional-client relationship, there is a problem about the implications for respect for the person. Those who uphold a principle of respect for persons may vary in how they interpret it and it is beyond the scope of this chapter to examine the principle in detail. There has, however, been a move towards calling the recipients of care 'clients' rather than 'patients'. This is supposed to reflect more respect for them as persons in the sense that 'patient' implies a passive role, when we should rather be thinking of the recipients of care in accordance with the principle of autonomy, as actively involved in decisions about their treatment. So far, so good. What is suspect about such moves is the suggestion that in order to show respect for recipients of a service, it is necessary to regard them as customers: the implication being that it is people who pay for a service who command respect. As Bernard Williams has pointed out, the relevant factor about people who want to receive healthcare is whether or not they are ill, not whether or not they have money (Williams, 1969).

COMMERCIAL SPONSORSHIP

On commercial sponsorship the UKCC (1990: 2) has this to say:

> The same principles set out ... in relation to advertising, that is independence of professional judgment based on the needs of patients and clients, unfettered by undue commercial influence, should equally apply to any commercial sponsorship arrangements.

What is envisaged here is the kind of situation where a nurse's salary is paid for by a commercial company. It has become more common for persons in all kinds of occupations to seek funding for their posts in such ways.

For the UKCC the important consideration is that such sponsorship should not compromise the independence of the nurse's judgment. (The need for professional judgment uninfluenced by commercial considerations is also emphasized by Clause 16 of the Code of Professional Conduct (UKCC, 1992)). Whether it does will depend on the degree of distance between the sponsor and the nurse's work. For example, if the sponsorship also entailed wearing a particular logo, then it would be ruled out in accordance with the argument in the preceding section. Similarly, if the sponsorship involved recommending one and only one particular brand of products not patients, the nurse's independence would be undermined.

In some cases, however, sponsorship of particular posts is compatible with there being no particular promotional message passed on to patients and clients. In such cases, perhaps the argument that it promotes the interests of all can be made out. A nurse is provided with employment; patients are provided with care; the public purse is relieved of some pressure. The argument against this is that, despite the apparent harmlessness of such arrangements, their increasing number reinforces the idea that health is not a public responsibility; that it is up to private concerns to finance it. In the long term it is difficult to see this as being in the interests of all, for a large concession is being made to the culture of publicity, which is an inappropriate one for the provision of healthcare. Our consideration of the debates surrounding advertising, then, has highlighted arguments from a moral point of view that support the stance taken by the UKCC and cast doubt on the applicability, in the healthcare context, of the standard justifications of advertising.

REFERENCES

Berger, J. (1972) *Ways of Seeing*, Penguin Books, Harmondsworth.

Carroll, M.A. and Humphrey, R.A. (1979) *Moral Problems in Nursing: Case Studies*, University Press of America, Washington DC.

Evans, D. (1990) Ethics and advertising. *Bulletin of Medical Ethics*, **59**: 21–4.

Gallie, W.B. (1955–6) Essentially contested concepts. *Proceedings of the Aristotelian Society*, **56**, 167–98.

Gillon, R. (1985) Autonomy and consent, in *Moral Dilemmas in Modern Medicine* (ed. M. Lockwood), Oxford University Press, Oxford, pp. 111–25.

Green, R.M. (1990) Medical joint-venturing: an ethical perspective. *Hastings Center Report*, **20**(4), 22–6.

Melrose, D. (1982) *Bitter Pills: Medicines and the Third World Poor*, Oxfam, Oxford.

Miles, M., Morrison, V., Weeks, J., Crimmin, M. and Shand, W. (1989) Letter to *The Times*, 11 November.

Oxford English Dictionary (1971) Oxford University Press, Oxford.

Pyne, R. (1988) On being accountable. *Health Visitor*, **61**, 173–5.

United Kingdom Central Council (1984) *Code of Professional Conduct for the Nurse, Midwife and Health Visitor*, 2nd edn, United Kingdom Central Council for Nursing, Midwifery and Health Visitors, London.

United Kingdom Central Council (1985) *Advertising by Registered Nurses, Midwives and Health Visitors: an Elaboration of Clause 14 of the Code of Professional Conduct,* United Kingdom Central Council for Nursing, Midwifery and Health Visitors, London.

United Kingdom Central Council (1990) *Statement on Advertising and Commercial Sponsorship and the Position of Nurses, Midwives and Health Visitors and the Health Care Environment,* United Kingdom Central Council for Nursing, Midwifery and Health Visitors, London.

United Kingdom Central Council (1992) *Code of Professional Conduct for the Nurse, Midwife and Health Visitor,* 3rd edn, United Kingdom Central Council for Nursing, Midwifery and Health Visitors, London.

Williams, B. (1969) The idea of equality, in *Moral Concepts* (ed. J. Feinberg), Oxford University Press, Oxford, pp. 153–71.

<table>
<tr><td>16</td><td># No room to breathe? Are nurses being stifled by the conflict between the handmaiden and the patient's advocate?</td></tr>
</table>

16	**No room to breathe? Are nurses being stifled by the conflict between the handmaiden and the patient's advocate?**

Jane Pritchard

SETTING THE SCENE

Legislation passed after the Second World War unified the provision of health services in the UK under state control. A generation was born and bred in the secure embrace of an unlimited availability of healthcare. The private hospitals existed alongside those in the public service and were increasingly regarded as élitist. Some care, which was privately paid for, took place in public hospitals. Doctors and other healthcare practitioners were able to run sideline consultancies alongside their NHS work. During the 1970s and 1980s, private health insurance was increasingly provided to employees as part of their employment 'package'. This confused the political arguments tremendously. Those who passionately supported State-run healthcare from a personal point of view, were pressed by employers to take short-cuts through the NHS waiting-lists by 'going privately' in order to reduce the time they were off-sick or working below par. The 'facts of commercial life' challenged the nation's attitude to the provision of State healthcare. At the same time, the costs of providing healthcare were increasing with the enthusiasm stemming from scientific discovery sometimes distorting the distribution of resources between 'care' and 'cure', 'cure' receiving the lion's share. These developments were used by the Conservative governments of the 1980s in preparing the ground for the NHS and Community Care Act 1990. However, the impact of this legislation on nurses should be assessed in the light of changes instigated by the Nurses, Midwives and Health Visitors Acts 1979 and 1992.

In order to understand change it is necessary to grasp the general political climate of the health service which has evolved. Certainly the establishment of 'free' healthcare for the nation can be seen as promoting a certain attitude within the population. Similarly, the high status enjoyed by doctors is partly due to a willingness to give them so much responsibility for the nation's health.

The post-war legislation, setting up the health service as the 'great provider', encourages a child-like reliance on hospital services for the provision of care. While it is perfectly reasonable for a civilized society to establish free healthcare for all as a legal right, the provision of such a service can be disempowering if it is not carefully handled. For example, if a person feels that they do not have a choice but must accept the doctor's recommendation, this is disempowering. Indeed, it is a strong person who goes against the doctor's advice even if the doctor is wrong. Similarly, to be continually told that drinking milk, for example, is 'good for us' can be disempowering because it takes courage to swim against the tide of popular culture.

But does the danger of disempowerment justify questioning the overall benefit of having a National Health Service? When so many of the world are dying, quite literally, for want of any medical care, it is difficult to conceive of the possibility that harm might result from the availability of too much healthcare. Could it be that the belief that a cure is available leads to a recklessness that, in turn, leads to what could be classed as an abuse of healthcare? For example, has the availability of antibiotics made people careless of catching cold and developing chest infection? The possibility of abortion has often been accused of promoting more unwanted pregnancies: that is to say, abortion has been blamed for making people careless about contraception.

Recognizing a general erosion of responsibility has consequences – for an increasing reliance on doctors and nurses, hospitals and the State to right all wrongs and make us better is prohibitingly expensive. In reality, there is a finite pot, if not a reducing one, available for healthcare.

Without suggesting that the new NHS legislation is the right, proper or only way to allocate limited resources, it is still appropriate to look at the effect of the new structure on how healthcare provision is viewed. The temptation to regard patients and treatments as products and to regard the workers as the means of production is a real one. Budget control seems to be firmly placed at the top of the organizational structure. Pressure on productivity and profitability, in practice often hiding behind expressions of cost-efficiency and enhanced customer care, makes it hard for some traditional activities, such as the time to talk to a patient as well as the time to find out what the patient wants, to survive. This, though, is only one side of a double-bind. A combination of the Patients Charter, marking a new emphasis on delivering what the customer (formerly the patient) wants and a tendency for the courts to push nearer to require informed consent to be given for treatment, gives the impression that there is more communication taking place between patient/customer and health staff. Is this an illusion? In fact, the conversation may be serving different ends: that is, to satisfy the requirements of legal and professional standards requirements, rather than to obtain information about the patient to enhance their treatment.

In which ways are these overall changes relevant to the role of nurses? The issues of the cost-reductions of healthcare and the dangers of people failing to take responsibility for their health are directly related to the development of a new role for nurses which will become increasingly controversial as the scope of the change is recognized.

THE COMPOUNDING OF A HANDMAIDEN

Being a handmaiden to the doctors is a traditional role afforded to nurses. Curiously, the 1990 legislation compounds this traditional role by facilitating certain approaches to personnel employed in the new structures set up in the health service which effectively stifles attempts to embrace any other approach.

The NHS and Community Care Act 1990 contains the means whereby State-owned hospitals can be purchased by NHS Trusts. Under this Act the government can lend money to a board of management and a new NHS Trust comes into existence. The process is not dissimilar to the sale of a nationalized industry, although no shares are issued. In almost all cases the Trusts have been set up with the assistance of government loans. Services to be provided by the Trusts, service 'providers', are stipulated by NHS contracts whereby the local health authorities 'purchase' the health needs of the locality. Similar provisions enable doctors to purchase their practices and become GP fund-holders; again the change of ownership may be facilitated by a government loan. This procedure is rather like borrowing money from a building society or bank to help purchase a house.

The statute consciously creates an atmosphere of an open market where the buying and selling of expertise is encouraged. It insists, too, on the Trusts having freedom to negotiate new contracts of employment with their staff. To underline the shift, the legislation stipulates that trades-union officials cannot be part of the governing Trust board. This is particularly important for nurses because of the grading system (Hodgson, 1993: 43). A recent case confirmed that there is no continuity of employment on the takeover of NHS staff by Trust hospitals although Hodgson seems to suggest otherwise (Hodgson, 1993: 45). In reality this means that nurses employed by the NHS at one grade are being employed by the Trusts under a new contract at what are effectively lower grades. In contrast, if staff working for a company in industry were retained by a new management in a takeover it would be usual for staff to enjoy the protection of continuous employment. In the latter case, the legal entity, the company, would remain the same notwithstanding that the owners of the shares in the company had changed hands. When staff change from being employed by the government to being employed by an NHS Trust Hospital, the employer is a totally new legal entity.

The Trusts have limited liability in the same way as limited companies established under the Companies Acts. In this sense the term 'Trust' is a misnomer, as trustees usually have unlimited liability. Time will tell what effect this limitation has on the ostensible accountability of the Trusts.

The clear intention is that with ownership of the Trusts comes responsibility and accountability for the services provided. Tight financial accountability is also imposed whereby the chief executive of the Trust has designated personal responsibility to make sure the Trust can meet its obligations and, particularly, whether it has the means to keep up loan payments to the government on the 'mortgage' for the purchase of the hospital when the Trust was set up.

The present concern with these changes is to consider what effect they may have on the staff employed by the Trusts and the impact of the legal contract on the psychological perspective emerging in the new NHS.

In readiness for the changes, surveys have been, and are continuing to be, carried out to assess the tasks done in the health service and by whom. This approach supports the notion that the patient and the various treatments need to be treated as units of care provision; they are the products of the new health industry. Closely allied to this is the attitude that staff are seen as the means of production. Doctors have traditionally enjoyed high status in a health service impressed with scientific advances, 'fancy' cures and operating techniques. In contrast, the provision of care by nurses has been viewed with less esteem. How will these two groups fare when looked on by cost-conscious Trustees?

Something between 'automata' and 'super heroes' is what the Trust legislation demands of professionals. The new commercial structure cannot tolerate too much discussion about what should and should not be done; rather it requires professionals to deliver the required commodity in the shortest possible time and at the least expense. This is new to health service professionals perhaps, but certainly not new to professionals such as solicitors and accountants all of whom have been required for many years to account to their customers (and their employers, as the case may be) for the time and money spent on attaining the desired end.

If this is the legal structure, what is the effect on nurses? Clearly there is no time for the 'handmaiden' to be promoted to a less servile position. We have seen that the position on contracts has in fact worsened her position. Furthermore, the insistence that a graded job takes no account of the experience and expertise of the particular nurse doing the job provides a clear message – one nurse is the same as another, whether she has been qualified for one month or 20 years. In this respect they are all handmaidens regardless of maturity, rather like the wives of successful men in the golf club are always collectively known as 'girls' regardless of age. There is no incentive built into this structure to improve or expand the areas of responsibility for nurses; there is no place here for autonomous professionals.

ASPIRATIONS TO BE THE PATIENT'S ADVOCATE

If the picture of the handmaiden is drawn from the NHS and Community Care Act, what vision springs from the Nurses, Midwives and Health Visitors Acts of 1979 and 1992? Certainly the strict atmosphere of economy and minimalism spawned by the Trust hospitals hardly provides a fertile ground for the development of the role of patient's advocate. Nevertheless, this role would seem to be at the heart of the aspirations for nursing promoted by the UKCC (Young, 1994: 177). In fact, there are historical precedents for seeing the nurse as the patient's advocate. While the dauphin died in 1712 because doctors indulged him in too much blood-letting, the nurses managed to keep alive the dauphin's younger brother by refusing to allow the doctors to blood-let and keeping him warm and comfortable (Kenyon, 1992: 232).

In the introduction to the chapter entitled, 'Illness and Ageing' (Kenyon, 1992: 230) Olga Kenyon writes:

> Women's medical knowledge was more frequently appealed to in the past than was men's. Wives such as Margery Parson were asked for remedies by their family. Nuns such as Hildegard of Bingen were famous for preparing herbal remedies for the community. Women acted as midwives until men proclaimed themselves as experts even in this field in the 19th century. Women studied medicine and acted as surgeons in medieval Italy, but were increasingly marginalized by university faculties of medicine.

University doors closed to women (who shall, for the purpose of emphasizing the applicability of Kenyon's words, be called nurses) in the Middle

Ages would seem to be creaking open under the provisions of the Nurses, Midwives and Health Visitors Acts 1979 and 1992. These Acts established the UKCC and effectively transferred responsibility for the education of nurses, *inter alia*, from colleges of nurses who had hitherto trained them, into the ivory towers of universities. With this transition which necessarily is taking several years to complete, came a change in emphasis: nurses would no longer be trained to do a specific task but would be more broadly educated so as to be better able to carry out designated tasks in an appropriate way. The differences between education and training can be debated for a long time but a side argument is that 'workers' are trained, while 'professionals' are 'educated'. Thus this move is part of a clear bid for independent professional status for the three groups affected: namely, nurses, midwives and district nurses. In practice most professionals, from lawyers to health professionals, require to be both trained and educated before they are competent enough to be let loose on clients/patients.

This example indicates how legal structure effects change in the working lives of nurses. While it is too early to assess rigorously the effect of the new education as opposed to the earlier-style training on the quality of practice, rumour already suggests that there may be too little emphasis on equipping student nurses to feel competent on the wards on registration. While the need for both education and training in sufficient parts may be regarded as idealistic in the present political climate of cost-consciousness in health and education, it is important to recognize that the aspirations embodied in the statutes referred to – the Trust legislation on the one hand and the slower-moving education legislation on the other – are incompatible, perhaps even in conflict. What seems likely is that the cost-efficiency driven structures of the Trust hospitals will win any struggle in the short term. The long term, however, is not so easy to predict.

Once it is accepted that the supply of finance is finite, the argument is about prioritizing and the allocation of resources. This is a more sensible approach, for it is important for people's general health that energy is spent on realistic pursuits rather than impossible dreams. While it is easy to complain about change and simply assume that less money means a worse service, the crucial test is in obtaining a voice that is heard on how those funds should be spent. Nurses have been ignored by health governance for so long that finding a way to be heard is the first battle to be confronted.

INEVITABLE CONFLICT

There are thus conflicting views of what the role of nurses might currently be. Hunt describes a conflict where the role depicted by the health-service management for nurses is something between 'a technical assistant and a shop assistant' for the products being marketed by the new trusts. This is contrasted to the Project 2000 vision of the 'new nurse' as an ideal carer (Hunt, 1992: 94):

> In some ways Project 2000 may be regarded as trying to 'return to source', to reconnect with this lost ideal, but in a new way. That ideal is the nurse as healthcare *par excellence*, addressing the well along with the unwell, dealing with people rather than with their bodies, caring for people in the context of their families and friends, helping people to overcome certain life problems with their own judgment and understanding.

There is a clear tension between these two roles. Hunt points out that there has been no indication from government that it will empower nurses to put into practice the aspirations of Project 2000, even though the Project itself was a reasonably foreseeable consequence of the Nurses, Midwives and Health Visitors Act 1979 which established the UKCC. Governmental support for the new provider/supplier ethos of the NHS and Community Care Act 1990, however, has been displayed in abundance. The Patient's Charter is one example (HMSO, 1992). This document is of uncertain legal status but is 'evidence of intention', namely that the government is supportive of stimulating an expectation among patients that they have rights and can make demands. The Charter is supportive of 'the customer is always right' theme.

The Patient's Charter was made without significant reference to the professionals who must deliver the 'customer service'. No regard was given to the practicality of the promises made. Rather, the Charter contained 'outputs' that the government identified as being to the satisfaction of customers.

However, there is a more personal view of the conflict as to what role a nurse has. If the two roles are imagined as simultaneously aspired to and internalized by a single nurse, the inevitable tension becomes evident. The traditional view that sees the nurse as the doctor's handmaiden is widespread. Student nurses often see this role as inevitable – even the male ones! As the handmaiden servility is nurtured, independent opinion is likely not merely to be ignored, but may be regarded as insolence and insubordination. The more modern notion that the nurse must speak up against the doctors and managers and demand consideration for the patient's interest and, more particularly, preferences, while being quite attractive, as it makes a hero of the nurse in a way that has never happened before, is undesirable in so far as it threatens to reshape the 'perfect forceps-giver' into the voicepiece of the rights-oriented, complaining patient/customer (Young, 1994: 173). This belief that she must speak up and be counted as advocate for the patient squeezes the nurse's individuality from another direction. It brings her no closer to independence. The role of patient's advocate is disempowering to both nurse and patient.

To talk to a nurse about seeking her own professional autonomy is, further, to burden her and to exacerbate her position by adding a third role: that of the self-governing professional. Her autonomy is stifled by the conflict between the handmaiden and the patient's advocate.

A POSSIBLE RESOLUTION: THE NURSE IN CHARGE OF HEALTHCARE AND ADVICE?

The tide would seem to be turning from the preference for cure over care. The astronomical cost of the discovery and practice of techno-logical medicine is finally being questioned. The refusal of some Trust hospitals to provide fertility treatment is an example. Where resources are finite, a preference can be shown for the care of people who are alive, rather than creatures who may be helped into life by technolog-ical developments. Another question focuses on the ethics of a society that allows some treatments to be available for the rich but not the poor. It is not appropriate here to discuss this further. The present undertaking is to seek a role for nurses which is compatible with both the priorities of the Trust legislation and the aspirations of the UKCC. It would be beneficial for the overall status of nurses if that role could cover an area basically separate from the curing role of doctors. This is no easy task and there may be other candidates than the role now pro-posed.

The traditional role of nurses assisting doctors in operations may continue in an atmosphere of nurse autonomy and greater status than they currently enjoy. For this enhancement of status to occur, the role would have to be acknowledged as specialist. The continuance of this role would be very different from that of the nurse educator (see below). It might represent a fork in the nursing profession rather like law is forked today, with barristers doing the majority of court work and giving opinions on the law whereas solicitors do everything else! It is solicitors who primarily have contact with the client. Another possi-bility is that it may be more appropriate for the job of assisting doctors in the operating theatre to be done by trainee doctors, in an appren-ticeship role of watching and learning from their more experienced professional colleagues. If trainee doctors carry out this work it would confirm, too, that the proper domain of doctors is that of 'cure'. Other advantages would be to settle, once and for all, the male/female, doctor/nurse differential: there would be junior and senior doctors in a very uncomplicated way. The other important function of doctors at present is diagnosis. Nurses have never had a part in this aspect and no change is here proposed in terms of 'scientific', that is, testable diagnosis.

What is left for nurses to do if helping doctors to cure the sick is taken away? The education and care of the well is left and that is an equally important role. The nation, since the forming of the National Health Service, has been raised in the belief that when their bodies let them down somebody will be available to put them right. Health 'cuts' should not be introduced so rapidly that the foundations of people's expectations, with regard to care, are undermined.

People have to be given back responsibility for their own health. Brought up differently, they will have to be nurtured into that autonomy. Dietary information will be the beginning. In giving care for those ailments which doctors cannot cure and thus should have no part in, cold and all manner of viral complaints, nurses would provide education about the 'dos and don'ts' of healthy living. In this she will not be the patient's advocate but will empower the patient to speak for herself.

The scenario portrayed here is necessarily simplistic because of the limitation on space. A great deal has been written about the many versions of health without cure. They currently bear a label of 'alternative', 'complementary' or even, 'quirky' (Kushi, 1977). In bridging the gap in the health service between doctors and nurses by giving equal status to cure and care, this proposal allows Western medicine to link arms with the medical knowledge of the East (Kushi, 1977).

It is relatively straightforward to see how this central role for nurses can be reconciled with the legislation leading to the education of professionals, rather than the training of assistants. However, it needs to be reconciled with the underlying motives of the government in relation to Trust hospitals if this proposal is to be given serious consideration. The following quotation from Loveridge and Starkey (1992: 8) identifies the tension that exists between government and doctor in relation to prioritizing resources:

At the same time the emphasis placed on the defence of the individual autonomy of their [Royal Colleges and NHS] members has tended towards encouraging a curative approach to healthcare management in which the doctor has retained his or her personal scope for judgment rather than a preventative or community-based perspective. This is a perspective which the new contracts offered to the profession by the Department of Health evidently seeks to redress.

Happily for the present purpose it provides an excellent starting point from which to persuade government and Trust Boards that it is expedient to pay attention to care rather than devote all resources towards cure. There is no reason why this proposal for nurses to have a role as carer and educator should not match very well with cost-efficiency drives by Trust management. Indeed, 'investing time to save time' by teaching patients to care for themselves might prove the value of nurses beyond everyone's wildest dreams!

CONCLUSION

Whether or not the role of health carer and advisor be augmented to provide the nurse with a clear and independent professional role proves popular or practical, what is certain is that there needs to be a considerable shift in policy for the nurse, once more, to be comfortable at work. This chapter has shown that the conflict resulting from two clashing pieces of legislation makes her present role untenable. Ironically, the legislation that oppresses her is successful only because the nurse herself takes on responsibility to solve the conflict by struggling to perform her dual role. The aspirations embodied in the statutes were better fulfilled if nurses could put them into practice without conflict. In this way, all the interested parties could find motivation in carving out for nurses a more appropriate role.

Note: According to Gregory Bateson, the 'double-bind' situation is a 'situation in which [a person] cannot make a move, or make no move, without feeling pushed and pulled, both from within himself and from the people about him, a situation in which he can't win, no matter what he does' (133). Here R.D. Laing is quoted in Capra (1989).

REFERENCES

Capra, F. (1989) *Uncommon Wisdom*, Flamingo, London.

HMSO (1979 and 1992) *Nurses, Midwives and Health Visitors Acts*, HMSO, London.

HMSO (1990) *NHS and Community Care Act*, HMSO, London.

HMSO (1992) *The Patient's Charter*, HMSO, London.

Hodgson, J. (1993) *Employment Law for Nurses*, BKT Information Services and Quay Publishing, Lancaster.

Hunt, G. (1992) Ethics, ambivalence and ideology, in *Project 2000: The Teachers Speak* (eds O. Slevin and M. Buckenham) Campion Press, Edinburgh.

Kenyon, O. (1992) *800 Years of Women's Letters*, Alan Sutton Publishing, Stroud.

Kushi, M. (1977) *The Book of Macrobiotics*, Japan Publications, Tokyo.

Loveridge, R. and Starkey, K. (eds) (1992) *Continuity and Crisis in the NHS*, Open University Press, Buckingham, p. 237.

Young, A.P. (1994) Law and professional conduct, in *Ethical Issues in Nursing* (ed. G. Hunt), Routledge, London.

Nursing, education and values: a sociological perspective | 17

Mairi Levitt

A SOCIOLOGICAL PERSPECTIVE

What does sociology have to offer to a consideration of nursing values? Broadly speaking sociologists may focus on values, or anything else in society, both at the level of everyday behaviour and communication (the micro-level) and at the level of social systems and institutions (the macro-level). While different sociological perspectives tend to begin with either a macro- or a micro-level analysis, it will be argued that both are necessary to an understanding of values. For example, the macro-level analysis can provide information on social structures and institutions and their effects on the work of nurses, while the micro-level can uncover and open to scrutiny the taken-for-granted beliefs and attitudes which operate in the health services.

At the micro-level a key concept is culture: that is, the way of life of a particular group, the values or ideals they share and the norms they follow (Bocock, 1992). Despite there being many different individuals who qualify as nurses, the nursing journals are able to make some assumptions about the shared interests and concerns of nurses in general and the UKCC is able to draw up a code of conduct and advisory documents directed at the profession as a whole (UKCC, 1992). At the level of culture, sociologists will be interested in interaction between people and their taken-for-granted values and attitudes. They might focus on the language and terminology used between nurses, doctors and patients. What does the way people communicate tell us about the relative status and power of nurses, doctors and patients and their value orientations? Sociologists often focus on the 'underdog', those with less power and control whose views are less often heard. In any given situation the underdog might be the nurse, the student nurse or the patient.

Nurses do not live in isolation from the rest of society but operate within particular economic and political structures. A consideration of macro-level structures leads to the question of how they affect the health services where nurses work and their status and power relative to other occupations. Statistics on gender and class inequalities in Britain can provide useful information which an individual nurse's experiences might not provide; for example, on the link between the social class into which a baby is born and the likelihood of the baby dying within the first year of life (Social Trends, 1993: 96). However, statistics on their own can only produce a snapshot of inequalities in some areas but cannot explain why these inequalities exist. To take another example: the reasons why there are currently more women nurses in Britain than men can only be addressed with knowledge of gender and the labour market, together with an understanding of cultural beliefs on suitable work for women and men and their roles within the family. Although we like to think of ourselves as unique individuals, we are influenced by other people and by the culture and social structures in which we live. Individual values have some connection to the type of society in which the person lives. Durkheim, a founding father of sociology, wrote about the 'cult of the individual' as a feature of industrial societies, arguing that the development of the division of labour with increasing specialization of the workforce led to people viewing themselves as individuals first (Durkheim, 1964: 172). He compared that with a simpler society in which there would be little specialization other than by gender and age and people would see themselves as part of the group (Durkheim, 1964: 179). He argues that the shared morality of complex societies is centred around individual rights and the main threat to social order is a lack of regulation and excessive egoism (Durkheim, 1964: 353ff). A similar view about the link between values and the wider social structures is being put forward when the 1980s are labelled as 'uncaring' both at the level of individuals and of political and economic structure. The interconnection between individual or group values and social structures will be examined next.

INDIVIDUAL VALUES AND SOCIETY

If society is viewed as a system of interconnecting parts, the connection between individual values and the wider society exists because values have a social function; for example, individuals feel obligations towards their children and this has a social function of taking some of the burden of child-care from society at large. What might be the social function of nursing values? These values may have a role in maintaining social order, in establishing the identity of nurses *vis-à-vis* other occupational groups and in legitimizing relationships of power and subordination. Put like that the functions sound rather far-removed from everyday interaction. However, a hospital functions with large numbers of workers fulfilling different roles, performing different tasks in a complex organization (maintaining social order). Such an organization would collapse if individuals within it continually had to start from scratch and negotiate their roles rather than be a staff nurse, a consultant, a porter or whatever. These workers do not usually need to consciously think about establishing their identities because name badges, uniforms and ward routines do this for them, as illustrated by the occasional fake doctor who dons a white coat and stethoscope and with an authoritative manner can gain access to patients and even operating theatres.

Any social group shares taken-for-granted commonsense understandings of 'the way things are done here', which enables the organization to function from day to day. Anyone with memories of a teacher who could not keep control in the classroom will know what can happen when these understandings break down. Commonsense can be defined as 'the uncritical and largely unconscious way of perceiving and understanding the world' (Gramsci, 1971: 322). While 'commonsense' can include understandings which seem to apply only to a very specific situation, for instance 'the way Dr X likes his ward round to be conducted', it will reflect, at the micro-level, the wider values of society as a whole: in this particular example, the hierarchy of status and the ideology of professionalism.

All the roles people perform carry expectations but those occupations described as professions tend to be seen as requiring special qualities. The next section looks at the values inherent in the notion of a professional and their relevance to the individual and everyday practice.

PROFESSIONALS

Professional occupations are often seen as special in some way: they have unique characteristics which set them apart from other types of occupations and have important functions which explain their wealth, prestige and power. One approach to the identifying of professions has been to list their 'traits', usually skill, theoretical knowledge, long training and education, altruism and a code of conduct. Higher-status professions always have the listed traits but lower-status occupations, including social work and nursing, may not qualify (Johnson, 1972: 58). The categorizing of occupations in this way tends to be an uncritical listing of the way occupations would like to be seen and a justification for their economic rewards and social status (Johnson, 1984).

It is to the benefit of those included in the definition 'professional' if society as a whole accepts the benign view of the professions as intrinsically altruistic and providers of a service to the whole community.

A less-optimistic, more critical view could focus on other functions of the professionals: the professional as reality definer who has the power to define health and illness, to create dependent clients, to preserve status and rewards by restricting access to their position and maintaining a monopoly over tasks which could be opened up to others (Whittington and Boore, 1989: 111). Do occupations seek to be seen as professions to service others more effectively or to increase their own rewards and status? Perhaps the two are inextricably intertwined.

Nursing has been engaged in a struggle to be recognized as a profession hindered by the view that 'all that is required is to be female and to have a "vocation" to care' (Whittington and Boore, 1989: 110). The medical hierarchy is assumed to be based on qualifications and skills which justify the inequalities of status, pay and conditions of service. An examination of this commonsense indicates that skills traditionally exercised by men are valued more highly than those ascribed to women. 'Womanly' skills can be seen as an extension of the maternal role, caring and serving others; they are poorly rewarded in jobs such as nursery or care assistant, secretary and infant teacher. Porter's study found resentment among nurses about their 'handmaiden' role but an acceptance of the occupational superiority of doctors as 'the unproblematic and exclusive results of a meritocratic process' (Porter, 1992: 519). The assertiveness of individual nurses in interaction with doctors did not challenge the structural inequalities.

When a critical view is taken of the exercise of power by professionals, the 'lower' professions, as measured by rewards and status, might appear to be on the side of the angels. However, it is not only the higher-status professions that have sought to exclude others from their power. Weber used the concept of social closure to describe ways in which different groups in the stratification system seek to preserve their position by the use of strategies which close off entry to those below them (Weber, 1968: 342). An example would be closing off the group to those from particular ethnic origins or those with the 'wrong' family background. Witz applies this concept to medicine and presents a model of occupational closure (Witz, 1992: 45). In medicine, men used exclusionary strategies to restrict access to medical practice and demarcationary strategies to police and control the boundaries between the occupation of medicine and related medical occupations. The restricted access, by educational criteria, helps to maintain the high status of doctors in general and, with additional criteria, the hierarchy among doctors. Educational qualifications appear to be a fair way of deciding access because they are open to all. However, there is a clear link between the achievement of those qualifications and other social factors such as class background (Social Trends, 1994: 52). Lower down the status hierarchy, midwives and nurses engaged in their own strategies. According to Witz, they resisted the medical men's demarcationary strategies and at the same time tried to exclude 'usurpers' seeking to enter their area of expertise by establishing the credentials necessary for entry, systems of registration, training and examinations (Witz, 1992: 117).

Given the interconnections between individuals and social structure, how could professions enforce values which differ from the mainstream? Durkheim saw a role for the professions in reinforcing the shared values of the occupation but argues that professional values 'can only be a special form of common morality' (Durkheim, 1957: 39). Changes in the 'common morality' of British society which particularly affect nursing are changes in the role of women at home and work, partly supported by sex discrimination legislation, and a less deferential attitude to traditional authority figures, partly supported by rights legislation. These changes affect women in nursing, their attitudes to those in authority over them and their patients. To take examples from two empirical studies: Porter found 'many instances where nurses were prepared to challenge medical orders ... [which] may indicate a changing relationship between these occupations' (Porter, 1992: 520). Ryan and McKenna (1994: 122) in a study of nursing and medical students concluded that:

> Clearly changes in the status of women, changes in healthcare delivery and nursing's bid for professional status all pose a severe threat to the traditional dominant/subservient relationship between nurses and doctors.

The contention here is that the actions of individual professionals can only be understood in the context of the social structure in which they operate and the constraints imposed on the professions from outside. The next section examines the social context within which individual nurses have to work: in other words, how aspects of society in general affect the recruitment of nurses, their training and their work.

THE SOCIAL CONTEXT OF NURSING

Nursing as a career

What features of society as a whole influence the recruitment of nurses? Although in Britain nursing has a workforce which is 90% female, men hold more than half the posts of chief officer and director of nurse-education posts (Porter, 1992: 511). This pattern of horizontal segregation is found in other occupations where women predominate, such as teaching and social work; women are concentrated in the lower-paid, lower-status jobs and underrepresented in top posts. Despite some advantage in terms of promotion, male nurses are part of a profession which is in a weak position in terms of power *vis-à-vis* doctors (Porter, 1992: 517).

In nursing, unlike other occupations such as the police, there has not been a problem of recruitment of minority ethnic groups in the past, although this may be changing (King Edward's Hospital Fund, 1990). However, there is evidence of racial inequality and discrimination in the lack of black women in higher level posts; their overrepresentation in specialisms seen as less prestigious such as psychiatric nursing and geriatric care and black women being channelled into SEN rather than SRN training (Baxter, 1988: 16; Bryan, Dadzie and Scafe, 1985: 40). The King's Fund Equal Opportunities Task Force concluded that the service given to the NHS by black and ethnic minority nurses 'has been under-valued and their talent has been squandered' (King's Fund, 1990).

In terms of social class, nursing has maintained a hierarchy in which higher-status training and work attracts more women from middle-class backgrounds. The strong link between social class and educational qualifications ensures that the more qualifications the occupation demands, the more it will recruit from higher social classes. Thus differences of race, gender and social class are reproduced in the nursing workforce and, as will be discussed next, in people's health and healthcare.

Health and healthcare

The Patient's Charter implicitly acknowledges the influence of social factors on healthcare in the section on respect for cultural and ethnic backgrounds. However, generally the emphasis is on individual rights: the right to information, choice and the right to complain (NHS, 1991).

Underlying these themes is a model of the individual as a free, independent person able to make rational decisions about their own education and health and that of their children. In reality the degree of knowledge, control and choice is structured by social and economic factors. For example, there is evidence that higher social classes in Britain make better use of health services, as well as having the choice to use private health if this appears advantageous (see Note). The middle classes make more use of NHS preventive medicine, including screening services, ante-natal and post-natal care and dental treatment and GPs have been shown to spend more time in consultations with middle-class than with working-class patients (Reid, 1989: 151; Social Trends, 1994: 97). Babies from unskilled manual homes are twice as likely to die in the first year as babies from professional/intermediate homes (a category in which registered nurses and other medical profes-sionals are included) (Social Trends, 1993: 96). The link between poverty and ill-health is well documented (Blackburn, 1991). A drive for greater equality by race, gender and region, as well as social class, is surely an essential part of putting into practice both the values of caring and the interests of the patient.

Structural inequalities are constantly reproduced and reinforced by individual actions and interactions. The problem with a blanket injunction to 'care' for all patients is that it might encourage the nurse to be gender, class and ethnically 'blind', claiming to treat everyone as individuals. This can become treating everyone the same, ignoring particular needs or not monitoring the differences in treatment that unconsciously occur. Studies of school classrooms have revealed that teachers who claim to treat boys and girls equally in practice, or not to think of pupils as boys or girls at all, spend more time and give more attention to the boys and even assess their work differently (Spender, 1982: 54–85). When teachers tried to correct the imbalance and give as much attention to the girls, not only were they unable to achieve this aim but the boys complained that the teacher was 'only interested in the girls', something which no probationary teacher would want to be reported and perhaps believed. However, these findings have made people aware of gender differences and stimulated debate (Shaw, 1989: 186). It is more difficult to measure such inequalities in a hospital ward where patients spend less time and have more widely differing needs.

The importance of a sociological understanding for nurses' ethical practice is shown by two examples. One focuses on values at the macro-level: the link between practice and social structure; the other, on values at the micro-level and the link between practice and taken-for-granted cultural beliefs.

VALUES IN PRACTICE

A code of conduct, however carefully constructed, cannot be translated into practice without the necessary societal and organizational structures and the will of individual nurses. The ethical statements of an organization are of interest in revealing the values to which the organization wants to be seen to subscribe. It cannot be assumed that they reflect everyday practice; nor can it be assumed that social structures will facilitate their practice.

It is easier to illustrate this problem by looking as an outsider at another health system. An article on 'the Center for Human Caring' at the University of Colorado School of Nursing enthuses about students learning nursing in a caring environment and practising it with their patients (*Nursing Times*, 1992). In a society in which more than 30 million people have no medical insurance, including about 11 million children, but the most technologically advanced care in the world is available to those who can afford it, the 'care' can only be an oasis in an 'uncaring' structure (Kronenfeld, 1993: 2–3). Does the School of Nursing encourage the nurses it trains only to look inwardly at their own practice, not at the system within which they operate? It is more difficult to stand back from one's own system and acknowledge the gap between ideology and individual experiences of healthcare.

The second example focuses on shared cultural beliefs in a small-scale study of the experiences of 32 Asian women in post-natal wards in east London (Woolett and Dosanjh-Matwala, 1990). The study revealed a contrast between the women's views and those underlying hospital practice (Woolett and Dosanjh-Matwala, 1990: 184). The medical staff made assumptions about 'normal' maternal behaviour which led to 'strained' relationships with women who had different ideologies about the needs of mother and child. In particular the staff stressed the importance of early bonding between mother and child, a theme central to recent psychological theories in Britain and the USA and one which fits in with the small, isolated nuclear family prevalent in those societies. The uncritical reproduction of psychological theories in textbooks for nursing students encourages their simplistic application as 'procedures which must be followed'. What are the patient's interests (mother and child) in this situation and how far is flexibility possible on a busy ward? Making the ideology inherent in hospital procedures explicit would be one possibility; in this instance the belief that the establishment of a close, exclusive mother/child relationship at an early stage is a priority. A sociological or historical understanding will show that belief to be historically and culturally specific.

Having argued that to understand and implement nursing values it is necessary to take a society-wide perspective, the final section considers what effects the integration of nursing into higher education institutions may have.

NURSING AND HIGHER EDUCATION INSTITUTIONS

Both the NHS and higher education are coping with increasing demands, new management structures, calls for greater efficiency and new measures of 'quality' to be summarized for the public in league tables. The charters for patients, parents and students share common themes of individual rights, open access to information, increased choice, respect for cultural or ethnic backgrounds and the right to complain (NHS, 1991; DFE, 1993, 1994).

The integration of nursing courses into higher education will not necessarily raise the status of nursing because as access to higher education widens the relative position of nurses may not change.

Teaching is now an all-graduate profession, whereas, in Britain, entry to training courses was possible with only 'O'-levels 20 years ago. However, there has not been any concomitant change in their status. Altschul asks 'if nursing is jumping from the frying pan into the fire in joining the academic bandwagon at this time when all the former benefits of tertiary education are fast disappearing' (Altschul, 1992: 1392). These benefits were available because higher education was for an élite, so universities had time and resources for research as well as teaching and students had smaller classes and relatively higher grants. Universities have been seen as arenas for the expression of controversial, unorthodox views, where freedom of expression and the encouragement of critical thinking are fundamental to the educational enterprise. Whether or not the ideology was realized in practice, it was different from that underlying nursing education with a behaviourist, medical model of teaching and learning.

In the UKCC Code of Professional Conduct, the first priority is to 'safeguard and promote the interests of patients and clients' (UKCC, 1992). One theme common in medicine and teaching is that the professional tries to act in the patient/pupil/students' best interest but that lack of resources frustrates their attempts. In an examination of values in one 'new' university, staff expressed dissatisfaction with the provision of resources for teaching, preparation and research and the lack of time to spend with students (Henry et al., 1992: 7). Staff saw themselves as open, communicative, collaborative, having integrity, being trustworthy, responsible and moral in their relationships with others but undervalued and controlled by the larger organization that did not allow them professional autonomy (Henry et al., 1992). The tendency to attribute positive qualities to oneself makes the negative qualities (i.e. being controlled and not assertive or valued) more interesting. Are those who feel they lack control and autonomy themselves in a position to be advocates for others?

If nurses should care for their patients and put their interests first, in what situations are they most likely to do so effectively? Presumably if they enjoy their work, feel valued themselves, are respected by and feel respect for those with whom they work and have a degree of autonomy and control over their situation. A study of nurses in Finland found that those who agreed with the statement 'I have power enough to enable me to improve the quality of nursing practice' were better motivated and rated elements of patient autonomy as an 'essential nursing responsibility' more highly than the nurses who saw themselves as powerless (Raatikainen, 1994: 426, 428). If these answers translate into action then training to produce 'powerful nurses' would be in accordance with the first aim of the UKCC Code of Professional Practice (1992). Students would need the confidence to put their training into practice when they meet 'ritual' action on the hospital ward. For example, nurses may 'assess pain and the need for analgesia on gender, nationality and type of operation' not on patient report (Wilson and Startup, 1992: 1481), a following of procedure without considering that purpose of administering analgesia is to relieve the pain that only the patient is experiencing.

The university model of encouraging freedom of expression, the challenging of received 'truth' and debate of different perspectives would seem to be of value to a dynamic health service in which methods of treatment, technology and theoretical frameworks are changing and new demands and ethical dilemmas are being generated (DOH, 1994). The main question is whether institutions of higher education can deliver what is required of them.

Note

Those people covered by private health insurance in 1991 numbered 7.4 million (Social Trends, 1994: 105). These figures were not broken down by social class but earlier figures from the General Household Survey suggest that between one in four and one in five professional people are covered compared with two in a 100 of those in semi-skilled or unskilled manual occupations (Reid, 1989: 149). Private education caters for around 8% of secondary age pupils. The most prestigious schools have the most socially selective intake. This pattern is mirrored in higher education, where the proportion of students from higher social classes increases, the more prestigious the institution (i.e. 'Oxbridge', old universities, new universities.). Figures are in Reid (1989), Chapter 8.

REFERENCES

Altschul, A.T. (1992) Is British nursing education jumping out of the frying pan into the fire? *Journal of Advanced Nursing* **17**, 1391–2.
Baxter, C. (1988) *The Black Nurse: an Endangered Species*, National Extension College for Training in Health and Race, Cambridge.
Blackburn, C. (1991) *Poverty and Health*, Open University Press, Milton Keynes.
Bocock, R. (1992) The cultural formations of modern society, in *Formations of Modernity* (eds S. Hall and B. Gieben), Polity Press with Basil Blackwell and The Open University, pp. 230—68.
Bryan, B., Dadzie, S. and Scafe, S. (1985) *Heart of the Race: Black Women's Lives in Britain*, Virago, London.
Department for Education (1993) *The Charter for Higher Education*, DFE, UK.
Department for Education (1994) *Our Children's Education: The Updated Parents' Charter*, DFE, UK.
Department of Health (1994) *The Challenges for Nursing and Midwifery in the 21st Century: A Report of the Heathrow Debate*, May 1993, Department of Health, London.
Durkheim, E. (1957) *Professional Ethics and Civil Morals*, trans. C. Brookfield,

Routledge and Kegan Paul, London.

Durkheim, E. (1964) The Division of Labour in Society, Free Press, New York.

Gramsci, A. (1971) *Selections from the Prison Notebooks*, Lawrence and Wishart, London.

Henry, C., Drew, J., Anwar, N., Benoit-Asselman, D. and Campbell, G. (1992) *EVA Project Report of the Ethics and Values Audit*, University of Central Lancashire.

Johnson, T. (1972) *Professions and Power*, Macmillan, London.

Johnson, T. (1984) Professionalism: occupation or ideology? in *Education for the Professions Quis Custodit ...?* (ed. S. Goodlad), The Society for Research into Higher Education and NFER-NELSON, London.

King Edward's Hospital Fund for London (1990) *Racial Equality: The Nursing Profession,* Equal Opportunities Task Force Paper.

Kronenfeld, J.J. (1993) *Controversial Issues in Health Care Policy*, Sage Publications, Newbury Park.

National Health Service (1991) *The Patient's Charter*, The Department of Health, UK.

Nursing Times (1992) Darbyshire, P. The Core of Nursing, Vol. 38: 36, 44–45.

Porter, S. (1992) Women in a women's job: the gendered experience of nurses, *Sociology of Health and Illness*, Vol. 14, No. 4, 510–27.

Raatikainen, R. (1994) Power and the lack of it in nursing care. *Journal of Advanced Nursing*, **19**, 424–32.

Reid, I. (1989) *Social Class Differences in Britain*, 3rd edn, Fontana Press, UK.

Ryan, A.A. and McKenna, H.P. (1994) A comparative study of the attitudes of nursing and medical students to aspects of patient care and the nurse's role in organizing that care'. *Journal of Advanced Nursing*, **19**, 114–23.

Shaw, J. (1989) Gender and primary schooling, in *The Social Context of Schooling* (ed. M. Cole), Falmer Press, East Sussex, UK.

Social Trends 23 (1993) HMSO, London.

Social Trends 24 (1994) HMSO, London.

Spender, D. (1982) *Invisible Women: The Schooling Scandal*, Writers and Readers Cooperative Society, London.

United Kingdom Central Council (1992) *Code of Professional Conduct*, UKCC, London.

Weber, M. (1986) *Economy and Society*, Bedminster Press, New York.

Whittington, D. and Boore, J. (1989) Competence in nursing in *Professional Competence and Quality Assurance in the Caring Professions* (ed. R. Ellis), Chapman & Hall, London, pp. 109–39.

Wilson, A. and Startup, R. (1991) Nurse socialization: issues and problems. *Journal of Advanced Nursing*, **16**, 1478–86.

Witz, A. (1992) *Professions and Patriarchy*, Routledge, London.

Woolett, A. and Dosanjh-Matwala, N. (1990) Postnatal care: the attitudes and experiences of Asian women in east London. *Midwifery*, **6**, 178–84.

Truth-telling in palliative care: a nursing response

Kevin Kendrick and Pauline Weir

The truth is rarely pure and never simple.

(Oscar Wilde)

We are all going to die. In a world of few certainties the absolute nature of human mortality remains constant. Fear of death or perhaps more fundamentally, what the process of dying will involve, is both common and primal to us all. To a large extent this reflects a biological instinct to survive; it is needed for the continuation of the human species. This theme is further compounded by a societal trend to treat all things relating to death and dying as taboo. With a poignant piece of writing, May (1969: 106) offers a penetrative and powerful reflection, steeped in the kind of language that explains why talk of death and dying is frowned on in most sections of the social milieu:

> Death is obscene, unmentionable, pornographic ... death is a nasty mistake. Death is not to be talked of in front of the children, nor talked about at all if we can help it.

Those of us who have direct contact with dying patients may find it difficult to identify with May's evocative demand that talk of death be avoided. Nursing, as a profession, has always viewed honesty as an important virtue and placed it high on the moral agenda. This has been reinforced and propagated by the stereotypical myth of the nurse as an 'angel' (Holloway, 1992; Kendrick, 1994). Such an image is supported by an almost gut reaction against the possibility that a nurse could ever justifiably tell a lie. Yet dilemmas of practice do throw down challenges to the notion that truth can always be upheld as a universal virtue. Reflecting this theme, Kendrick and Kinsella (1994) state: 'The truth is often hidden behind a veil of secrecy and mystique – lifting it can create both light and shadow.'

What we must ask is 'if telling the truth causes harm can we be morally justified in telling a lie?'. This question holds particular resonance in the delivery of palliative care; examining the moral quagmire which such a query creates forms the focus of our discussion. We begin by considering the impact notions of duty have had on truth-telling in the delivery of healthcare.

A SENSE OF DUTY

Many of the current phrases used in healthcare swell with an implicit demand to conform with the ethos of duty. Terms such as 'accountable' and 'responsible' may be part of an agenda that is concerned with nursing's continual search for professional credence and credibility (Kendrick, 1995), but the underlying theme is concerned with a passivity and alliance to the demands of duty. Research suggests there is a semantic divide between the reality of practice and the words used to describe it (Mackay, 1989, 1993). Thus, there may be rhetorical talk of 'accountable and responsible practice' in the ivory towers of academia, but the frenetic experience of ward life still suggests a compliant acceptance to both duty and hierarchy. These themes are graphically supported by Mackay (1993: 158) who comments on the dynamics of the ward round:

> The structures within which nurses and doctors work ensure that a deferential relationship is perpetuated. The ward round is a good example. The nurse in charge holds the patient's notes for the doctor; when asked, she will offer perhaps a few words about the patient for the doctor's consideration, she prepares the patient for examination and is silent as he examines the patient and decides what action is to be taken. The nurse gives a reassuring smile to the patient and moves with the doctor to the next patient. It is a structured interaction which emphasizes the power between the nurse, the doctor and the patient.

Scenes such as this seem more in keeping with the images offered by the 'Doctor in the House' film genre of the 1950s and it is disquieting to discover such dynamics through the findings of contemporary research. What this does emphasize, however, is the allegiance which nursing holds to duty. This has tremendous impact when applied to truth-telling and two principles which have traditionally been used to analyse and justify decisions in healthcare practice; these two maxims are:

- a duty to do good (beneficence);
- a duty to do no harm (non-maleficence).

DOING GOOD AND AVOIDING HARM

Most nurses would agree that it is an intrinsic part of their remit to do good; similarly, avoiding harm is also a central element of care-giving. However, there are important differences between the two principles; Beauchamp and Childress (1983: 107) support this theme by stating:

> Our duty not to push someone who can swim into deeper water seems stronger than our duty to rescue someone who has accidentally strayed into deep water. It is also morally imperative for us to take substantial risks with our safety in many cases in order not to endanger others, but it is less obvious that even moderate risks are morally required to benefit others.

What emerges from this is that the duty to do no harm is more stringent than the positive principle of to do good. Translating this to a nursing context, there is more emphasis on the practitioner to ensure that any act or omission does not cause patients or colleagues harm than there are on being proactive to promote good. Applying this to pragmatic themes, Johnstone (1989: 78) argues:

> We have a stronger duty not to force a colleague to work (or even to 'rescue' a colleague from working) in an area or care for a patient where that person has sound and just moral or personal reasons for refusing to do so; we may even risk censure by arguing with a nurse supervisor or superior against sending our colleague to the contentious area. We would obviously not have such a strong duty to come to the aid of colleagues who were refusing an assignment just because they 'did not like it' or wished to go off to the beach instead.

The principles of beneficence and non-maleficence run into difficulty when applied to issues of risk/benefit analysis. Sometimes healthcare delivery is not simply a matter of doing good and avoiding harm – interventions involve causing a degree of harm. A simple example is offered by considering the initial pain caused when an intramuscular injection is first plunged into tissue. Hopefully, however, the harm caused is usually validated by the therapeutic effect of the drug, there-fore the net effect is balanced in favour of beneficence. A similar approach can be taken towards the dilemmas involved with truth-telling in palliative care.

It may be said, with reasonable certainty, that truth and honesty are central themes in relationships between patients and practitioners. In most cases, to deal in anything other than the truth can violate trust and destroy any hope of a therapeutic association. However, returning to a question raised earlier in the chapter, if revealing the truth creates more harm than good, can a nurse be morally justified in telling a lie?

CASE STUDY

Consider the following scenario based on a real event from practice; all names used are fictitious:

John is 15 years old. He has been suffering with early-morning nausea and vomiting, violent headaches and an inability to concentrate on his school work. His general practitioner thought this was a virus which would pass in a week or two. However, the symptoms got progressively worse and included faints and a feeling of numbness down the left-hand side of John's body. He was immediately referred to the regional neurological centre for investigations.

The result of these investigations was devastating: John was found to have a particularly aggressive, malignant tumour. Unfortunately, the growth was fixed to vital structures which meant that surgery was not a viable option. John's parents, Jane and Michael, were extremely upset by this news. The consultant neurologist was gently honest and said that the most that could be done was to make John as comfortable as possible in the time left to him. Jane and Michael were enraged. Why could nothing be done for their son? 'There must be something you can do – he's only 15'. The dreadful reality was that nothing could be offered to John and his parents except the fervent hope and desire that palliative care could keep him pain-free and comfortable.

Five days after hearing the news of John's prognosis, Jane and Michael ask to see the senior sister, Pam Ferris. Looking drawn and exhausted, Jane starts to plead with Pam: 'Sister, Mike and I have had a chance to think things through about John. It's really nice that you feel able to say his illness will be closely watched and everything done to make him comfortable. That reassures us, but something else is really bothering us.'

Jane starts to cry and Pam sits quietly waiting for her to carry on in her own time. Mike interjects: 'The point is that we don't want John to know about his illness. At the moment he still thinks that he has a virus. He really couldn't take the news that there was nothing more which could be done ... So if he asks what is wrong he mustn't be told the truth. He just couldn't take it. For goodness sake, he's our little boy.'

Jane and Mike cling to each other, both weeping bitterly. Pam leaves them at what she feels is an intensely private moment and ponders the dilemma which the team now face; do they really have the right to tell a 15-year-old boy that he is going to die when the people who love and know him better than anybody else plead against it? Do health professionals have a moral mandate to override such knowledge?

COLLUSION: FIST OF STEEL OR VELVET GLOVE?

The type of dilemma which Pam is being asked to engage in is sometimes known as 'collusion'. It involves an understanding that the news of a poor prognosis be kept from the patient. The mores that inform interaction between people would not normally tolerate this form of dynamic. However, such views are confronted when relatives or significant others put forward the sort of powerful sentiments which have occurred in the previous scenario. Relatives who seek collusion often argue that they are in a much better position to understand what their loved one can and cannot take.

Reflecting on the reasons why relatives put forward requests such that the truth of a poor prognosis be kept from the patient, Kendrick and Shea (1995: 9) comment:

> A prognosis which indicates that death is inevitable confronts the most primal elements of the human condition. It is understandable that relatives sometimes request or even demand that such devastatingly 'bad news' be kept from a loved one. The essential reason for this is to try and protect the dying person from the ravages inherent to such an announcement. Underpinning this is a firm belief that it is in the dying person's 'best interests' not to know that death is approaching.

What emerges from this is a convincing mandate from John's parents to keep the truth from him. Initially this can take both a direct and indirect form. If John were specifically to ask what was wrong with him, the nurse being questioned could either omit to tell the truth by, for example, conveniently side-stepping the issue, a common ruse being: 'I'll get the doctor to have a word with you.' Alternatively, the nurse may choose to take the more direct route and lie to John by saying, for example, 'These viruses can take an eternity to clear up.' Approaches of this nature are usually offered under the guise of a patriarchal impulse intended to protect the patient from the truth. Despite the good intent that may support such themes, a host of ethical indicators highlight the harm that can emerge from such reasoning.

TRUTH AS A CASUALTY

The very nature of collusion means that truth will be a casualty. If practitioners and relatives enter into a covert understanding which alienates a dying person from knowledge of the prognosis, the threads of a therapeutic bond become violated and torn. What can emerge from this is a scenario born of deceit and disingenuous encounters. The intent underpinning collusion is often to protect the dying person from the news of an inevitable death from a pathology which cannot be cured. Unfortunately, once such a position is taken it can have dire repercussions for the dynamics between all those involved with the dying person. Reflecting these themes, Kendrick and Kinsella (1994) state: 'Once we have entered into the dangerous scenario of collusion it leads to a constant striving to avoid tumbling down the slippery slope into a swirling vortex of lies, misrepresentation and fabrication.'

Returning once more to the earlier scenario, Jane and Mike would love to protect John from the news of the brain tumour and what it will inevitably mean. However, the loss of autonomy and trust which can result from collusion can hardly be justified: the opportunity for John to reflect on his life and make sense of it should not be taken from him under the guise of beneficence. In a seminal work on medical ethics, the moral theologian Bernard Haring (1974: 45) explores the ethical issues surrounding collusion:

> Loving care for the dying is one of the supreme expressions of our respect for the human person and of truthful relationship with him … To deceive a dying person about the most crucial personal and awesome fact of his life, his approaching death, is to treat him like an object. It can mean robbing him of the most decisive act of freedom.

The use of the word 'object' gives the thrust of Haring's argument definite focus and direction. What this establishes is that in colluding against the truth, relatives and practitioners deny the dying person the status of being a valued subject. In logical sequence, this inevitably means that the patient becomes an object. This shift in perception and emphasis has a long history in the way that dying people are treated (Menzies, 1970; McIntosh, 1977; Hanson, 1994). The cliché which is often used to highlight this shift from valued subject to object is when a practitioner refers to the patient as, for example, 'the CA in the side ward'.

This part of the chapter has dealt with the difficult ethical themes involved with collusion. We have discovered that the beneficent base which is used to support collusion crumbles when faced with the affront it can cause to honesty, openness, autonomy and trust. Commenting on the destructive aspects of deceit, Korsgaard (1986) cites Immanual Kant who stated: 'Whatever militates against frankness lowers the dignity of man.' Practitioners sometimes use language as a veil to hide from their own vulnerability and fear of mortality (Bond, 1982; Maguire, 1985). This flailing in the shadows of semantics is understandable, but denying someone access to the truth about the nature of a terminal illness not only shatters any basis for an open dialogue but threatens the therapeutic themes which palliative care can offer.

In the final section of this chapter, we take these themes further and consider the notion of truth-telling in relation to the difficult and direct question of: 'Am I going to die, nurse?'

'CARE TO BE HONEST'

No matter how experienced we become, the question: 'Am I going to die, nurse?' is never easy to answer. There is nothing vague or ambiguous about the question. We do not have to use mirroring skills or explore the cues to make further inferences; the question is simply put and very direct. Indeed, this focused approach can catch us off guard. There is nowhere to hide when a dying person makes such an enquiry and the choice is clear: we either lie or tell the truth.

There are usually two main reasons put forward to support lying:

- adherence to the principle 'do no harm';
- patients do not want to know the truth.

As we have already seen with the problem of collusion, the notion that healthcare delivery can ever be 'free of harm' is Utopian. If a person has the courage to ask so plainly about their mortality, then it deserves to be answered in a similar fashion. This does not mean that revealing the truth to a person about their impending death will be easy, either for the patient or the nurse, but it does free the dying person to face death with an open, informed gaze. Such an approach is supported by Hebblethwaite (1991: 78) who argues: 'There is a recognition that "the truth" will almost inevitably be painful and almost nothing can make it painless, but we must be careful not to underestimate anyone's inner resources.'

In relation to the second premise in defence of lying, there is little doubt that some patients do not want to be told the truth about their impending mortality. However, Bok (1978) revealed that 80% of patients wanted to know the truth about their condition and prognosis. Supporting this approach, Gillon (1985: 105): states: 'There are difficulties to overcome, but avoiding deceit is a basic moral norm, defensible from several moral perspectives.' Similar themes are echoed by Faulder (1985: 89) who states: 'In asking patients to trust them it would seem only fair that doctors should reward that trust by dealing honestly with them.' All this must be tempered by the notion that news of a poor diagnosis should always be revealed as gently as possible and in a way which is dictated by the patient.

The consequences of not dealing truthfully with a dying person can be catastrophic. Sometimes practitioners enter into the fragile world of word games to try to avoid a direct confrontation with the truth. Over the years we have heard many vague and evasive responses to the question: 'Am I going to die, nurse?' For example: 'We are all going to die, the big question is when'; 'I thought the doctor told you that it was a tumour. I never heard the word cancer mentioned'; 'What sort of a question is that to ask when you are looking so well?'

Commenting on the way in which nurses sometimes hide behind words, Kendrick (1994) states: 'We do not "disguise the truth", "tell fibs" or offer "white lies". Such terms are mere rhetoric. We either lie or tell the truth. Terms such as "to be economical with the truth" are a moral smoke-screen and do not negate the moral weight of a lie.'

If we do decide to keep the truth of impending death from a patient, it can violate any of the therapeutic themes which have been established. To be the victim of lies and deceit at the end of life can volley the dying person into a disenfranchized state where those who were thought to be trustworthy become the conduits of subterfuge. The only substantive reason that would justify a dying person being left in a state of unknowing is a clear expression of not wanting to hear about a terminal prognosis. To impose such news on someone who did not want to be privy to it profanes autonomy and trust in much the same way as withholding such information does to the individual who expresses a desire to know.

NURSING A TRUTHFUL DIALOGUE

The key task of this chapter has been to examine the main moral issues which emerge from the question: 'If telling the truth causes harm, can we be morally justified in telling a lie?' We have seen that the pragmatic considerations which emerge from this question cannot simply be viewed as a matter of doing good and avoiding harm. In relation to truth-telling and palliative care, revealing to patients that their death is fast approaching may evoke feelings of horror and disbelief. However, there may also be a feeling of relief – that at least something has been found which can be labelled and seen as the cause of illness. Professional experience often reveals that patients find the 'not knowing' more unbearable than the harsh reality that life is coming to an end (Hanson, 1994). Being honest about a prognosis which indicates that life will end does give the patient a tremendous blow. However, such news, if offered gently and with a velvet glove, is easier to take than the devastation of trust and honesty which lying and deceit means for the dying person.

It is extremely difficult to envisage a situation in palliative care where lying could ever be morally justified. We have argued that the therapeutic relationship between the nurse and a dying person becomes shallow, defiled and even irreconcilable once lying and deceit have entered it. Reflecting these themes, Kendrick (1994: 677) states: 'The patient's vulnerability adds another dimension to the importance of truthfulness – to lie to such a person hacks at the structures on which so many frail defences are placed. To expose patients to such an affront can rarely be justified within a process so intrinsically concerned with caring.' The alternative to honesty and openness is a scenario of hushed whispers, hidden agendas, collusion, deceit and lying. Surely such elements can never be reconcilable with the central themes of nursing.

REFERENCES

Beauchamp, T.L. and Childress, J.F. (1983) *Principles of Biomedical Ethics*, Oxford University Press, Oxford.

Bok, S. (1978) *Lying: Moral Choice in Public and Private Lives*, Harvester Press, East Sussex.

Bond, S. (1982) Communication in cancer nursing, in *Recent Advances in Cancer Nursing*, (ed. M. Cahoon) Churchill Livingstone, Edinburgh.

Faulder, C. (1985) *Whose Body Is It? The Troubling Issue of Informed Consent*, Virago Press, London.

Gillon, R. (1985) *Philosophical Medical Ethics*, John Wiley, Chichester.

Hanson, E. (1994) *The Cancer Nurse's Perspective*, Quay Publishers, Lancaster.

Haring, B. (1974) *Medical Ethics*, St Paul Publications, Slough.

Hebblethwaite, M. (1991) Shall we pretend it isn't happening? *Journal of Advances in Health and Nursing Care*, **1**, 2.

Holloway, J. (1992) The media representation of the nurse: the implications for nursing, in *Themes and Perspectives in Nursing* (eds K. Soothill, I.C. Henry and K. Kendrick), Chapman & Hall, London.

Johnstone, M.J. (1989) *Bioethics: a Nursing Perspective*, Bailliere Tindall, London.

Kendrick, K. (1994) Should nurses always tell the truth? Honesty versus deception in health care. *Professional Nurse*, **9**, 10.

Kendrick, K. (1995) Nurses and doctors: a problem of partnership, in *Interprofessional Relations in Health Care* (eds K. Soothill, L. Mackay and C. Webb), Edward Arnold, London.

Kendrick, K. and Kinsella, M. (1994) Beyond the veil: truth-telling in palliative care. *Journal of Cancer Care*, **3**, 211–15.

Kendrick, K. and Shea, T. (1995) With velvet gloves: the ethics of collusion. *Palliative Care Today*, **IV**, 1.

Korsgaard, C.M. (1986) The right to lie: Kant on dealing with evil. *Philosophy and Public Affairs*, **15**, 336.

Mackay, L. (1989) *Nursing a Problem*, Open University Press, Milton Keynes.

Mackay, L. (1993) *Conflicts in Care: Medicine and Nursing*, Chapman & Hall, London.

Maguire, P. (1985) Barriers to psychological care of the dying. *British Medical Journal*, **291**, 1711–13.

May, R. (1969) *Love and Will*, Dell, New York.

McIntosh, I. (1977) *Communication and Awareness in a Cancer Ward*, Croom Helm, London.

Menzies, I. (1970) *Communication and Stress: a Nursing Perspective*, Macmillan, London.

19 Professional values with specific reference to midwifery

Jeanne Siddiqui

IDENTIFICATION OF VALUES

According to Raths, Harmin and Simon (1966), the process of valuing, or holding values consists of three sub-processes: (a) prizing one's own beliefs and behaviours; (b) choosing those beliefs and behaviours; and (c) acting on those beliefs. The noun 'value', signifies worth, merit, account, benefit, calibre, desirability and eminence. These meanings are expressed in relative terms, whereas the verb 'value' usually indicates price or cost. Professional values, while indicating all the meritorious aspects already mentioned, also carry a cost in terms of professional practice.

Values, like beliefs, may be influenced by what is fashionable. Indeed, values, like customs, are embedded in cultural heritage, experience and personal belief systems. They are part of a person's self-concept; those beliefs or behaviours that are held as important (valuable) make the individual. Sartre (cited in Anderson, Hughes and Sharrock, 1986: 98), novelist and philosopher, referred throughout his literary work to the essence of man. Sartre maintains that we are all in the process of 'becoming' and that man makes his own history by the values he holds: 'The taking of choices and the construction of being in our lives is the exercising of freedom and responsibility.

Values are often adopted because of the moral good their actions cause. The two main perspectives used to determine values are the consequentialist and deontological ethical theories. The consequentialist theory is the prominent feature in utilitarianism. Utilitarians propose that the moral rightness of an action should be judged by its consequences which should lead to a generally accepted goal or value such as pleasure, knowledge, health, beauty and friendship. These values are said to be non-moral because they are generally accepted as the consequences of good, proper human action.

The deontologist would argue that because the consequences of an action are good, it does not follow that the moral rightness of an action is always proved. For example, if the action involves telling a lie to spare someone from distress, the utilitarian would justify that although telling lies is generally not a good thing, the consequences of telling the truth would be more damaging or cause harm, so in the interests of ensuring the greatest happiness for all concerned, the utilitarian would rationalize the action. The deontologist, however, would hold that telling lies is never justified and that to tell the truth is morally right regardless of the consequences; so truth-telling should be adopted as a general value. An important feature of the utilitarian perspective is that there is intrinsic value in some conditions that does not vary from person to person, such as health and freedom from pain; therefore these are the conditions we ought to produce in human life (Beauchamp and Childress, 1989). This idea of intrinsic worth is often applied to professional values that are identified as good and lead to 'good practice'.

Values may vary from culture to culture, from group to group and from person to person and identifying shared values may be a difficult task. However, real problems may arise when attempting to apply values, principles, theories and rules to particular actions, particularly during a climate of professional or organizational change. For example, when asked about the recent government recommendations in the Patient's Charter (DOH, 1992), a consultant obstetrician (Siddiqui, 1995) commented:

> I really do feel that it is all a façade, I really hate much of what is happening in the NHS now. I hate all this business in the wards, this 'named nurse', 'welcome' over the doors. When did you welcome anyone to a sick ward? Would you put 'welcome' up in funeral parlours?

This response indicates that this practitioner does not share the newly emerging 'business' values which demonstrate commitment to consumer satisfaction.

COMMITMENT TO VALUES

Values that are based on abstract concepts such as autonomy, advocacy and accountability are prized as personal and professional principles; however, the realization of these values in practice may be fundamentally flawed by a conflict in their interpretation. Jenny (1979: 177) examined the ethical obligation of nurses to act as advocates for patients:

> Although some nurses interpreted the advocate role as an affirmation of traditional protective obligation, others believed that the role required a more assertive stance concerning patients' rights.

Other commentators have identified that the nature of the advocate role is not straightforward. Chadwick and Tadd (1992: 22) comment:

> This notion of advocacy, either as a defender of patient rights or as patient representative, also appears to be fraught with difficulty and contradiction.

The significance of a professional value such as advocacy is in the commitment practitioners have in promoting it in practice. While values may be adopted by a profession as an ethos, the members of that profession may hold varying depths of belief and commitment to it. Practitioners may be at variance with the degree they would be prepared to go in practising values or upholding principles. This potential inconsistency may negate the moral worth behind a value. Much of the conflict surrounding professional values, such as advocacy, occur because of the dichotomy of the role of the nurse or midwife. The United Kingdom Central Council for Nursing, Midwifery and Health Visitors in the *Code of Professional Conduct* (1992) implicitly encourages a deontological approach: 'Act always in such a manner as to promote and safeguard the interests and well-being of patients and clients' (Clause 1).

This directive indicates a 'duty to care', yet it may be compromised by the following utilitarian standpoint which can be drawn from the same document: 'Work in a collaborative and co-operative manner with health-care professionals and others in providing care and recognize and respect their particular contribution within the care team' (Clause 6).

This lack of clarity from the UKCC is compounded by the fact that in the past, nurses and midwives have been educated and socialized in an environment where compliance and obedience to the doctor was the rule.

If advocacy was valued equally by all the health professionals, the difficulty in practising this value would be negligible. However, in the author's research, varying degrees of commitment to advocacy are displayed, particularly if the client disregarded medical advice. One general practitioner (Siddiqui, 1995) commented:

> Well, I think advocacy comes into it, but after all we are there to advise what is best. If we left it up to the patient to make all the decisions, we would be failing them ... they expect us to come up with the answers.

This response is interesting, for the respondent clearly feels that his advice is the most important element in the caring relationship. In contrast, the British Medical Association (BMA, 1986: 29) takes a different view:

'Doctors offer advice, but it is the patient who decides whether or not to accept the advice'.

A different perspective was articulated by a midwife respondent (Siddiqui, 1995):

> I think advocacy is very important because pregnancy can place the woman in a very vulnerable position. Women often find it difficult to voice their opinions. The midwife can then step in and after talking to the woman can act on her behalf and put forward her views. I think it is really important. Sometimes a woman can be intimidated by the doctor and may have difficulty really saying how she feels.

Realistically, expressing concern about the autonomy of the client is much easier than advocating for it. In the recent past, practitioners may have adopted a stance of 'bystander apathy' in relation to professional values. An example of this is often seen in ante-natal clinics when a woman requests a home confinement. This choice may be denied her by the consultant obstetrician because he feels it is safer to have the baby in hospital, even though no valid evidence exists for this reasoning for all women. The midwife may avoid advocating for women's choice in these circumstances, even though she knows she ought to, because the consequences might cause conflict with the obstetrician. The vulnerable client and the principle of advocacy become less valued than maintaining a peaceful collaboration with the doctor.

Another example of inconsistent commitment to values is with regard to breast-feeding. Midwives are taught that breast-feeding is the best and safest method of feeding an infant, therefore it should be valued as being good. However, breast-feeding rates in Britain remain disappointingly low and many mothers claim that conflicting advice and midwives' attitudes reflect a lack of commitment to the value of breast-feeding (Rajan, 1993).

SUPREMACY OF VALUES

Caring and respect for others may be considered a universal value for all health workers and, by its implication, caring has the notion of being 'good' or moral. Thompson, Melia and Boyd (1988: 68–9) discuss the conflict that may occur within multidisciplinary teams where one group may have held professional supremacy over the other members of the team in the past:

> As the emergence of different professions has been marked by the formal differentiation of rules and the demarcation of different

areas of responsibility or functions within healthcare, so each has developed its own peculiar set of values.

Burnard and Chapman (1988) cite examples of interprofessional conflict relating to moral or ethical issues such as euthanasia, abortion and genetic engineering. More commonly, conflict may occur related to values that are more abstract and demand reflection by the individual regarding what stance to take. Conflicts occur related to values that, while not life-and-death issues, can make all the difference to the 'quality' of care received by the patient. In the book and film *One Flew Over the Cuckoo's Nest* (Kesey, 1962) the vulnerable patient was disempowered by the senior nurse in the establishment. Instead of other nurses challenging this behaviour, it was a fellow patient who could not reconcile the conflict of his value of respect for persons with the behaviour of the nurse. The nurse seemed to value her own status or power above that of her clients.

It may be that the motives for the action spring from a moral or 'good' perspective (the duty ethic) and the individual professional may rationalize the action and condone it according to a utilitarian perspective. This may lead to double standards and confusion within and outside of the profession. Women undergoing termination of pregnancy for reasons of congenital abnormality provide a good example of this kind of double standard arising from inconsistent values. These women may be treated differently from other women undergoing therapeutic abortion for personal reasons. The former are often cared for by midwives in a delivery suite with compassion and empathy. The latter are cared for in gynaecological wards, placed on routine operating lists and quickly discharged home. The subliminal message is that it is acceptable and even encouraged to terminate a pregnancy when the risk and cost to society is of another handicapped member, while to make the same choice based on personal values is deemed less noble.

While caring and respect for others may be considered universal values for all health professionals, conflicts arise when personal values are used to judge the moral actions of others. It is important to identify our personal values and to know how they influence our interaction with others. It is also vital to recognize the value systems of others and understand the effects of imposing one set of values on a person or persons whose values are in conflict with another. This is even more important when working in multiprofessional teams where supremacy of values may be dictated by authoritative knowledge. Cultural snobbery may be substituted for values and people with strong values are held to be unique, eccentric or radical depending on the amount of discomfort their values cause to their peers: Florence Nightingale, Joseph Lister, James Ballantyne and contemporaries Wendy Savage and Graham Pink are a few examples of people who challenge care that has previously been accepted as models of good practice. The well-known surgeon and epidemiologist, the late Denis Burkitt, renowned for his research into cancer, argued that the most important ingredients for successful research may not be high intelligence, ample funding and a sophisticated back-up. His epigram, written when signing copies of his books, reflected his values and provides a refreshing change from the usual positivist outlook of the medical profession (BMJ, 1993):

Attitudes are more important than abilities.
Motives are more important than methods.
Character is more important than cleverness.
Perseverance is more important than power.
And the heart takes precedence over the head.

If all health professionals are to completely experience the essence of caring and increase their level of understanding of human beings, the social sciences and humanities must be held in equal value by doctors, nurses, midwives and other health professionals. The medical profession must abandon its reductionist model of education based on cause-and-effect principles; and midwifery and nurse education must similarly review the models of care that are focused on processes and problems rather than the individual.

Nursing and midwifery education has promoted professional values and attitudes which have reinforced these caring professions as being subordinate to medicine by the continuation of a bureaucratic hierarchical structure. Stein (1978, in Soothill, Henry and Kendrick, 1992:165), states:

The value system into which nurses are socialized can be seen to emphasize hierarchy of authority, ritualistic behaviour and excessive role portrayal in everyday clinical practice.

This adherence to a philosophy, whereby everything must be judged in an objective and controlled way, has led to the problematic ethical issues faced by doctors, nurses and midwives when man and his world are in conflict. Values or moral principles (ethics) by their very nature are formed on the basis of the behaviour of mankind and of what is acceptable in the world and society in which they live.

Anderson, Hughes and Sharrock (1986: 83–4) examine the claim of 'scientific' knowledge that it had somehow wrenched itself free of subjectivity:

All knowledge begins in the consciousness, in subjectivity, even science. The 'impersonal', 'objective' rules of scientific procedures and argument are just as rooted in consciousness as any other form of knowledge.

It is therefore important to place in context the demands of supremacy of values based on a claim of scientific knowledge.

Dewey (1960: xx–xxi) in his reconstruction of philosophy states:

> The present reach and thrust of what originates as science affects disturbingly every aspect of contemporary life; from the state of the family and the position of women and children, through the conduct and problems of education, through the fine as well as the industrial arts, into political and economic relations of association that are natural and developing with such rapidity, that they do not lend themselves to generalized statement. Moreover, their occurrence presents so many and such serious practical issues demanding immediate attention that man has been kept too busy meeting them piecemeal to make a generalized or intellectual observation of them. They came like a thief in the night, taking us unawares.

One of the major difficulties facing midwives today is attempting to practise according to a philosophy that is opposed to the medical control and interventionist methods of obstetrics. Tew (1990: 20) points out that: 'One philosophy cannot take precedence over the other unless its practitioners likewise take that precedence'.

The message is clear: if midwives wish to empower women through the care they give, the philosophy of the profession must be supported by action. Many professional values demand a standard of practice that is based on principles that have **moral** implications. For example, it may be held morally right to value the principle of respect for life and support the notion of respect for persons but if the concept of respect for person is unclear, there will be conflict in the values relating to the respect for human life.

Henry (1986: 26) illustrates how important the practical application of a concept is if it is to be acknowledged as part of a professional philosophy:

> The concept of care, like the concept of the person, does not have a formal definition and it is, therefore, difficult to ground in any formal foundational knowledge. However, it may be possible to ground both concepts in commonsense knowledge.

In other words, we construct our own meaning and this becomes accepted through social recognition because of the language we use. Henry continues to explore the concept of persons and proposes that the ascription of personhood depends on an understanding of several concepts, one of them being 'human'. The term human is descriptive but includes a norm or standard to its use. The description refers to being a member of a biological species and the semi-normative element to the value we place on having human features.

Sometimes we use the term 'person' to mean the same thing as 'human' when in fact they are not synonymous. According to Teichman (1985) the term human-being is used as a starting point for the term person. Wittgenstein (cited in Winch,1958) holds the view that the understanding and meaning of terms and concepts are not to be found in logical analysis but in their use within the particular 'language game' to which they belong. In fact, the two terms, human and person, may be used by different groups to mean different things by emphasizing the different elements. So, for example, biologists may use the descriptive element of the term 'human' as indicating classification to the 'human species' by identification of certain physiological features while, in contrast, midwives and nurses tend to use the term 'human' in an altogether different context, emphasizing the semi-normative element of the term, for example, 'He's only human' indicating fallibility. In this example, the language places 'value' on the 'person' traits and so demonstrates the confusion between the term 'human' and the concept of the 'person'.

Once we begin to place a value or price on certain features of humanity, it is easy to see how our values and principles may alter. We only have to look at the determination with which medical science is working in the fields of genetics to see that the goal is human perfection and by implication anything other than this is valued less.

CONCLUSION

Ayn Rand (1964: 21), a contemporary philosopher and novelist, analyses the concept of 'value'. She maintains that values arise from and are necessitated by the distinctive nature of living organisms:

> A value is that which one acts to gain or keep. A value is the object of action; it is that which can be secured only by action. Values presuppose the existence of an entity to which things are a value, an entity capable of acting to achieve values, an entity capable of initiating goal-directed behaviour. Values further presuppose the existence of ALTERNATIVES, in the face of which action is necessary. If there are no alternatives, then no goals and hence no values are possible.

When examining professional and personal values, it is important to see them in practice, i.e. contextually. The significance is in the commitment we have to our values and beliefs and these should be measured by the extent of our actions, not the length and wordiness of our written philosophies. Therefore a philosophy of practice must make clear the factors which influence our actions. It should provide a direction-giving statement, which may in part be idealistic and may represent the longer-term intentions and goals; it should reflect the shared values of all the participants which have been identified through appropriate research. An example of this type of research was carried out by Henry *et al.* (1992) through an ethics and values audit (EVA) which examined the values and principles of educationalists, managers and students in a university setting. They suggest that similar research may be used to the advantage of health professionals, particularly during times of organizational change.

Clearly, many changes are taking place in midwifery practice. Midwives, however, cannot rely solely on the whim of political support or depend on the vocal minority of those women who are brave enough to demand choices. Midwives must identify their true beliefs about their profession. They must value them and demonstrate their depth of commitment to these values by acting in accordance with them through the principles of care.

REFERENCES

Anderson, R.J., Hughes, J.A., Sharrock, W.W. (1986) *Philosophy and The Human Sciences*, Croom Helm, London.

Beauchamp, T.L. and Childress, J.F. (1989) *Principles of Biomedical Ethics*, 3rd edn, Oxford University Press, Oxford.

British Medical Association (1986) *Philosophy and Practice of Medical Ethics*, BMA, London.

British Medical Journal (1993) *Obituary: Denis Burkitt*, April.

Burnard, P. and Chapman, C.M. (1988) Professional and ethical issues in nursing, in *The Professional Code of Conduct*, HM & M Nursing Publications, John Wiley, Sons, Chichester, pp. 25–6.

Chadwick, R. and Tadd, W. (1992) *Ethics and Nursing Practice: A Case Study Approach*, Macmillan, London.

Department of Health (1992) NHS Management Executive, *The Patient's Charter and Primary Health Care*, EL (92) **88**, 30 Nov.

Dewey, J. (1960) *Reconstruction in Philosophy*, Beacon Press, Baston.

Henry, C. (1986) The concept of the person, Unpublished PhD thesis, Leeds University.

Henry, C., Drew, J., Anwar, N., Campbell, G. and Benoit-Asselman, D. (1992) *The EVA project: Ethics and Values Audit*, University of Central Lancashire, Preston.

Jenny, J. (1979) *Patient advocacy – another role for nursing?* International Nursing Review, **26**, 176–81.

Kesey, K. (1962) *One Flew Over the Cuckoo's Nest*, Picador, Pan Publications, London.

Rajan, L. (1993) The contribution of professional support, information and consistent correct advice to successful breast feeding. *Midwifery*, **9**(4), 197–209.

Rand, A. (1964) *The Virtue of Selfishness,* New York Publishing, New America Library, New York.

Raths, L., Harmin, M. and Simon, S. (1966) *Values and Teaching*, Merrill, Columbus Ohio.

Sartre, J.P. (1905–80) cited in *Philosophy and the Human Sciences* (1986), (eds R.J. Anderson, J.A. Hughes and W.W. Sharrock), Croom Helm, London, pp. 97–9.

Siddiqui, J. (1995) Conceptions of midwifery – a study of forms of knowledge and values foundational for midwifery, Unpublished MPhil Thesis, University of Central Lancashire.

Soothill, K., Henry, C. and Kendrick, K. (1992) *Themes and Perspectives in Nursing*, Chapman & Hall, London.

Stein, L. (1978) The nurse-doctor game, in *Readings in Sociology for Nursing*, (eds R. Dingwall and J. McIntosh), Churchill Livingstone, Edinburgh.

Teichman, J. (1985) The definition of person. *Philosophy*, **60**, 175–85.

Tew, M. (1990) *Safer Childbirth: A Critical History of Maternity Care*, Chapman & Hall, London.

Thompson, I.E., Melia, K.M. and Boyd, K.M. (1988) *Nursing Ethics*, 2nd edn, Churchill Livingstone, Edinburgh.

United Kingdom Central Council for Nursing, Midwifery and Health Visitors (1992) *The Code of Professional Conduct*, UKCC, London.

Winch, P. (1958) *The Idea of a Social Science and its Relation to Philosophy*, Routledge & Kegan Paul, London.

Wittgenstein, L. (1889–1951) cited in Winch, P. (1958) *The Idea of a Social Science and its Relation to Philosophy*, Routledge & Kegan Paul, London.

PART III

Managing and Delivering Care

Keith Soothill, Catherine Williams and Jon Barry (Chapter 20) argue that nurse turnover is not merely a problem for management but can also have an effect on the delivery of care. The issue of nurse turnover is much more complicated than is generally recognized and, at present, available information is not being properly or fully used to answer the important questions. They also discuss how specialized surveys can, when combined with information routinely collected on computer by personnel departments, produce useful insights into this often puzzling phenomenon. The views not just of nurses working within the NHS but also of those who have left it can provide interesting perspectives.

David Worthington's purpose (Chapter 21) is to introduce nurses and prospective nurses to the concept and potential value of nurse supply modelling in the current planning context. A clear discussion of this technical topic focusing on some of the important issues related to the practical application of nurse supply modelling leads to an assessment of its likely role and value to the nursing profession and to the health service, now and in the future.

The increasing consolidation of Project 2000 has presented the profession with a structure which is revolutionizing the nature of nurse education. However, this change also has implications for a number of traditional groups responsible for certain aspects of care-giving. Emily Griffiths (Chapter 22) considers the role of the nursing auxiliary with particular reference to recent changes. The introduction of the new support worker presents a stark innovation to the traditional role of the auxiliary. Griffiths presents a research-based chapter which vividly illustrates the feelings of auxiliary nurses working at a grassroots level.

Elizabeth Hanson (Chapter 23) tackles the sensitive issue of stress levels among persons with cancer. This chapter is firmly based on research findings and illustrates the importance of understanding the concepts of stress if an effective basis for care is to be achieved. The very notion of cancer is fraught with fear about death, suffering and the unknown in general. If we are even to approximate towards an understanding of the fear and anxiety which persons with cancer suffer, it is necessary to consider the mechanisms involved in stress formation. The rationale Hanson presents can help to achieve this in the delivery of care.

The current transformation of the NHS means a re-evaluation of the various strategies of response by workers to management initiatives. Paul Bagguley (Chapter 24) considers the organizations that represent the nurses' interests and the changing contexts in which they are operating. Hence, his main focus is on nurses' professional organizations and trade unions. While providing a review of the current situation, he also indicates how hazardous it is to comment on possible developments, as the situation is changing so rapidly.

Finally, Stephen Ackroyd (Chapter 25) focuses on the varying effects of traditional and new management on nursing while emphasizing that the management of public services has always been a very different type of activity from management in most parts of the private sector. He argues that a participative management pattern, where nurses have a central role, does most to preserve and promote the best aspects of public services. Ackroyd maintains that this model is preferable to the forms of management, largely based on private sector service, which are being actively promoted by government policy at the present time.

Understanding nurse turnover | 20

Keith Soothill, Catherine Williams and Jon Barry

INTRODUCTION

Concern about nursing turnover has a long history but different emphases emerge at different times. More than 20 years ago the influential Briggs Report (1972) noted how 'often it has been assumed that wastage rates among nurses and midwives are abnormally high compared with those found in other walks of life' (para. 418). However, when it came to examine the evidence, the complexity of the issue soon began to emerge. Certainly the focus in the 1972 Report was on 'wastage' with the suggestion that 'a high wastage would be a significant indicator of dissatisfaction' (para. 418). Paradoxically, by the late 1970s, it was the concern about a stagnant workforce with insufficient turnover which some (e.g. Redfern, 1978) began to recognize as an equally serious problem. In contrast, by the mid-1980s, concern about the problems of recruitment in the NHS (e.g. Dickson, 1987; Hancock, 1986) became linked with worries about the high level of turnover among nurses already employed (Price Waterhouse, 1988; Martin and Mackean, 1988; Waite, Buchan and Thomas, 1989).

Concerns about recruitment became especially acute at a time in the 1980s when there were fears of a projected shortfall of 18-year-olds eligible to enter nursing. Then, it appeared impossible to overcome the problems of a high leaving rate by training more nurses. While mutterings about the dangers of a 'demographic timebomb' were widespread, there were alternative scenarios of the future also being expounded. So, for example, Grocott (1989) argued that nurse wastage was not going to be a major problem because, while the numbers of new learners were certainly declining, the total workforce was actually increasing; in other words, more previously qualified nurses were going back into nursing.

Few, however, anticipated the emerging issues of the 1990s and so, for example, the concern among the unions about the significantly increasing numbers of 'bank nurses' or on-call staff and agency staff produces a different agenda from the traditional concerns about recruitment and retention. As Maggie Dunn, chair of the nursing unions' negotiating team, recently proclaimed, 'What we are seeing is the casualization of the nursing workforce' (*The Guardian*, 22 September 1994). Certainly there are significant shifts and it is difficult to predict the future. The government's recent evidence to the Review Body for Nursing Staff calling for no national pay rise is accompanied by a plea to allow NHS trusts to award local pay rises linked to performance. Hence, it is clear that the on-going repercussions of the National Health Service market on the nursing workforce are still far from exhausted.

Hopefully, this brief introduction has highlighted that the problems in relation to nurse recruitment and turnover can quickly fluctuate. Indeed, following the recognition of a new problem there is often confusion as to whose problem it is and, more insidiously, a scapegoat is usually found to blame. It is often seen that the nurse is the problem. However, the starting point must be that nurse wastage and nurse turnover needs to be recognized as a complicated issue. We argue that, without a proper understanding of the problem, effective management is impossible.

We begin with a brief discussion of nurse wastage and offer ideas about how it might be defined in different situations. We follow this analysis by examining whether wastage is a major problem today and, if so, which aspects are most important. Finally, we discuss the implications of our findings for nurse managers.

IDENTIFYING THE PROBLEM

Before a manager can decide whether nurse turnover is a problem and, if so, what to do about it, it is essential that they are clear about what wastage actually means. Unfortunately, a clear definition is not always obvious.

In the academic literature, nurse wastage has mostly been used as a general term to describe the number of nurses leaving in some given time period. That is, it has been taken as another word for nurse turnover. However, we feel that the phrase 'nurse wastage' which was a particularly pervasive term when we first started to study the phenomenon a decade ago encompasses more than the narrow definition of nurse turnover.

'Nurse wastage' became a popular phrase not only among health authority planners but also among journalists, social scientists and, in particular, nurses themselves. In fact, wastage is an emotive term. In the dictionary the meaning of waste is peppered with pejorative terms such as: unproductive, desolate, useless expenditure (Chambers, 1988). To waste is quite simply a bad thing. Why is such an emotionally loaded term sometimes used?

Language has been called 'the garment of thought', and it is important to try to tease out the underlying thinking when words are used. Words used judgmentally imply that one group is making a judgment of another group. And here is the rub for nurses. Nurses always seem to be the ones who are being judged. The language is instructive. Ask what 'nursing wastage' means. When talking about the topic to acquaintances, many thought that nursing wastage meant all the equipment, dressings, etc. that nurses wasted! Certainly the term 'wastage' is one which nurses readily internalize. It has intimations of sin, guilt and letting down the service. Nursing still retains enough of the notions of a vocation to suggest that nurses who leave are rejecting their calling. So all this adds to the pressure nurses already suffer in trying to conform to the popular image of the caring, all-giving nurse without being regarded as a waste if she takes a break from nursing or turns her ambitions to the apparently greener grasses of other occupations.

The crucial problem, though, is that 'wastage' has too readily been seen as a problem created by nurses leaving – they're to blame – rather than generating any attempt to begin to consider more fundamental structural reasons which may actually create the problem. Certainly, though, before considering who's to blame, one needs a mechanism by which to calculate the problem.

When a nurse leaves, however, there are at least two kinds of repercussions. First, there is the obvious loss of the training and experience that the nurse has already gained; and second, there is the cost of recruiting new staff. Incidentally, there are some other, less obvious, forms of wastage that can still take place while a nurse is still in post. For example, wastage could also be considered in terms of absenteeism or lack of commitment due to becoming disillusioned with the job. Sickness, absenteeism and low morale are exhibited by nurses who, in broad terms, either cannot leave or choose not to. That is, potential work is being wasted because a nurse is not happy with what they are doing. Another 'hidden' form of wastage occurs when a shortage of specialized nurses causes unqualified or non-specialized nurses to be employed in these specialized positions. This type of wastage, while difficult to measure, may be an increasing problem at the present time when the saving on scarce resources seems paramount. Almost inevitably, the result of this is to reduce the standard and efficiency of working. However, while these other forms of wastage are of undoubted, perhaps increasing, importance, here we will largely restrict ourselves to considering only the first two forms of wastage mentioned above – that is, looking at wastage in terms of wasted training and the cost of recruiting new staff. We return to these ideas after we have looked at the standard ways in which health authorities (HAs) calculate summaries of wastage.

CALCULATING THE PROBLEM

At present, most health authorities calculate wastage in six-monthly or yearly periods. This is done by dividing the number of leavers in the period by the average number of nurses employed during the period. Finally, this figure is multiplied by 100 to give wastage as a percentage. However, this is not the only way to summarize nurse wastage numerically. For example, Bartholomew (1976) suggests using the time taken for some fraction of a cohort of nurses (say, all those in post on 1 January 1995) to leave employment or, conversely, the proportion of a cohort who survive for some specified period (e.g. 80% of the above January cohort may have stayed for at least one year). One advantage of Bartholomew's suggestions is that they give a feel for whether the main turnover takes place among a small or large proportion of the nurses. (So, for example, in our own work we identified most of the leaving activity took place among 10% of the sample, while there were nearly 90% who exhibited a high likelihood of staying in the job.) With the standard method normally used it is impossible to determine this.

Matters become even more complicated if we recognize the very different kinds of 'wastage' which can take place. So, for example, as Grocott (1989) emphasizes, we can consider wastage in at least three strata. Grocott suggests that wastage can be divided into district (those leaving the district health authority), regional (those leaving the regional health authority) and national (those leaving the NHS altogether) levels. With the recent advent of NHS Trusts, the permutations become even more complex. However, Grocott makes the useful point that, as far as the NHS is concerned, a nurse is not wasted if she joins a health authority in another district or region (whatever local difficulties a move may cause) and similarly, as far as a region is concerned, a nurse is not wasted if she moves to a health authority within the same region. Though again with the introduction of Trusts, the situation has changed as it is the Trust that has to shoulder the financial costs of 'wastage', particularly if they have funded the cost of a nurse's training for a specialty.

Certainly, Grocott's type of analysis has been helpful in disentangling these various levels and he uses this approach to challenge whether there really is a problem of wastage. Indeed, as mentioned above, Grocott claims that the total workforce within nursing is increasing and the cries of the possible dire effects of a 'demographic timebomb' whereby nurse recruitment may be in jeopardy owing to the decreasing numbers of 18-year-olds in Britain may well be exaggerated. Whether one accepts his full argument, it still stems from his analysis that the problem of nursing wastage is a relative one. There are, for example, widespread geographical differences with some areas experiencing a shortage of nurses and other areas an abundance. Nevertheless, Grocott's work has enabled a fresh look at our first form of wastage: namely, wastage in terms of wasted training.

While Grocott's arguments may hold for our first definition of wastage, they do not satisfy the second: for any move there is still the cost of recruiting and possibly retraining the newly arrived nurse. This assumes that the nurses leaving are to be replaced and nowadays much of the hidden cost is in terms of re-allocating work in ways which may in fact antagonize and alienate the workforce. While the problem of nurses leaving the job or even the profession has claimed most attention, it also needs to be recognized that a stagnant workforce with no turnover might also be undesirable. There is much force in the argument that a certain amount of wastage should be tolerated or even encouraged. From the nurses' viewpoint there is less recognition that a very low turnover can itself produce problems; in such circumstances, promotion opportunities may rest only on the scope offered by 'natural wastage' such as retirement. Hence, the issue of nurse turnover becomes complex when we recognize that a suitable balance needs to be maintained between the two extremes of, on the one hand, a stagnant workforce where there is no serious scope for the introduction of new ideas of helpful practices (for the patient) and, on the other, a rapidly changing workforce where staff morale is low and the possibilities of good practice becoming routinized are negligible.

ESTIMATING THE NATURE OF THE PROBLEM

Grocott's work challenging whether there is indeed a wastage problem of too many nurses leaving and proposing instead that the total workforce has been increasing is a vivid example of how there are shifts in locating the nature of the problem. In fact, what seems to happen is that a general problem is posited and so, for example, the potential problems associated with the so-called 'demographic timebomb' were heralded with the recognition that this problem could be further amplified by the introduction of Project 2000 – where the aim is for learners to spend more time actually learning, as opposed to doing and to be supernumerary to the operation of the wards. However, evidence gradually began to emerge that regions and specialties were being affected differently as these impending shifts began to get closer. So, for example, as Pilkington (1989) pointed out, recruitment was a problem in some city regions such as London but in more rural areas the problem was often that there was insufficient finance to employ nurses. Five years later the lack of finances in relation to the employment of nurses is being proclaimed as an all-encompassing one. So London, previously struggling with a recruitment problem, is now struggling even more in the hospital sector with a finance and resource problem. This cyclical pattern of portraying differences of problems between locations and then the similarities of problems throughout the service partly reflects reality and partly reflects how media and professional interest fluctuates. However, it also needs to be seen as part of the wider process in the deterioration in the working conditions and the power of the nursing profession over the past decade and a half which is discussed more fully by Stephen Ackroyd in Chapter 25.

The government's view of turnover/wastage among nurses remains complex and often contradictory. Indeed, only reluctantly during the latter part of the 1980s did they begin to acknowledge a crisis in the health service of which nurses' concerns were a part. Certainly one consistent theme of the government has been in trying to restrict the growth of the public sector and arguing that increasing costs in this sector have been damaging to the economy. As a consequence, there was no fundamental support or affinity with the difficulties and concerns of the nursing profession during the early days of the 'Thatcher revolution'. However, increasingly, since the mid-1980s the government has been forced to acknowledge that nurses' claims – in both pay and other issues – cannot just be swept aside. While industrial action is a tactic which excites much controversy within the ranks of nursing (see Chapter 24 'Nurses and the New Industrial Relations'), it is implicitly recognized by the government that industrial action by nurses may well receive sympathy and tacit support among the public in ways which most other public servants cannot – or have learned not to – expect.

In order to throw light on some of the emerging conflicts and contradictions, the Review Body for Nursing Staff, Midwives, Health Visitors and Professions Allied to Medicine was set up in 1983 to publish a yearly report. At that time, the problems of the nursing profession were much less in the public view. Curiously, despite the fact that around half a million nurses are employed within the National Health Service, many issues surrounding nurse turnover had not been considered in a systematic way for over a decade since Mercer's work published in 1979 but with the field-work actually carried out in 1975–6. In fact, the Review Body commented in its second report in June 1985 that: '*In the management's view* only a very small proportion [of nurses] left the NHS for reasons of dissatisfaction' (our emphasis). This was said at a time when some local health authorities were beginning to recognize that they were experiencing difficulties in the recruitment and retention of nurses. We felt that it was clearly time to hear what nurses had to say.

Our work (Mackay, 1988a, b, 1989; Barry, Soothill and Francis, 1989; Williams, Soothill and Barry, 1991a, b, c, d, e, f, g; Soothill, Barry and Williams, 1991; 1992; Peelo, Francis and Soothill, Chapter 2 in this volume) has been to identify some of the problems facing nurses, to recognize some of the recurring themes that emerge when you talk to nurses or ask them to respond to questionnaires and, more recently, to consider in detail the views of some nurses who had left the health authority over the past three years.

REASONS FOR LEAVING

There are considerable advantages of following through the same set of nurses in a longitudinal study rather than the more usual cross-sectional research design when nurses are questioned about their attitudes at one particular point in time. As we argue elsewhere (Williams, Soothill and Barry, 1991), nurses' attitudes are dynamic rather than static. In other words, the situations of nurses change over time, in both expected and unexpected directions, reflecting both conditions internal to nursing (such as changes in pay and conditions) or events external to nursing (such as a partner moving job to another area, having a baby, etc.). As a consequence, their view of their situation will change as new evidence of their life chances emerges. More specifically, we found in a study considering the outcome of stated intentions that people actually change their mind about whether or not they intend to leave (Soothill, Barry and Williams, 1992) and similarly that they are likely to shift their views as to whether they regard nursing as a vocation, a career or just a job (Williams, Soothill and Barry, 1991f).

While we have emphasized that attitudes may change over time, it is also fair to point out that the health authority in the north-west of England which was the location of the study may not necessarily be representative of the variety of experiences of nurses in Britain although the authority did have about the average level of turnover at the time of the original study. Caution is always appropriate in transferring results across time and place but the material we found is both illustrative and useful as a demonstration project.

Health authority records indicated whether or not the nurses in our sample had left within the three-year follow-up period.[1] However, it was more difficult to trace the physical whereabouts of nurses for the purpose of probing more systematically their reasons for leaving.

Ninety persons returned the questionnaires we despatched. An analysis of their responses (Williams, Soothill and Barry, 1991a) gives the flavour of how nurses disperse into a range of activities when they left a particular health authority. In fact, two-thirds (66%) remained in nursing when they left. Of the total sample, 40% left to move to other health authorities within the NHS for a wide variety of reasons, from promotion to discontent. A further 26% decided that nursing outside the NHS was the

---

1 In fact, this exercise was not as easy as this brief sentence suggests and the outcome for a number could not be traced (see also Barry, Soothill and Francis, 1989).

best option for them. Of the remaining one-third (34%), most were not now in paid employment and were childrearers, students, retired, ill, disabled or registered unemployed. Some of these outcomes, such as retirement and ill-health, are inevitable. However, leaving for reasons of ill-health may not be straightforward. Some, for example, who have suffered from the after-effects of illness felt that they could have worked in a different area of nursing and that no effort was put into finding them alternative work or part-time work until they were completely recovered. Similarly, leaving for childrearing can have different meanings. This type of loss to nursing is acceptable providing the parent has chosen to be a full-time parent rather than feeling that she has been coerced into that position by lack of adequate childcare facilities.

The smallest group of 11% represent those who had left nursing altogether and had moved into other occupations. These former nurses were doing a variety of activities from setting up a snail farm, secretarial work, gardening, painting, dressmaking, running a child-minding service to working in shops.

While the follow-up shows the diversity of activity after leaving, the most striking aspect of the follow-up study was that in essence all the groups were saying remarkably similar things. They were expressing dissatisfaction at staff shortages, lack of resources, the workload getting in the way of them doing their work properly, the lack of personal development opportunities in their own training and careers, the management of the NHS, non-existent childcare facilities and difficulties for parents in coping with shiftwork and an overall feeling of not being appreciated and being devalued both financially and by their managers and government.

This sad and rather depressing tale of woe emerged not only from responses to the questionnaire but also from a series of interviews conducted with a sub-sample of the 90 persons who had returned completed questionnaires. Out of the 39 leavers interviewed, none could recall having had a formal leaving interview conducted by the authority and only one or two had had an informal leaving interview. There seemed to be a total lack of interest on the part of the health authority in the reasons why these nurses had left. In fact there were reasons entered on the computerized personnel records that we had access to (perhaps given by the person's line-manager) and these were often at serious odds with what nurses said at the interview. This discrepancy is not altogether surprising, for even efficiently conducted leaving interviews may still produce differences between the reasons given to the health authority for leaving and those which may be given to more intimate associates. Indeed, asking nurses why they are leaving is a delicate methodological problem regarding the quality of information one might receive. While many personnel departments of health authorities may be improving the quality of their leaving interviews, personnel managers will be deluding themselves if they think that improving the procedures will resolve the issue entirely. A variant of this problem is what we term the 'official' and 'unofficial' reasons for leaving.

Official reasons are indeed the reasons given to officials. The reasons given in their letter of resignation are usually safe, polite reasons that would not offend or jeopardize a future reference. In contrast, the unofficial reasons, which are more likely to be expanded at length to close intimates, may paint a rather different picture. Again, there is a danger in believing that these accounts represent some kind of 'objective truth', for one needs to appreciate that one often needs to justify one's actions to loved ones. Actions are not always so straightforward and rational as one so often tries to portray them. Hence, the usual pattern is to 'gild the lily' so that one emerges in one's own account in a somewhat better light than, say, an account given by a disinterested bystander who knew all the facts. Nevertheless, unofficial reasons given to intimates are much more likely to contain the genuine passion which may accompany leaving decisions. Such passion has usually been sanitized from the official letters of resignation which nurses know may remain on file. We felt that by gaining confidence and trust in terms of guaranteeing anonymity and confidentiality, our interviews got much closer to revealing the unofficial reasons for leaving which may usually only be given to the nurses' more intimate associates.

Certainly the unofficial reasons told at the interviews we conducted with nurses were much more passionate and often described shocking attitudes from those senior to them and the experience of poor conditions at work. The interview study complemented the responses to the questionnaire. The top three reasons given for leaving in the questionnaire were centred on working conditions and combined 'workload preventing nurses giving their best', 'staff shortages' and 'the constant struggle with underfunded resources' (see Table 20.1). The second group of three issues focused on the personal prospects of the individual and encompassed 'wanting to widen experience', 'wanting a new challenge' and a general concern about 'a lack of promotion prospects'. Issues around management, stress and child-care were also prominent as reasons for leaving and aspects requiring improvement.

A crucial point to recognize is that the problem of pay was rarely mentioned. This is curious, for the focus on nurses' pay has been a paramount issue in the last decade. Indeed, pay had been readily identified by government, opposition politicians, trade unions and the media as the main focus of concern. This is partly because of the simplistic way that concerns about employment conditions are analysed, with pay being the common denominator that all parties involved in a dispute can readily understand. However, our research has consistently shown that there are a range of issues requiring attention which run even more deeply within the nursing profession than the familiar sore of low pay. There are problems in

Table 20.1 Top ten reasons for leaving nursing

	Overall	Top reasons			
	% (N = 90)	1st (%)	2nd (%)	3rd (%)	Total (%)
Workload prevents giving of best	40	4	10	67	21
Staff shortages	37	3	9	10	22
Constant struggle with underfunded resources	31	3	0	7	10
Wanting to widen experience	31	11	6	0	17
Wanting a new challenge	31	2	8	6	16
Lack of promotion prospects	29	2	2	7	11
Management style of organization	27	0	4	0	4
Hours not suiting home life	26	4	3	7	14
Stress too high	24	6	7	2	14
Bad atmosphere at work	24	8	1	2	11

writing about and researching areas of concern which impinge on matters being raised in the public arena. In brief, if one denied the supreme importance of pay, then one might be seen to be undermining a reasonable and understandable grievance which needed to be rectified. However, there is no doubt that the belief that meeting pay demands – but they are never met in full and in the case of nurses the most significant recent settlement raised another set of issues which emerged in the re-grading process – will produce a solution is misguided. Our research shows quite clearly that there are structural and operational concerns within nursing which go beyond the concerns of pay. Incidentally, discussions with nurses do suggest that a residual embrace of the notion of nursing as a vocation makes many nurses their own worst enemies with regard to pay-bargaining. They recognize that, for some of their colleagues, pay is a problem but for themselves they are often unwilling to push the point. Hence, their expressions of concerns about the job focus much more readily on how others are potentially harmed rather than how they are disadvantaged. Nevertheless, as Bagguley emphasizes (see Chapter 24), the new grading structure introduced in 1988 has caused considerable dissatisfaction among nurses. He argues that the nursing profession within the NHS is much more deeply divided in terms of their levels of pay and the determination of their pay and conditions than was previously the case. While these differences may be becoming more visible as the aims and objectives of the nursing profession are increasingly being called into question, our research shows how the very different reasons for leaving illustrate a considerable range of concerns which need to be addressed. The striking feature about Table 20.1 is that no particular reason totally dominates. It is the wide dispersion of reasons rather than a specific concentration which is most worthy of comment.

INTERVIEWING NURSES

Interviewing nurses who had left was often a distressing experience. While objectively the respondents may be accused of exaggerating the situation, there could be no denying how they subjectively felt. The passion displayed was quite disturbing. A midwife in her late twenties said:

> My first reason [for leaving] was understaffing ... the staff was diminished, we missed meal breaks because no one came in to relieve you, coffee breaks in the mornings just didn't exist ... It's not worth going to work, working as hard as you do, staying late, not getting time back and getting all that aggro at work ... I just thought I can't exist like this.

A recently qualified RGN answered the interview question angrily:

> Well, you'll have heard it all before, not enough resources, nor enough time, not enough back-up ... you've not enough time to do your job properly. The current way that I am being treated has knocked all the stuffing out of me because I'm not allowed to do my job properly.

What is important to emphasize is that these kinds of criticisms, of which the above two give just an indication, are concerned with upsetting elements of the job which are preventable. In other words, they are not talking about matters which are an inherent part of the job like bedpans, faeces and vomit. Nurses seem to accept these unalterable facts of human frailty. In contrast, they are criticizing aspects of the job that can and should be changed. The criticisms of the job are ones of NHS finance and management. Hence, they are concerned with unpleasant features of the job which are in principle avoidable. In short, money, management training, drive and initiative could alleviate many of these kinds of problems in a remarkably short time.

In considering why people leave, it is also instructive to consider the complementary question of why people decide to take up nursing (Williams, Soothill and Barry, 1991b). In fact, we asked our sample of leavers: 'What made you decide to take up nursing as a profession?' We gave them a list of ten possible reasons, asking them to tick as many as applied. Interestingly again, not one person ticked 'the money' reason indicating the general attitude of nurses to their pay. More than half (56%) of our sample were under 30 years of age, so this is not a throwback to the era when it was thought that if nurses were paid too much, then the wrong sort of person would come into nursing, but an up-to-date statement that none of our sample chose their career for money. The two factors ticked by most people were 'opportunity to work with people' (64%) and 'to be part of a caring team' (62%). These clearly reflect that the two main factors that decided these people to take up nursing are based on an interest in the content of the actual work. Nursing is very person-centred and demands considerable interpersonal skills. In fact, these two factors link in with the top three reasons our sample gave for leaving: 'workload prevents giving of best'; 'staff shortages' and 'constant struggle with underfunded resources'. While at first glance a relationship may not be immediately obvious, it became increasingly clear when the questionnaire returns were supplemented by the interviews we conducted that many of our sample quite simply felt they were no longer part of a caring team, nor were they able to give their patients what they needed and wanted. The heavy workload, staff shortages and lack of resources were getting between the nurse and the patient and also between the nurses themselves. The individualistic philosophy so enthusiastically encouraged during the high point of the Thatcher years is totally disruptive in operation on the wards:

> It was really happy and we had a real good team. That's what's missing, a team; everyone's individuals on a ward now, we're not part of a team ... there's no loyalty. I mean they haven't even got loyalty to each other, so how can they have loyalty to a team ... so it's dog eat dog, a matter of survival.

It is ironic that at a time when the importance of intra- and inter-professional working is being more widely recognized (e.g. Soothill, Mackay and Webb, 1995), the practitioners see the opportunities for team-working as diminishing. Curiously, however, the scope for the thrusting, ambitious individual within nursing – perhaps willing to overthrow to some degree the traditional values of working as a team – seems equally limited and limiting within the NHS. So it is noteworthy that the second group of three reasons in the top six (see Table 20.1) focus on issues around the personal prospects for a career in the NHS for the individual nurse. The concern was again vividly captured during some of the interviews. A young man who had left nursing completely indicated some of the frustrations:

> I said I'd love to get a job on here and I would love to do my speciality training. But first of all you get told that sorry that we've got no more money on the unit for new staff nurses, but if just by chance you did get on, then they would never let you go on the specialty course because they don't second anybody and if you do get on a course, a job's not guaranteed, so where is all the career structure? If you've any sense of the future you want some sort of plan for the next few years, don't you?

Similarly, a specialist health visitor left:

> Because I felt stunted and restricted because of a loss of opportunities and inability to go on study days ... It was really bad management, lack of career opportunities or even lack of interest from managers

to pursue your career opportunities. You know, sort of keep everybody down, that's what came across to me.

Earlier we noted how our leavers from the health authority we were studying moved to a variety of destinations. Not surprisingly, there were some differences in reasons given for leaving by the various groups (Williams, Soothill and Barry, 1991a). So, for example, 'workload' was the primary reason for leaving the NHS for those still in nursing but now working outside the NHS. Among those in the unpaid group, retirement was the main stated reason for leaving. But behind this apparently benign reason there can be a multitude of accounts. Certainly a number had retired early because they were fed up at work and disillusioned by the problems within the health service. Among those who had taken a job outside nursing, a higher proportion had indicated 'stress too high' as a reason for leaving. Nevertheless, what seems to bind all the groups together is not the work but the broader issues surrounding the job. This is encapsulated by the saying: 'Nurses love their work but hate their job.'

What of those who had left this health authority but remained working within the NHS? For these people the main reasons for moving health authorities were centred on career and personal development: 'wanting a new challenge', 'wanting to widen experience', and 'lack of promotion prospects' characterized the reasons cited by these nurses. Is this response saying that the nurses staying within the health service are willing to put up with all the issues cited so frequently by others, providing they get their own promotion, wider experience and challenge within the NHS? In fact, the analysis shows that the other reasons are also real issues for them, but that career issues were more significant to those who continued to work within the NHS.

DECIDING TO STAY

The importance of a career is reinforced by the 'stayers' we interviewed.[2] These nurses, who had originally intended to leave but had continued in post during the three follow-up years, generally remained discontented, although for some their situation had positively improved. The two who were at the time of the study the most discontented were two enrolled nurses. One quite simply said: 'Money and lack of opportunity ... are keeping me here now.' She felt that as an enrolled nurse, there was little

2 Recognizing that the 'leavers' were perhaps giving a somewhat distorted picture, we interviewed nine nurses who had altered their original intention of leaving the health authority and were still in post at the end of the three-year follow-up period. We were interested in what had persuaded them to change their mind about leaving.

opportunity within the health service but that the possibilities for someone of her age (in her late thirties) outside the health service were even more limited. She had applied for a variety of jobs outside nursing but the pay was always less. The other unhappy enrolled nurse had also applied for a number of other jobs and said: 'If someone came along with an interesting offer, then I'm afraid my loyalties to nursing would not have the same power as they used to have.'

Both these nurses had worked for the health service for some considerable time and, while disillusioned and dissatisfied, neither had finally left. They were both single and felt restricted by their mortgages. In effect, they felt trapped in their jobs.

In contrast, two other enrolled nurses among the stayers expressed all the familiar dissatisfactions about shortages and resources but were now quite content within themselves. The major difference between these two and the unhappy two were that the happy pair had both got places on a conversion course. They were buoyant about their improved prospects. They felt enormously lucky they had got a place on a conversion course, as one of them indicated that there had been only ten places and 300 applicants on her course. So these women had achieved major career development and, although both were aware and remained passionate about staff shortages and other issues, they now intended to stay in NHS nursing.

The other five 'stayers' who were interviewed had also achieved promotion and had good prospects ahead of them. They were now in management positions and conveyed a feeling of satisfaction in their progress, although the future for some was still negotiable. One woman who, three years earlier had been intending to leave this health authority but had stayed, remained clear about her intentions:

> I'm quite busy and I'm enjoying every minute of it. [The health authority] has been very good to me, but I've worked hard for [this health authority] and I like what I'm doing. But I'm looking for further development now, and I want a full-time management post ...
> I have a degree of loyalty to [this health authority] because they've been good to me but ... you have to put yourself first these days ... I want an I [grade]. I'll go elsewhere in the end if they don't give it to me.

So, quite straightforwardly, if the health authority gives this woman what she wants with regards to promotion, they will keep her. If not, she will go. The message could not be clearer, although the outcome may be more problematic.

By looking at those who had unexpectedly chosen to stay we can see that most of them had achieved promotion, which contributed to their decision. In contrast, the first two had not progressed in their career and were both unhappy, feeling trapped after looking round for alternatives. There is little doubt that career progression – or lack of it – appears to seriously affect the way people view their job and alters what they are willing to tolerate or not tolerate.

CURRENT ATTITUDES

The evidence from our study indicates the ambivalence that many nurses and former nurses feel about their job. Many really do love the notion of nursing and the opportunity it gives them to work with people and help them recover, die or prevent ill-health. Few who left wanted to leave nursing. But the confines of the job often seemed to get in the way of allowing them to do what they want and need to do.

The opinions of people leaving a workplace are a valuable resource and a window into the working environment. The aim of the study was to see the situation from the nurses' perspective. So whereas managers, for example, often maintain that there are indeed enough staff to do the required work, this is not how it has generally been seen in recent years by nurses. However, we are not concerned here with the truth or otherwise of their assertions. Sociologically the familiar point is made, as W.I. Thomas suggested in the early 1920s, that: 'if men define situations as real, they are real in their consequences'. Hence, while managers may perhaps deny some of the stark assertions made, the belief in the reality of their assertions on the part of nurses is undoubtedly important in the increasing demoralization of the nursing workforce.

Certainly perceived staff shortages, lack of resources and all the other major causes of turnover highlighted in our study need to be faced and not just sidelined as issues raised by a few malcontents. The message is too widespread. Sadly, empirical work by academics, however rigorous and well-designed, is often too readily dismissed as out-of-date or out-of-touch with what is actually happening. However, in the study of nurse turnover and retention, various studies over the past decade have been producing very similar results (Price Waterhouse, 1988; Martin and Mackean, 1988; Waite, Buchan and Thomas, 1989).

It is difficult to estimate the extent to which current problems with nursing are transitory or permanent. Certainly we have identified certain features of concern which, though expensive to eradicate or improve, are at least in principle possible to confront in a positive manner. However, it is sometimes hard to dismiss the notion that discontent may also be rooted much deeper in our extremely materialistic society. In a society which glorifies consumerism and the constant change of personal belongings, toys, stereos, fridges, cars, etc. it is not surprising that this attitude also seeps into employment. The new car is always going to be better, more fun and give more satisfaction, as is the new job. Reality is often different. New cars are involved in accidents and breakdown, as are new jobs. Hence, there is the argument that, until our society moves away from gross consumerism into valuing what you have and enjoying familiarity instead of looking to the shiny, new alternative, high turnover in jobs will continue to be the norm. In this way we need to recognize that understanding nurse turnover also requires an understanding of the wider processes operating in society.

Furthermore, the recent changes which have been taking place in the NHS have been associated with serious problems of morale within the whole arena of healthcare. While essentially these problems are caused by pressures on resources, both financial and human, there have also been efforts to improve the quality of care by an attempt to engender a spirit of competition within the NHS through the creation of hospital Trusts, independent organizations which are in competition with other hospitals, as well as through the distinctions being made between the purchasers and providers of services. This has been all happening within the context of more subtle pressures. In brief, recent governments have mounted sustained attacks on the established and emerging professions. Hence, the power of the professional groups to determine their own conditions of work, their own standards of service and to monopolize their area of competence has not been appreciated by governments which wish to assert the primacy of 'the market' (Mackay, Soothill and Webb, 1995). There is certainly little to suggest that the concerns of the nurses in our study do not continue to reflect current concerns of this professional group.

There are also considerable regional differences which need to be considered. Our own study, which focused on talking with nurses who all lived and worked in north-west England, indicated how the local geographical context may be crucial. Generally, these nurses did not feel that there were jobs which were 'up for grabs' owing to staff shortages. Indeed, quite the opposite. A father of two children under five years, who had worked as a welder for four years, then did his RMN training and worked in the psychiatric field for two years and had just completed his RGN training, was finding it very difficult to find a job:

> The only thing is that they're short of money as usual, and they're only employing staff on temporary contract. For some staff they're only on weekly contracts, so they don't know where they are, so morale is low because of that ... They're desperately short of staff, but they won't employ any others because they've no money.

The current situation is extremely paradoxical, confusing and ambiguous. While the NHS Regional Planners' Group (Conroy and Stidson, 1988) suggested that staff shortages would replace finance as the most significant block to providing an efficient service, certainly in north-west England finance remains the main factor. In brief, the nurses are there, the money isn't. This shortfall of money affects recruitment and retention in terms of providing meaningful careers for the majority of nurses within the workforce and, more immediately, in providing sufficient posts to counter the concerns of nursing staff and their unions. In London the number of nursing staff has fallen significantly[3] and numbers have fallen in Scotland and Wales in a year by 1% and 0.8% respectively. In contrast, nursing numbers for the rest of England increased by 0.7% in 1992–3 (*The Guardian*, 22 September 1994). Clearly, some adjustments are taking place. How sophisticated are the current shifts is difficult to evaluate. As Maynard (1994) has recently observed: 'The skill mix across hospitals appears to vary greatly but it is not clear whether this is a product of the local labour market, case severity, tradition or God.'

In many ways we seem to be caught in an Orwellian newspeak which is difficult to disentangle. Certainly there is a belief among nurses that staffing levels are being pruned to the minimum and that establishment figures are being driven to fit in with unrealistic financial targets rather than with patients' needs. As a result, vacancies may deliberately not be filled. The Orwellian touch is that when vacancies are not filled and the posts are eradicated, there is no staff shortage as the job does not exist any more.

The use of language is fascinating and we have pointed to how the pejorative term 'nursing wastage' rather than the more neutral 'nursing turnover' has connotations which tend to place the blame for staffing difficulties on the nurse. We have portrayed some of the current concerns and discontent of nurses which often lead to a movement both to posts within nursing and to paid and unpaid employment outside it. We have hinted that the concerns about adverse demographic trends, while important, are sometimes used as a diversionary, screening tactic to avoid facing other more fundamental issues. Maynard (1994) is even more sceptical, saying that: 'claims about an oversupply of nurses are as ill-founded as the 1980s' threat of an imminent nursing recruitment crisis. Don't be conned.' However, his message is not one of enlightenment but a call for enlightenment: 'The most remarkable thing about the supply of nurses and the demand for them is how little is known about it.'

Managers are constantly being asked to restrict and cut back expenditure, yet we tend to forget that this can produce a downward spiral in morale which is difficult to reverse. Low morale, whether it leads to turnover or

---

3 In figures submitted to the nursing pay review body as part of the government's evidence, the number of nursing staff in inner London had dropped by 10.9% over 12 months, from 27,970 in 1992 to 24,920 in 1993. In outer London, numbers dropped over the same period by 3.4%. However, a note attached to the figures said the London data had been affected by 'coding problems' and must be treated with caution (*The Guardian*, 22 September 1994).

not, causes a drop in standards and lowers efficiency in nursing care. If more money, time and energy were spent addressing the issues that cause nurses to leave and move to another authority, into the private sector or out of nursing altogether, then it is possible that we could help to prevent people leaving work they really enjoy because they cannot now stand the job:

> I can't imagine ever having a job that would give me the satisfaction that I used to have in nursing. I can't think that there is a job on this earth that would ever do that for me.

This was said by a woman who, despite wanting to be a nurse from childhood, has now left nursing altogether and has no intention of going back. She was unusual in deciding never to return to nursing, but typical in continuing to love its ideals. Nevertheless, perhaps she comes close to identifying some of the current conundrums within nursing as we grapple with the ideal and the realistic. Certainly at the moment the ideals of the nurse and the realism of the manager are failing to coalesce satisfactorily.

In relation to nurse turnover, our prescription is a modest and realistic one. Managers should have an understanding of the way that turnover operates in their health authority. For example, is there a high level of turnover among some nurses and less among others, or is there a steady turnover among all nurses? There needs to be a much greater recognition that there are a number of aspects that managers can control. For example, the provision of crèche facilities may encourage mothers with young children to remain in nursing; an increased availability of job-share and part-time working would help many nurses; and, perhaps most importantly, managers could communicate better with nurses and show that they do understand the problems and stresses that those working on the front-line have to face. However, there are some aspects which relate to turnover that managers cannot and, perhaps, should not control. For example, nurses may want to travel for extensive periods or experience the challenge of working at a new health authority. Turnover, for reasons such as these, can help retain nurses' enthusiasm for their work. In brief, turnover is not always negative.

Hence, we conclude on an optimistic note by observing that there are some aspects of running a health authority that managers should be able to control, while recognizing that there are other aspects that they cannot and perhaps should not. The main problem is that the potential areas for understanding and control are not always currently being managed successfully.

REFERENCES

Barry, J., Soothill, K. and Francis, B. (1989) Nursing the statistics: a demonstration study of nurse turnover and retention. *Journal of Advanced Nursing*, **14**, 528–35.

Bartholomew, D.J. (1976) The statistical approach to manpower planning, in *Manpower Planning* (ed. D.S. Bartholomew), Penguin Books, Harmondsworth.

Briggs, A. (1972) *Report of the Committee on Nursing*, Cmnd. 5115, HMSO, London.

Conroy, M. and Stidson, M. (1988) *2001 – The Black Hole*, The NHS Regional Manpower Planners' Group.

Dickson, N. (1987) Best foot forward. *Nursing Times*, **83**(1), 40–1.

Grocott, T. (1989) A hole in the black hole theory. *Nursing Times*, **85**(41).

Hancock, C. (1986) The staffing equation. *Nursing Times*, **82**, 40–2.

Mackay, L. (1988a) Career woman. *Nursing Times*, **84**(10).

Mackay, L. (1988b) No time to care. *Nursing Times*, **84**(11).

Mackay, L. (1989) *Nursing a Problem*, Open University Press, Milton Keynes.

Mackay, L., Soothill, K. and Webb, C. (1995) Troubled times: the context for interprofessional collaboration? in *Interprofessional Relations in Health Care* (eds K. Soothill, L. Mackay and C. Webb), Edward Arnold, London.

Martin, J.P. and Mackean, J. (1988) *Can We Keep Nurses in the Health Service? A Study of Nurse Retention in Two Health Districts*, Institute for Health Policy Studies, University of Southampton.

Maynard, A. (1994) Numbers nonsense. *Nursing Management*, Vol. 1, No. 6, 7 Oct.

Mercer, G. (1979) *Employment of Nurses*, Croom Helm, London.

Pilkington, E. (1989) A growing sick list of morale, *The Guardian*, 29 November.

Price Waterhouse (1988) *Nurse Retention and Recruitment: A Matter of Priority*. Report commissioned by chairmen of Regional Health Authorities in England, Health Boards in Scotland and Health Authorities in Wales.

Redfern, S.J. (1978) Absence and wastage in trained nurses: a selective review of the literature. *Journal of Advanced Nursing*, **3**, 231–49.

Soothill, K., Barry, J. and Williams, C. (1991) Why do they go? Probing reasons for nurses' leaving: An exploratory study. *Journal of Advances in Health and Nursing*.

Soothill, K., Barry, J. and Williams, C. (1992) Words and Actions: A Study in Nurse Wastage, *International Journal of Nursing Studies*, Vol. 29, No. 2, 163–75.

Soothill, K., Mackay, L. and Webb, C. (eds.) (1995) *Interprofessional Relations in Health Care*, Edward Arnold, London.

Volkart, E.H. (ed.) (1951) *Social Behavior and Personality: Contributions of W.I. Thomas to Theory and Social Research*, Social Sciences Research Council, New York.

Waite, R., Buchan, J. and Thomas, J. (1989) *Nurses In and Out of Work*. IMS Report No. 170, Institute of Manpower Studies, Brighton.

Williams, C., Soothill, K. and Barry, J. (1991a) Love nursing, hate the job, *The Health Service Journal*, Vol. 101, No. 5238, 18–21.

Williams, C., Soothill, K. and Barry, J. (1991b) Targeting the discontented, *The Health Service Journal*, Vol. 101, No. 5239, 20–1.

Williams, C., Soothill, K. and Barry, J. (1991c) Why nurses leave the profession: Part I, *Nursing Standard*, Vol. 5, No. 39, 33–5.

Williams, C., Soothill, K. and Barry, J. (1991d) Why nurses leave the profession: Part II, *Nursing Standard*, Vol. 5, No. 40, 33–5.

Williams, C., Soothill, K. and Barry, J. (1991e) Why nurses leave the profession: Part III, *Nursing Standard*, Vol. 5, No. 40, 33–6.

Williams, C., Soothill, K. and Barry, J. (1991f) Nursing: just a job? Do statistics tell us what we think? *Journal of Advanced Nursing*, Vol. 16, 910–19.

Nurse supply modelling

David Worthington

INTRODUCTION

Concern about the availability of an adequate number of suitably qualified nurses is a perennial problem for the National Health Service. For example, in 1993 the RGN general secretary argued that the internal market was leading to a failure of hospitals to be properly concerned about the future supply of qualified nurses, (Hancock, 1993). At the same time the director of the Institute of Health Service Management offered the personal view that: 'Within the next decade the pool of potential nursing students will shrink dramatically and the younger generation will have easier access to universities. Nursing will be competing in a much tougher labour market', Rowden (1993).

In the late 1980s the area of concern was the same, although the context was different. Nursing's 'demographic timebomb' had been clearly identified as a major problem for health service managers to solve, see for example Hancock (1986). The problem was essentially that while there is no anticipated drop in the demand for nurses, (indeed service plans and Project 2000 proposals may well mean an increased requirement), by the early 1990s the pool of school leavers from whom most nurse trainees are recruited will have fallen by about 35%.

Whatever the context, the problem is not straightforward because the supply of nurses from nurse training is augmented by two other major sources: namely the retention and return of previously qualified nurses. While these sources complicate the problem they may well also contribute to its eventual solution.

In this context, nurse workforce planning is a vital activity for the health service. In a discussion of whether or not there is a shortage of nursing skills Martin (1990) concludes that:

Supply modelling is required that focuses on different specialisms and is linked to education/training provision. The value of investment in such work is justified by the size, complexity and cost of the nursing workforce. Until this sounder information base is available the question of skills shortages can only be answered at local levels and by anecdotal evidence.

In reviewing the situation the NHS Management Board (1987) emphasized the dual role of demand and supply modelling in strategic planning. It noted the wide variety of methodologies in use and provided guidance on 'minimum expectations on the use of manpower planning methodology'. This included the proposal that 'use of common methodologies should be the long-term aim', but recommended for the moment that:

a) there should be a supply model in use in each region which does not have to be the same in every region;
b) there should be a demand model for strategic planning purposes in use in each region which should be common to each district in the region, but may differ between regions.

However, serious interest is still relatively new and nurse workforce planning is evolving in the face of real practical problems. The purpose of this chapter is to introduce nurses and prospective nurses to the concept of nurse supply modelling in the context of nurse workforce planning. It explains the general concept of nurse supply modelling and goes on to describe some of the major issues which impact on its practical application. It then identifies the possible practical roles of the present generation of nurse supply models and describes key areas of concern for the future.

NURSE SUPPLY MODELLING

The nature of nurse supply models

The general purpose of nurse supply models is to allow a manager to investigate the supply consequences of possible management actions. Such a 'model' is in fact almost always a piece of computer software which allows the user to input data that corresponds to the management actions. The model then predicts the consequences of those actions using mathematical relationships designed to reflect what is known about the dynamics of the situation.

However, as in many other fields, nurse supply models are unable to incorporate the actual operational decisions that may be under consideration. For example, if management wishes to examine the effects of reducing wastage on the supply of nurses, a supply model could be reasonably expected to calculate the effects of different wastage rates. However, it would be very unlikely to show the effects of actual management actions, for example opening a crèche. Current supply models, in the main, only consider management actions indirectly in terms of the rates they will cause rather than the detail of how those rates will be achieved.

The problems involved in modelling in any greater detail in a systematic way make the current approach appropriate. However, this leaves a certain amount of responsibility with the manager to judge what rates can be achieved and how. This may lead to some other modelling exercises; however, in general this is better kept separate from the main supply model.

The structure of nurse supply models

In general terms, nurse supply models all have the same basic structure, as shown in Figure 21.1. The situation is modelled in terms of a number of stocks and flows. For example, at the national level the four most important stocks are: qualified nurses working for the NHS, qualified nurses in the UK who are not working for the NHS, trainee nurses and the rest of the UK population. In the main these stocks change due to flows between them, e.g. qualified nurses leaving the NHS or trainees newly recruited from the rest of the UK population. If the starting stocks are known and future flow rates can be predicted, then a supply model should be able to predict future stocks reasonably accurately.

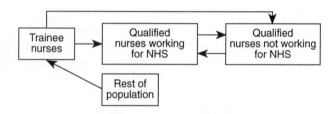

Figure 21.1 The basic structure of nurse supply models.

While Figure 21.1 summarizes the main principles of nurse supply models, it does not itself represent a realistic model. For example, because flow rates will usually depend on the ages and grades of the nurses involved, most practical models subdivide the major stocks by age groupings and by grade. The resulting model is still a network of stocks and flows and hence the principles are unchanged. However, a realistic model will normally be much more complex than in Figure 21.1.

While models along the lines of Figure 21.1 are usually too simple to be of practical value, it is also important to avoid over-complicated models. In reviewing manpower planning models in general, Edwards (1986) suggests that: 'simple techniques should be used ... The aim should be to encourage interaction with the models to gain an understanding of the quantitative aspects of the manpower system; none of these is beyond the capabilities of a good spreadsheet package (with graphics) …'.

Types of models

Different supply models are appropriate in different circumstances. The circumstances can be reflected in terms of the timescale under consideration, the level within the organization (e.g. hospital, region), or simply the available data.

One important distinction is between 'prescriptive' and 'what if' models. In the former the model tells the manager what rates will be required to achieve chosen targets. In the latter the manager chooses the rates and the model calculates the consequences. In the context of manpower supply modelling 'prescriptive' models can be very thought-provoking and can generate some useful solutions. However, given the ingenuity of managers and the complexity of the problem, the flexibility of 'what if' models is probably more useful in the long term. They will usually require a greater degree of involvement from the manager, but should provide a better level of understanding and a higher level of credibility.

Manager participation

Management participation is a sound principle in any modelling work. In the context of nurse supply modelling it is clearly essential that managers are involved to offer their judgment on what rates might be achievable and perhaps to accept responsibility for attaining those rates. For the successful use of nurse supply models a three-way interaction is therefore desirable, involving the manager, the analyst and the model.

While this mode of usage is obviously preferable, it can be very time-consuming and various shortcuts can be envisaged. For example, supply models have been designed that are intended to be sufficiently user-friendly for a manager to be able to use them directly without the need for an analyst. In other studies, 'one-way interactions' have been tried in which the manager tells the analyst the parameter values, but does not fully understand what the analyst and the model are doing with them. However, such shortcuts are very risky, given the form of the models and the present lack of experience in running and interpreting such models that exists among NHS managers. For example, data problems often require the analysis or the model to make additional assumptions in order to obtain results. Many results from the model may be relatively insensitive to these assumptions; for others they may be critical. Such a judgment would usually require inputs and awareness from both analyst and manager. In fact, one of the major benefits of some supply models is that they can act as a catalyst between managers and analysts.

Data imposed limitations

As with many other areas of modelling, data availability rather than the ability to manipulate it provides the major constraint on what is possible. Thus in some cases, the absence of data means that particular desirable features have to be omitted from the model, while in other cases sampling errors associated with the available data makes a high level of aggregation necessary. Both these problems tend to encourage models that are relatively simple and aggregated.

One particular implication of this form of constraint is that, while in theory stochastic models of manpower supply systems can be devised, such models can rarely provide much more information than can be obtained from deterministic models.

MAJOR ISSUES FOR NURSE SUPPLY MODELS

The idea of using nurse supply models to investigate the supply consequences of alternative management actions is clearly good in principle. Indeed, a number of such models are now available and others are being developed. The Second Report of the All Wales Manpower Planning Committee (1987) provides a comparison of seven of these models.

However, if models of this sort are to be used properly, a number of important issues need to be appreciated. In particular it is important that nurse managers recognize the potential and limitations of the modelling process, the criteria that are likely to lead to successful applications and the respects in which they need to be improved.

Participation rates versus wastage rates

Existing models are based on one of two methodologies: 'participation rates' (PR) or 'wastage rates' (WR). It is important to understand the differences between these two methods, although, as will be argued later, they also have much in common.

Referring back to Figure 21.1, the major difference is essentially in how the flows of qualified nurses between 'working for the NHS' and 'not working for the NHS' are modelled. If we refer to the net flow from the former to the latter as the 'net wastage rate' then the two models estimate age-specific net wastage rates as follows:

WR model

Net wastage rate of nurses of age a years

$$= \text{wastage rate at age } a - \text{joining rate at age } a$$

PR model

Net wastage rate of nurses of age a years

$$= 1 - \frac{\text{participation rate at age } (a+1)}{\text{participation rate at age } a} \quad ;$$

Note that the following standard definitions are used:

$$\text{Wastage rate at age a} = \frac{\text{WTE leaving of age a during year}}{\text{WTE in post of age a at start of year}} \quad ;$$

$$\text{Joining rate at age a} = \frac{\text{WTE joining of age a during year}}{\text{WTE in post of age a at start of year}} \quad ;$$

$$\text{Participation rate age a} = \frac{\text{WTE nurses age a employed by NHS}}{\text{Total no. qualified nurses age a}}$$

(WTE = whole time equivalent)

It has been shown in Worthington (1988) that the calculations that the two types of model perform with these two different estimates are essentially the same. However, a major difference between their results can occur because the two estimates of net wastage rate can be very different, as explained below.

Long-term or short-term estimates of net wastage rates

In the WR model wastage rates and joining rates are estimated from recent data on the numbers of nurses leaving the NHS and joining the NHS, preferably by age and possibly also by grade. The level of aggregation will be determined by the detail and amount of data available. If the amount of data is small, a high level of aggregation may be necessary to reduce sampling errors. Thus for the WR model net wastage rates will reflect current trends, probably at most the trends of the last two or three years, depending on the amount of reliable data available. These current trends will obviously reflect recent opportunities for nurses outside the NHS, recent levels of morale within the NHS, recent attempts by the NHS to attract qualified nurses back into the NHS and recent policies within the NHS to reduce nursing numbers in some areas. If wastage rates and joining rates also have to be aggregated across age groups and so are not age-specific, they will reflect the current age-structure of the qualified nursing workforce.

The PR model on the other hand estimates net wastage rates from current participation rates. However, current participation rates are obviously a product of wastage and joining rates from the last 40 years or so. Again it is preferable to use age-specific rates if possible, otherwise the rate will also reflect the current age-structure of the total qualified nurse population.

Thus one basis for choice between the two approaches that could be put, rather unfairly, to managers is whether they wish to assume recent trends or trends based on up to the last 40 years for the nurse supply planning period they are considering. Without the aid of a crystal ball, this is likely to be a very speculative choice, particularly if the planning period is more than a few years.

An alternative and more constructive idea is that promoted by Trent RHA, (see for example Beaumont and Peel, 1987: namely, to offer the manager supply projections on the basis of both sets of estimates. This at least informs the manager about the possible degree of inaccuracy involved in the method. There is also perhaps the hope that the true future will lie somewhere between the two – although this is not certain. There is clearly a role for a modelling approach that will help the user to consider alternative realistic net wastage rates other than these possible extremes.

Participation rates can be misleading

One of the initially anticipated advantages of the PR models was that data on participation rates would help managers to identify the scope for attracting qualified nurses back to working in the NHS. For example, a 60% participation rate might indicate another 40% who might be attracted back to the NHS. However, because an unknown proportion of the qualified nurses identified as not working for the NHS have no wish to return to nursing within the NHS, the figures are misleadingly over-optimistic.

Other wastage rate models

The discussion so far has concentrated on WR models in which age-specific WRs have been used and these have been compared with PR models. In some models, wastage rates are aggregated across all age groups, while others use grade-specific rather than age-specific wastage rates.

Because of the lack of age-specific WR data, some supply models simply use an average WR which they apply to all ages of nurses together. Thus while the age structure of the nursing workforce will, in reality, change, this will not be reflected in a changing average WR. It is possible that in some analyses this simplification will not introduce significant errors. However, example calculations carried out by the author for two DHAs in the north-west of England suggested that ignoring the age structure led to overestimates in workforce projections over a ten-year period of approximately 6% and 13% respectively.

Perhaps more fundamental is the point that it is only possible to test the sensitivity of results to this particular assumption by using a model based on age-specific rates. This is especially worrying in a context where possible supply strategies may involve deliberately changing the age structure of the workforce.

Other WR supply models deliberately choose grade-specific WRs instead of age-specific rates. These models highlight an important problem: namely, that joining and leaving rates could depend on the grade structure of the nursing population as well as its age structure. While the results from these models will complement results obtained from those previously described, if presented alone they must be treated with caution for a number of reasons. As noted above they omit the effect of changing age structure. They also have to make some quite complex assumptions about grade-specific wastage, joining and promotion rates. The debate initiated through Project 2000 about restructuring and redefining the roles of nurses can only serve to further complicate this problem.

Cross-boundary flows

Although Figure 21.1 describes the main stocks and flows, there are others which we refer to here as cross-boundary flows. At a national level, examples would be qualified nurses leaving the UK to work abroad, or qualified nurses coming from abroad to work for the NHS. These will be relatively small and if they need to be modelled at all can probably be represented by simple net flow rates into/out of the system. However, at the regional level, cross-boundary flows are relatively larger in size and so may need to be modelled in greater detail. This is particularly so because, unlike international boundaries, the NHS has some influence on and interest in what happens on both sides of the regional boundaries.

At the district and hospital levels, cross-boundary flows again take on a greater importance. They will affect recruitment of trainees, the wastage rates of qualified staff to other districts/hospitals and the recruitment of qualified staff from other districts/hospitals. These extra flows can be incorporated into the supply models relatively easily. However, obtaining data on their current values can be quite problematic and estimating future values is likely to be little more than wishful thinking. The crux of the problem is that recent values, if available, will reflect recent policies of the district/hospital (e.g. to reduce staffing levels in the face of economic constraints or to increase training-school intakes in anticipation of new facilities) and also those of its neighbours. Simple extrapolation from recent values is therefore unwise. However, to do more than this a district/hospital has not only to consult its own schemes but also those of its neighbours. This is not an easy matter given the fluid nature of nurse supply schemes that are likely to exist. Clearly the situation requires district/hospital level models that are carefully co-ordinated between districts/hospitals.

Data requirements

All nurse supply models have some data requirements and even with an excellent model the popular adage 'garbage in, garbage out' remains true.

The basic requirement for all models is up-to-date numbers of staff in-post, preferably by age and by care group and possibly by grade. Even these basic requirements have posed problems for nurse supply modelling in the past. This has been particularly so for national figures as they are essentially the sum of local figures and hence need all local figures to be available and reasonably accurate.

WR models also require numbers of starters and leavers, again preferably by age and by care group and possibly by grade. Here it is important to know starters and leavers by source and destination, as people who simply change job within the NHS should not be counted as either starters or leavers. Some of the confusions that can be caused when this data is not available are well described in Grocott (1989).

One of the basic data requirements of the PR models is the total number of qualified nurses in the population, by age and by care group. The best source of this information at present is the national census database. However, this obviously needs to be updated for intermediate years which requires further approximations to be made. A second problem with this data is in the allocation of nurses to care groups. Many nurses hold qualifications in more than one care group and the census records this information in two ways. It counts numbers of nurses by most recent qualification and it counts qualifications. Unfortunately neither of these counts is precisely what is needed: the former can seriously misallocate nurses between care group, the latter will count actual nurses in more than one care group.

Some models also incorporate data on the pool of school-leavers from which the bulk of trainee nurses are likely to be recruited. In others this is important background information for the manager in considering possible future recruitment rates. Typically only approximate figures are available.

In the context of data requirements, one advantage that some districts and hospitals (and regions) will have is the quality and detail of the data they hold. Thus while the data available at national level is essentially the minimum of that available in all districts/hospitals, clearly many districts, hospitals and regions will have better data. Conversely, although data may be available in greater detail at the local level it will also be subject to greater sampling errors. Thus staff groups may have to be aggregated simply to reduce these errors rather than because of lack of detail in its collection.

Expertise

Ideally a nurse supply model would be a user-friendly piece of computer software which can be used easily and interpreted safely by nurse (and other health service) managers. However, the nature of the nurse supply modelling process currently prevents this possibility. In particular, the need to make the best of available data and then interpret the results in the light of the approximations in the data and the assumptions of the model will almost always require some additional modelling expertise. This may in time come from nurse managers who have become involved in the supply modelling activity, but will for the moment in most cases require some external input.

ROLE OF NURSE SUPPLY MODELLING

Role of local models

Despite the reservations outlined earlier, nurse supply models can make important contributions to the nurse workforce planning activity at the local level. To a large extent, the value extracted will depend on the quality of information and effort put into the exercise. Three types of use can be distinguished:

* as a management game;
* to improve understanding by providing 'ball-park' figures; and
* to identify management targets.

Management game

The process of using a nurse supply model requires nurse managers to provide relevant statistics on such items as current in-post staffing levels; recent joining and leaving rates; and possible planned training, recruitment and retention rates. Running the nurse supply model will then demonstrate to those involved the important influences that such factors are likely to have on future staffing levels.

Thus using such a model, even with inaccurate and incomplete information, will cause managers to recognize the important factors, to start to collect relevant information and perhaps to go on to monitor key rates with a view to controlling them (and hence the workforce size) in the future.

'Ball-park' understanding

Even though data is known to be inaccurate and there is a possible debate about modelling methodology, nurse supply models can still provide useful messages for management. For example, Figure 21.2 shows the result of using two different models to forecast the future supply over a ten-year period of registered mental handicap nurses in a district in the north-west. While the results of the two models differ and the target figures are only approximate, there is a clear message for local management that there is a potential overstaffing problem.

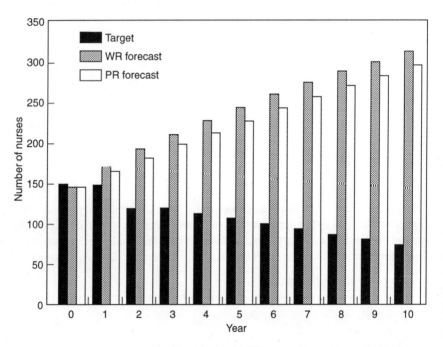

Figure 21.2 Forecast and target numbers of MH nurses for an example district.

Similarly, as described in Worthington (1990), applying nurse supply models to individual districts in the north-west has indicated that the likely impact of a 30% decrease in the number of 18/19-year-olds would not be as severe an impact on future workforces as is often anticipated. The model projected the effect to be only a 5% decrease in RGN workforces over a ten-year period.

Setting targets

If data is reasonably reliable and the model sufficiently realistic, then nurse supply models can help managers to set targets for training, recruitment and retention. For example, one might rerun the mental handicap model used to produce Figure 21.2 with alternative training, recruitment and retention rates until the projected workforce coincides with the target. These rates could then be used as management targets.

Role of national (and regional) models

In principle, nurse supply modelling can have similar value at the national (and regional) level as at the local level. However, many of the decisions that will affect the key rates in the models must be taken at local level, in the light of local circumstances. At the time of writing some such decisions will be influenced by the relatively short-term requirements of meeting contracts within budgets.

Moreover, the very different problems faced in different parts of the country mean that an average national (or regional) picture will hide many of the real problems that are at the local level, as well as some of the opportunities to solve them. It is thus important that any national (or regional) models are accompanied by local models that will enable localized problems and opportunities to be identified and investigated.

THE FUTURE

The major roles for nurse supply models have been outlined earlier. For them to succeed and to improve in these roles in the future there are three key areas of concern.

Data

As in many other areas of modelling the most important improvements will be caused by the increasing availability of better quality data. Accurate staff-in-post figures by age and care group for all districts is the first requirement and is already available in many parts of the country. Once age-specific WRs by care group are also available (which some parts of the country are already able to produce), WR models can then be used with reasonable confidence. However, this requires counts of joiners and leavers by source and destination respectively. In particular, joiners must distinguish internal flows within districts or hospitals (which can be excluded), flows of qualified staff from elsewhere, appointments of previously qualified staff who have not been working in the NHS, appointments of newly qualified staff trained within the district and appointments of newly qualified staff trained locally. Similarly, counts of leavers must distinguish internal flows within districts or hospitals (which can be excluded), flows of qualified staff to elsewhere and staff who leave the NHS. Clearly if this data is collected by locality, simple aggregation will also provide the data required for regional and national models.

The UKCC live register is capable of providing reasonably up-to-date data on numbers of qualified nurses by age, by qualification and by locality which may help to improve the accuracy and value of PR models. McClean *et al.* (1992) present some recent results for manpower planners derived from this sort of database. Also, the Nurses Central Clearing House is starting to build up a database on applicants to nursing schools that should shed greater light on future recruitment potential from and to individual geographical areas.

In addition to these standard data sources there is also an important role for local studies to improve understanding of the present situation and of possible future developments. For example, studies such as that of Barry, Williams and Soothill (see Chapter 20) can provide insight into local wastage rates, possible future levels and indeed into potential methods for controlling them.

Technical developments

A large number of nurse supply models have been developed over the last 15 years. This has in part reflected a natural tendency for local managers to wish to develop models specifically for their local problem as they see it. For the future, a more co-ordinated development is probably preferable. This should not only be more efficient but should also help to standardize and co-ordinate planning activities, particularly in adjacent areas.

Given the complementary nature of the WR and PR models via the concept of net wastage rates, a sensible technical development would be a single 'net wastage rate model'. Such a model would offer maximum flexibility to the user who could use the same model with input data expressed as wastage and recruitment rates, or participation rates or in fact using any other parameters from which future net wastage rates can be derived.

There is also the need to develop models that will reflect changes, for example as caused by Project 2000 and the introduction of purchaser and provider arrangements. Because the effects of such changes are potentially quite complicated, there is a natural tendency to build complex models. This should be avoided if possible, as complex models usually have quite demanding data requirements which can cause a major stumbling block for the potential user.

Support

Alongside these information and technical developments there is also the need to support and develop further expertise in nurse supply planning.

The data requirements described above must be clearly specified and should be carefully monitored by 'experts', perhaps at regional level.

The process of nurse supply planning also needs to be supported and co-ordinated. Thus modelling locally should actively involve local managers and nurse-planning 'experts' who are able to advise on the use and interpretation of the models and to co-ordinate the assumptions being made by districts or hospitals, particularly about cross-boundary flows. Such co-ordinated activity may also help to find regional solutions to local problems. Co-ordination is particularly important at the present time when market pressures are tending to encourage hospitals to take short-term contract-related decisions rather than longer-term strategic decisions that are required for sensible workforce planning.

CONCLUSIONS

Nurse supply modelling offers a powerful tool to nurse workforce planners. However, for it to be applied successfully, prospective users need to appreciate its potential and its limitations. Nurse supply modelling is an approach that is continuing to develop. It should become increasingly successful as data improves, as better models are developed and as nurse workforce planners become increasingly familiar with the approach and become better supported in their planning activities.

ACKNOWLEDGMENTS

Much of the original material for this chapter stemmed from a project carried out on behalf of Operational Research Services, Department of Health and Social Security during 1987. The work greatly benefited from a high degree of interest from a wide variety of NHS personnel. Much of the writing was carried out while the author was employed for five months at the University of Odense, Denmark.

REFERENCES

All Wales Manpower Planning Committee (1987) *The Second Report of the All Wales Manpower Planning Committee: Nurse Supply Modelling.*

Beaumont, K. and Peel, A. (1987) *The Trent Nurse Supply Model: User Guide*, Trent RHA.

Edwards, J.S. (1986) Manpower planning in 1986, in *Recent Developments in Operational Research* (eds V. Belton and R.M. O'Keefe) Pergamon, Oxford.

Grocott, T. (1989) A hole in the black hole theory. *Nursing Times*, 65–7.

Hancock, C. (1986) Project 2000: the staffing equation. *Nursing Times*, Aug. 20, 40–2.

Hancock, C. (1993) Valuable assets. *Nursing Times*, Oct. 27, 20.

Martin, L. (1990) Nursing skills: is there a shortage?. *International Journal of Manpower*, Vol. 11, 37–43.

McClean, S., Reid, N., Devine, C., Gribbin, O. and Thompson, K. (1992) Using a manpower database to analyse the nurse limbostock. *Journal of Advanced Nursing*, Vol. 17, 992–1001.

NHS Management Board (1987) Nurse manpower planning: letter to regional, district and SHA general managers, 6 March.

Rowden, R. (1993) The next decade. *Nursing Times*, Oct. 27, 21.

Worthington, D.J. (1988) *Nurse Manpower Planning (Supply Models and Quantitative Aspects of Recruitment, Retention and Return)*, Report for ORS, DHSS, England.

Worthington, D.J. (1990) Recruitment, retention and return: some quantitative issues. *International Journal of Nursing Studies*, Vol. 27, 199–211.

Auxiliaries in healthcare | 22

Emily Griffiths

INTRODUCTION

With the introduction of Project 2000 nurses has come that of the vocationally qualified support worker, who is ultimately to replace the auxiliary. There has been great concern for many years over the existence of auxiliaries and the extent of their role. Abel-Smith (1960) cites a chief nursing officer as early as 1949 calling for the need for a distinction in the duties of a trained nurse and those with lesser training. More recently, Seymour (1992) has suggested that nurses must actually start to provide hard evidence of the need for trained nurses. The debate in the intervening years has not been informed by research; the discussion on auxiliaries has largely concentrated on the limiting of their role and disassociating them from trained staff. It has been argued (for example, Draper, 1990) that the current changes are more to do with professionalizing nursing than improving patient care. In fact, despite the need for the nursing profession to be involved in the establishment of the support worker training (Northcott and Bayntum-Lees, 1993), the English National Board (ENB) has pulled out of a joint working body and the United Kingdom Central Council (UKCC) out of the Care Sector Consortium (Friend, 1991) who were overseeing the creation of the qualifications.

Historically, the institutionalized elderly have received most care from auxiliaries, often with few trained staff working with them. It has been suggested that not only will this continue (Royal College of Nursing, 1989) but that their numbers may also increase in other sectors (Jowett, Walton and Payne, 1994). Furthermore, there is an increasing number of elderly being cared for in nursing homes, outside the NHS, and it is recognized that here there may be only a minimum number of qualified staff. This is despite

Carr-Hill *et al*. (1992) finding that the quality of care is better the higher the grade that provides it and that auxiliaries provide better care when working with a higher grade. Hence, it is not surprising that concern should be expressed over standards of care in cases where auxiliaries dominate and about the nature of the relationship between trained and auxiliary staff (UKCC, 1994).

Despite the concern, however, it is clear that the role of the 'auxiliary' (or her equivalent – the term 'auxiliary' is used here throughout for simplicity) working on her own or with another auxiliary is likely to continue. Questions will similarly continue to be raised about supervision and education: that is, the way in which it is anticipated their work will be controlled. In the following, the auxiliaries' own perception of their work is considered. On the basis of this research* suggestions are made as to what the difficulties are in their providing care. The role of education and supervision is then considered by focusing on the extent to which trained staff help auxiliaries to improve their care through these strategies. This all then leads to asking how one can maximize the potential of the auxiliaries' contribution to care.

DOING THE JOB

Clarke (1978) described the atmosphere on long-stay and rehabilitation wards as that of 'getting through the work' with the emphasis on the provision of physical care and good intentions to talk to patients, which never reached fruition. Hardie and MacMillan (1980) similarly described the atmosphere on wards where many auxiliaries were employed as 'more of getting through the work and finishing on time than elsewhere'. This still appeared to be the key to understanding these workers' perception of the job.

In some respects they saw their work as like that in a factory, with a production line of patients to be washed, dressed, fed and toileted. Thomas (now doing his nurse training) described his experience: 'I remember on a psycho-geriatric ward having to get up 20 or 30 confused old men and going down the line, getting them washed, dressed, to the dining room, and then the next one. Just a drudge really – I hated it.'

It was not that they saw this as the best way to provide care, rather that they believed this was what trained staff expected of them. Norma commented: 'The auxiliaries get all the dirty work. I come on and am just expected to get on with it, without so much as a good morning!'

All the auxiliaries working with the elderly saw direct patient care as their most important duty, to be done as first priority. Housekeeping-type

---

* The research referred to took place in 1989, involving detailed interviews and participant observation with 54 auxiliaries from five hospitals, described at length in Griffiths (1991).

tasks such as tidying lockers or bagging-up linen were also a part of their job. On a ward where 'primary' nursing had been introduced, only the auxiliaries (renamed care assistants) did these housekeeping tasks. On other wards, trained staff or those in training helped the auxiliaries with this. These jobs were fitted in around direct patient care, with their execution constantly being interrupted by calls from trained staff to take someone to the toilet, pack their belongings and so forth.

Although it may be perceived that the auxiliaries were doing basic tasks, including washing, dressing and taking them to the toilet, observation showed there were constant opportunities to do more than the basic delegated task. For example, when the auxiliary on an orthopaedic ward was giving out drinks, she spotted a young man in his first attempt at using a wheelchair. The auxiliary explained what the doctor had said he could do and warned him not to overdo it. Another example was when an auxiliary was told to bed-bath a patient. To the observer he also required pressure-area care, bowel care, a shave and a change of position to help his breathing. The auxiliary bathed him but the other needs were left unmet. He was not assisted by another nurse for the rest of the morning.

What, then, was the criteria used by auxiliaries to decide what was their job? To an extent it depended on the experience of the auxiliary. While in the example above the auxiliary did not apparently identify the need for bowel care, on another occasion an auxiliary was seen to prepare a patient for an enema, and get a nurse to administer it, who then left immediately while she continued with the care. The actual giving of enemas was clearly not a part of auxiliary work, similarly dressings, paperwork, i.e. careplans and giving medication. Attendance of ward reports was sometimes only for trained staff. Giving patients information was a trained nurse's job, unless it was 'commonsense', but what usually happened to patients with certain conditions on that ward was a part of commonsense. Refusing access to trained staff and therefore to information was also seen on a maternity ward with the auxiliary deciding what was acceptable behaviour for the patient. A mother asked her to get a midwife to ask about feeding her baby and was told by the auxiliary it was 'up to her'. On other occasions, auxiliaries would find midwives for mothers when requested.

It appeared to the auxiliaries and the observer that at times many patient needs were likely to be left unmet (or unmet for some time) if not done by them. This was particularly upsetting to them if that task had been apparently safely done by them before. One auxiliary described how she would see patients requiring fluid by rhyles tubes and, having done it for years, would remind trained staff to do it or, if no one was about, give it herself and not report it.

Although, overall the auxiliaries were prepared, if they had some further limited training, to do more than they currently did, this was not always the case. Edith described how difficult it was on a rehabilitation ward as 'there was nothing to do but talk'. Attempts by the sister to introduce twice-daily diversional therapy had been met with reluctance by the auxiliaries. Edith said it was not that she felt silly, as some auxiliaries did, 'chucking a ball about', but that some real knowledge of the patient's medical condition was needed to do it properly.

There are two main points here. First, for auxiliaries the work has a production-line quality to it, but they see this as how the trained staff want them to work: that is, they are responsible for getting all the patients up and dressed and so forth by set times. Second, strictly limiting their role runs into difficulties in reality because patient needs occur simultaneously and an auxiliary is often more available to the patient than a trained nurse. Auxiliaries going beyond their role worked at times to the patients' advantage, but if the auxiliaries missed needs, trained staff did not always check up to identify and meet these needs themselves (or did not for some time).

THE PATIENT

The auxiliaries talked a lot about the job and very little about the patients. In their view the patients had two aspects: they were people whom they were concerned about, but they were also the 'work objects' to whom they had to do things as already illustrated. The latter will be enlarged on first. To continue with the metaphor of factory work, Beynon and Blackburn (1972) described how the factory workers they looked at became frustrated when the line was interrupted, slowing them down and how they gained satisfaction from achieving their targets. For the auxiliaries, one of the main interruptions to their work was caused by confused patients who were unpredictable and might disrupt their work with other patients or undo work already done, for example, by getting up after being put to bed or otherwise failing to co-operate. As Ada said, 'Sometimes the patients do things that are unexpected and put me all behind – and everyone think I'm very slow anyway and then I get irritable.'

Lucid patients could also 'put one behind'. On one ward a sister, who had only recently left, had encouraged patients to wait until the toileting rounds before asking for the commode. Extra requests – that is, those outside the routine – were seen as unreasonable. Therefore when a woman wanted to use the toilet before going to bed it caused an auxiliary to comment: 'You'd get finished early, but for her. She's spoilt.'

Although this attitude towards extra work might appear extreme, this idea of some care being seen as extra has been noted elsewhere (see Treacy, 1987, in her study of student nurses). Bedfast patients who required only washing and changing were described as 'good', since they caused the minimum amount of extra work and interruptions. Provision of care outside the usual order was also unpopular because it also slowed one down.

Hence Annette (who worked on a ward for the elderly, where primary nursing has recently been introduced), commented: 'It's okay Ann [ward sister] letting patients lie in or giving them baths before breakfast, but it only means we've got to finish off the rest of the patients after breakfast, while they do something else.'

There are then, as Payne notes, inherent difficulties which arise 'from the fact that the elderly people are different, having differing needs and standards than that of the institutional regime' (Payne, 1988: 11). That is to say, you cannot always 'do the job' and care for the patients at the same time.

Despite this, the auxiliaries did care about, as well as for, their patients. (This distinction between the 'task of tending and feeling for' another person is made by Dalley 1988). Only one of those interviewed had 'worked to grade' in the 1989 pay dispute, as this involved limiting what was done for patients. But caring about patients was problematic, particularly caring about confused people, for three main reasons. First, one could not have 'normal' dealing with confused patients. Hazel clearly illustrates this point:

> Where I was they were more confused than not confused. They'd no conversation, and when they did – sometimes you'd think, 'Oh my God, they're away with the fairies.' This might sound awful, but you weren't dealing with people.

Second, they could not always accurately judge a patient's mental state, particularly if they were deaf. The alternative was that they tended to treat everyone as confused or deaf, because most were. Interestingly, an American study (Wolanin and Philips, 1981) found that trained staff also had these kinds of difficulties.

Third, it was noted during periods of observation, that there was confusion between 'firmness' and 'bullying' of patients. To quote Hazel again:

> I think that auxiliaries there get a power that they have never had and get quite bossy. They're never talked back to ... I've heard it said, 'Do you want a bath Mrs So and So?', 'No, I don't!'. 'Well, if you think you are getting off' ... and they'd tell them off – I've heard it said.

But such behaviour was not limited to auxiliaries. For example, trained staff were seen 'encouraging' a patient to walk by 'threatening' them with a long-stay hospital which they knew the patient was afraid of, remembering it as the old workhouse. This shared behaviour between trained and auxiliary staff was also seen in relation to getting fed-up and irritable with patients and laughing at them (rather than with them). An example of the latter was when a staff nurse and auxiliaries were seen to spend some time repeating the name of a park to one confused patient, for their amusement, as it made her very agitated.

Therefore, despite the rhetoric of caring about the patients, the need to meet the routine and the characteristics of some patients cared for meant there were inherent problems in providing a high standard of care. In the light of these issues, the role of education and supervision in modifying their approach to work will now be considered.

LEARNING THE ROPES

Previous research has found student nurses learn on the wards, with minimum supervision, the 'real' as opposed to the school way of working (Treacy, 1987). Auxiliaries were assumed to an even greater extent to be workers practically from the start. When asked how much one needed to learn to do the job and how much was commonsense, a typical answer was that given by Mary: '50% commonsense, 50% learnt – or maybe 75% commonsense.'

Nursing is traditionally seen as 'women's work' and caring for children or parents at home might be seen as similar to an auxiliary's role on the ward. However, all the auxiliaries spoken to, who had recently started the job, rejected this view. Elizabeth, for example, found that the work at home was not helpful, other than teaching her not to be squeamish. Auxiliaries had to learn the hospital routine. Surprisingly and paradoxically, although it had to be learned, they still saw it as commonsense. An example was having to use two flannels to wash people with, one for hands and faces and one for 'down below'. This was not done at home but was still commonsense once you have been told. This emphasis on learning the routine of a ward, rather than learning to care for people, which might in fact be similar to work done at home, is almost identical to the description of student nurses' experiences (Melia, 1981; Treacy ,1987).

The auxiliaries described being shown what to do, mostly by other auxiliaries. When asked what they had been 'taught' when starting on a ward, each mentioned activities such as lifting or bedbathing. They generally saw themselves, however, as being expected to 'pick things up as they went along'. Two women had been 'orientated' on their first day, but had been too anxious to remember anything. One had worked for several shifts with the same staff nurse and felt that she had learned a lot from her. Overall, however, they had learned by watching. They did not watch trained staff in particular, but whoever was at hand, usually another auxiliary and questioned whoever was most approachable. Several had found their own mentors in this way. For one woman it was an auxiliary who had started only a few weeks before her. The new auxiliaries described how learning through watching was very difficult, as everyone did the same tasks slightly differently. There were also apparent contradictions. For example, one of the sisters insisted that dirty linen should not be put on the floor. The newcomer then found that everyone did just that. The auxiliaries on that ward rapidly concluded that two types of behaviour were required: one to 'get through the work', and one for when sister was around.

As for more formal teaching, this varied. Some, employed for ten years or more, had received lectures from a charge nurse, which they considered relevant to the total patient care they then gave. Of those more recently employed, many had had no formal teaching. Two had refused training as they felt they knew all that was relevant. Of those who had been on courses, many felt it was interesting but irrelevant and several were not sure what they had been about. One hospital had given auxiliaries competence booklets, but no one had completed them. When asked what was learned that was useful, Rita said the teacher had suggested things such as raising the beds to stop patients getting back in them! This and the talk by the physiotherapist were the only things mentioned. Clearly, auxiliaries, as well as student nurses, have difficulty with the theory/practice gap.

When asked what they needed to learn, the most frequently cited point was the meaning of abbreviations such as CVA. Several of the auxiliaries wanted to go on to do nurse training. Medical knowledge was of most interest to them and, notably, an understanding of the various illnesses. While in many respects auxiliary work could be described as nursing, nursing knowledge did not interest them. Knowing the routine was all the knowledge required for this job.

In discussion with a tutor at one of the hospitals visited, it was commented that the aim of the auxiliaries' course was to teach them what they were *not* to do. Another said that really the aim was to make them feel important and interested in their job. It may be that, as the auxiliaries felt, they do not need teaching. However, this is likely to be based on the assumption by trained staff (not shared by the auxiliaries) that they are closely supervised. The auxiliaries' view of supervision will now be considered in more detail.

ARE AUXILIARIES SUPERVISED?

At the time of the fieldwork, auxiliary nurses had been 'regraded' and had received the lower of two possible grades on the basis that they were supervised in their work. The auxiliaries did not feel that they were supervised and some (though only one of those interviewed) had 'worked to grade' for a short period. For example, some auxiliaries had refused to do a bedbath unless accompanied by a trained nurse. They had not continued to 'work to grade' for long, as they felt it was unfair to patients. The new auxiliaries, in particular, were surprised by the extent to which they were just left to 'get on with it'. However, this was also seen as one of the benefits of the job. Kate, for example, said she had worked for a time with a sister who was always checking up on her. It made her nervous and feel as though she was not trusted. Typically, auxiliaries worked together or on their own. There might be a trained nurse working in the same area as them, but not overtly observing their work.

Assuming that the supervision of the auxiliaries was not done, in that no one watched directly over them, it might be expected that they would be obliged to report back to someone on the work which had been delegated. However, as already mentioned, the paperwork associated with the nursing process was not used by the auxiliaries and even when the auxiliaries were present, attention at ward reports was focused on the medical condition of the patients and not on the nursing care required or received. The auxiliaries themselves felt, if they had the patient's medical diagnosis, that was all the information they needed. Only Thomas, who had worked in a hospice, had been encouraged by the sister to contribute to a ward report on spiritual or social matters, even if he had nothing to offer on nursing care. On one occasion during the participant observation, a report was given to an auxiliary who had just come on duty by a staff nurse. The auxiliary was specifically told to do various things, including encouraging a patient to eat her tea. Despite this, she still accepted the patient's first refusal to eat her meal. Again, it appeared to come back to the auxiliary's belief that nursing knowledge is irrelevant. They had the routine.

The auxiliaries themselves suggested they had little use for the knowledge of trained staff. When the researcher asked, in the first interview completed, what they might ask trained staff about, Alice and Barbara both looked surprised. They said that they did 'report' things to staff, but that they did not 'ask' them anything. The other auxiliaries gave similar replies. Trained staff knew about dressings, drugs and medical information and required auxiliaries to report any changes to them. Without them they would not know what was going on. Although the auxiliaries were aware of the need to report things, the majority of those observed in their work did not appear aware of what to look out for and therefore report, so that they could not fulfil their good intentions.

Although there may be no formal supervision and reporting back, trained staff are constantly acting as role models for auxiliaries and, through their management of them, showing them what the priorities are to be. To deal with the latter point first, it was commented that although trained staff might say it was important to talk to patients, as soon as you did, a job was handed out. This follows from the earlier point that auxiliaries believed trained staff expected them just to get on with it. Penny (now a student nurse) summed it up: 'It didn't matter if your standards were immaculate, so long as you were quick and remembered to wipe the lockers as well as their faces.' Penny considered herself unusually fortunate in having initially worked with a really good staff nurse, whom she had wished to emulate.

Gibson and McMillan (1992) suggest that the clinical facilitator provided a role model for the auxiliaries in their study, thereby improving their care. Bond *et al.* (1990) considered that this standard setting by the trained staff was critical in maintaining the level of care on the primary nursing ward studied. However, for the auxiliaries in this particular study there were difficulties with role modelling as the trained staff at times did not set an appropriate example – the problem of distinguishing between being 'firm' and 'bullying', inappropriate use of humour and shared understanding and frustration are mentioned earlier. Furthermore, trained staff did not appear to have appropriate skills to deal with some patients, particularly those who were confused. They therefore could not demonstrate these skills to the auxiliaries. An American study similarly found that dealing with such patients was one of the biggest problems faced by the unqualified staff. On teaching them appropriate interventions, an aide suggested they should teach all the nurses (Feldt and Ryden, 1992). Such teaching of appropriate intervention to all grades of staff would appear appropriate here.

Another problem appeared to be that giving patients a choice and interrupting the routine could be seen as a luxury for trained staff while the auxiliaries still had to ensure the 'work' was done. This seemed to be the case in the example already given, when the sister had let the patients stay in bed. Bond *et al.* (1990) note that the importance of auxiliaries in maintaining standards of care was recognized on the wards which gave particularly high standards of care. In the research described here it appeared that although they were in fact providing 'real care', it was seen as 'basic' and the auxiliaries' contribution not recognized.

CONCLUSION

The situation described is one where there is a strong culture among the auxiliaries about what their work is. Formal learning and supervision are not seen as relevant. Learning the routine is seen as different from learning that requires knowledge of nursing care. Those more recently employed saw their job more as carrying out discrete tasks than providing total patient care. It has been suggested elsewhere that where auxiliaries work in a role clearly subservient to trained staff, there is a risk of their 'potential alienation' (Robinson *et al.*, 1989: 31). The training provided for them and the way in which the grade of their job was allocated reinforces this. The difficulty appears to be that, particularly in the care of the elderly, auxiliaries are in fact the ones doing the nursing. The routine is often nearly all the care that patients get. A study of hospital domestics showed that, when they were encouraged to do only their cleaning, much valuable patient care was lost, decreasing their job satisfaction and also increasing the potential nursing care required (Tonkin and Hart, 1989). The effect of emphasizing these specific limits on the role of the auxiliary is likely to have a similar result. The loss of potential care from auxiliaries is, however, much greater.

The trained staff were not seen as having relevant superior knowledge concerning the work the auxiliaries did. In particular, it was not apparent in relation to the two main problems faced by auxiliaries, which are in providing care within the routine of an institution and dealing with people who could be difficult to care for.

It is therefore concluded that the most appropriate way to improve standards of care for patients (assuming that care will continue to be provided by auxiliaries) is not to place an emphasis on the lowly status of auxiliaries versus qualified staff and to attempt to limit their role, as in reality it appears exceptionally difficult to divide nursing care into discrete tasks. Rather, the real problems faced by auxiliaries should be seriously addressed. In this way we could usefully develop their genuine attempts to provide good care.

REFERENCES

Abel-Smith, B. (1960) *A History of the Nursing Profession*, Heinemann, London.

Beynon, H. and Blackburn, R.M. (1972) *Perceptions of Work*, Cambridge University Press, Cambridge.

Bond, S., Fall, M. and Thomas, L. with Fowler, B. and Bond, J. (1990) *Primary Nursing and Primary Medical Care: A Comparative Study in Community Hospitals*, Report No. 39, Health Care Research Unit, University of Newcastle upon Tyne.

Carr-Hill, R., Dixon, P., Gibbs, I, Griffiths, M., Higgins, M., McCaughan, D. and Wright, K. (1992) *Skills Mix and the Effectiveness of Nursing Care*, Centre of Health Economics, University of York.

Clarke, M. (1978) Getting through the work, in *Readings in the Sociology of Nursing*, (R. Dingwall and J. McIntosh), Churchill Livingstone, Edinburgh.

Dalley, G. (1988) *Ideologies of Caring*, Macmillan, Basingstoke.

Draper, P. (1990) Change in nursing, and the introduction of the support worker. *Nurse Education Today*, **10**(5), 360–5.

Feldt, K.S. and Ryden, M.B. (1992) 'Aggressive behaviour – educating nursing assistants. *Journal of Geronotological Nursing*, 3–12.

Friend, B. (1991) A misleading picture? *Nursing Times*, **87**(23) 19.

Gibson, K. and McMillan, W. (1992) Nursing auxiliaries: developing services for elderly people. *Nursing Standard*, **6**(31) 29–32.

Griffiths, E.J. (1991) A qualitative study of hospital nursing auxiliaries with specific reference to standards of care, unpublished M. Phil thesis, University of Lancaster.

Hardie, M. and MacMillan, M. (1980) The nursing auxiliary in the National Health Service, unpublished report, Edinburgh University.

Jowett, S. and Walton, I. with Payne, S. (1994) *Challenges and Change in Nurse*

Education – a Study of the Implementation of Project 2000, Berkshire National Foundation for Education and Research in England and Wales.

Melia, K. (1981) Student nurses: aspects of their work and training: a qualitative analysis, unpublished PhD thesis, University of Edinburgh.

Northcott, N. and Bayntum-Lees, D. (1993) Who Cares. *Nursing Times*, **89**(22), 40–1.

Payne, M. (1988) Caring in residential homes, *Conference Paper*, British Geriatric Society Annual Conference, London.

Royal College of Nursing (1989) *The Care of Elderly People – Provision after Griffiths and the NHS White Paper*, ACE/Focus Discussion Paper, Royal College of Nursing, London.

Robinson, J., Stillwell, J., Hawley, C. and Hampstead, N. (1989) *The Role of the Support Worker in the Ward Care Team*, Nursing Publicity Centre 6, University of Warwick.

Seymour, J. (1992) Pick and mix. *Nursing Times*, **88**, (33), 19.

Tonkin, G. and Hart, E. (1989) I love my work, I hate my job – a study of hospital domestics. *ESRC Report*, University of Birmingham.

Treacy, M.M. (1987) In the pipeline – a quantitative study of general nurse training, unpublished PhD thesis, University of London.

United Kingdom Central Council (1994) *Professional Conduct – Occasional Report on Standards of Nursing in Nursing Homes*, UKCC, London.

Wolanin, M.O. and Philips, L.R.F. (1981) *Confusion, Prevention and Care*, C.V. Mosby, St. Louis.

23

Stress and the person with cancer: an exploration of the concept of stress and the nurse's psychological support role

Elizabeth Hanson

INTRODUCTION

The lack of psychological care of persons with cancer by healthcare professionals continues to be a common source of distress for patients and family members alike. Anecdotal stories reveal the failure for the most part of professionals to treat patients and families as persons. This is indicative of the dominant perspective within healthcare: that is, the medical model in which illness is viewed as a malfunction of one or more of the body's components, entailing a set of measurable symptoms, signs and bio-chemical or physical abnormalities. The criticisms levelled at the medical model in relation to the care of patients and families within a hospital setting have been well-documented in healthcare literature spanning the last 15 years.

In contrast, a humanistic model has been espoused within the nursing literature with the aim of understanding human behaviour from the individual's perspective. The individual is the author of their actions and behaviour cannot be managed in the same manner in which natural phenomena can be controlled. Thus, a humanistic model serves as an appropriate framework to explore the nature of stress among persons with cancer and to describe the nurse's support role.

In order to assist students and qualified nurses to gain an increased understanding of psychological care of persons with cancer, a précis of the psychological concept of stress and key theories of stress will be undertaken, followed by a critical review of healthcare literature pertaining to psychological care of persons with cancer.

THE PSYCHOLOGICAL CONCEPT OF STRESS AND THE KEY THEORIES OF STRESS

The word 'stress' continues to be a buzz-word in the 1990s and is frequently hailed as the catalyst for a variety of illnesses ranging from myocardial infarction through to breast cancer (Lazarus, 1992). The *Concise Oxford Dictionary* defines stress in the following ways: 'constraining or impelling force'; 'effort, demand upon physical or mental energy'. The key psychological theories help to further elucidate its meaning.

The response-based model of stress

This first model, expounded by Selye (Selye, 1993; Tache and Selye, 1985; Selye, 1979; Selye, 1957), is commonly adopted by healthcare professionals as it focuses on clearly recognizable physical symptoms. Selye argued that it is necessary to look for a particular pattern of responses which can be taken as evidence that the person is stressed. The response is then treated as the stressor or its defining parameter. In this way, the occurrence of the response represents the occurrence of stress, which may act as a stimulus for producing further responses.

Selye's central tenet regarding stress is the notion of non-specificity of the physiological response of the body to any demand made on it. Thus, the physiological response is not dependent on the nature of the stress as there is a universal pattern of defence. He described this defence reaction as the 'general adaptation syndrome' (GAS). If the stress continues, resources dwindle, collapse and, at the end stages, disease states occur which represent the cost of the defence reaction.

Selye explained that the physiological response is maintained by two major psycho-endocrine systems: the sympathetic adrenal medullary (SAM) and the pituitary adrenal cortical (PAC). This assumes that there is an important functional balance between the two branches of the autonomic nervous system which govern the activity of the internal organs, for example, cardiac smooth muscle and digestive function. Selye summarized his perspective on stress by stating that stress occurs when the controlling mechanisms are strained in the maintenance of the internal environment of the vital areas. Thus, his definition is embedded in physical responses.

Selye illustrated his medical model by explaining the physiological reactions in humans during a stress situation, leading to the 'fight or flight' syndrome. Sympathetic nervous system activity leads to specific physiological effects such as increased catecholamine secretion, increased corticosteroid activity, increased blood-glucose levels, increased heart rate and blood pressure, dryness of the mouth and throat and dilation of the pupils. Using Selye's model, Cox (1978) argued that more general health effects can be seen as a response to stress. For example, headaches, ulcers, cardiovascular disease, amenorrhea and asthma.

In order to provide quality care to persons with cancer, it is essential that physiological indicators of stress are not assessed in isolation from the psychosocial, spiritual and existential factors which may also affect the individual. Selye's response-based model fails to reveal an interaction between physiological and psychological factors, creating a physiological bias. Clearly, both factors are involved, but Lazarus and Folkman (1984) believe that the most important factor to consider is the individual's perception of the situation as stressful or otherwise. Selye's model loses sight of the individual because it is a general theory, with the result that respect for the individual is sacrificed.

An explicit weakness exists in Selye's concept of non-specificity of the body's response to stress because specificity is evident. For example, heart and respiratory rates and catecholamine excretion rates differ as an individual may respond more or less to one stressful situation compared to another. It is also important that physiological indicators of stress are assessed in conjunction with the physiological effects of an individual's illness and/or treatment. For example, an increased corticosteroid activity may reflect the cancer patient's disease or specific effects of medication, as opposed to an indicator of stress *per se*.

Cox and Cox (1993) proposed more generalized responses to stress in the form of behavioural and cognitive effects of stress. For example, excessive eating, drinking or smoking, drug-taking, impulsive behaviour, lack of concentration, forgetfulness, trembling, excitability and restlessness. In my research study (Hanson, 1994a) of the taken-for-granted world of the cancer nurse in relation to stress and the person with cancer, cancer nurses noted the relevance of subtle changes in patients' behaviour. For example, 'going over the top' (overly high in spirits); withdrawing; being unusually chatty and being critical about everyday or non-specific matters. Most nurses mentioned insomnia as a common reaction to stress among cancer patients. Several nurses explained that patients may get up and ask for a cup of tea, smoke a cigarette or sit in the day room with the door closed. It was also explained that at night, symptoms such as pain and dyspnoea are heightened, making patients feel worse.

Cancer nurses also described the importance of body language to assess stress in persons with cancer. For example, crying, wringing hands, looking sad, looking worried, holding nurse's attention longer than necessary and fidgeting. Observation of 30 nursing admission assessments revealed that most cancer patients exhibited stress non-verbally (Hanson, 1994a). For example, frequent rubbing of hands; avoiding eye contact when talking; giving small smiles; rapid speech; repetition of words and using 'ah's' and 'um's' at intervals. One patient's voice was inaudible at times. Several patients tended to laugh loudly and quickly after they had finished talking. The non-verbal cues of some patients substantiated their implicit verbal reports of stress. However, in other cases, non-verbal cues were in direct contrast to a person's 'cheerful' verbal communication. It is important, therefore, that non-verbal and behavioural cues are assessed in conjunction with the individual's verbal communication and are not evaluated as distinct variables.

To summarize, the response-based model of stress expounded by Selye focuses on a physiological approach. While physiological and behavioural cues (including body language) are important considerations in the assessment of stress, it is essential that they are considered within the entire context of the individual with cancer.

The stimulus-based model of stress

A stimulus approach to stress is based on a medical/engineering model and considers external stressors in the environment that lead to a stress response. Welford (1975) suggested that stress occurs whenever the demand for adaptation made on an individual departs from a moderate level. This illustrates that low levels of demand on an individual can be equally as stressful as high levels of demand. Welford proposed that humans have evolved to produce optimum adaptive performance under conditions of moderate demand.

The focus of a stimulus approach to stress is to identify situations which can reliably be described as stressful to people. For example, Cox (1978) put forward the following demands in the work situation which can be viewed as stressful: excessive noise or complete silence; excessive heat or cold; poor illumination or glare; extremes of humidity and atmospheric pollution.

Holmes and Rahe (1967) attempted to quantify the degree of stress associated with major life events. They constructed a scale of 43 life events. Death of a spouse was consistently rated highest and was given a value of 100. All other events were given proportional values based on this value. For example, divorce 73, marital separation 65, jail term 63, personal injury or illness 53, marriage 50, fired at work 47, marital reconciliation 45 and retirement 45. The authors purported that people in the United States, Western Europe and Japan all tend to rate life events in similar ways.

In my research study (Hanson, 1994a), cancer nurses described their perceptions of the main causes of stress for persons with cancer which included the prospect of death and the effect on family and lifestyle. Similarly to the response-based model of stress, the stimulus model is a macro-theory which fails to account for individual differences in relation to their experience of stress. The cancer nurses gave further specific examples of individuals with cancer for whom these general factors had caused them to experience stress but for differing reasons. For example, the effect on the family was considered by the nurses to be a universal cause of stress for patients. A nurse recalled a patient who was worried about her disabled husband at home. Another nurse recounted how a patient was worried about her daughter who was heavily pregnant and without work, to the extent that she was unable to give herself time to recuperate from chemotherapy. From these examples it can be seen that the experience of stress varies according to the individual. This leads into the third model of stress.

The transactional model of stress

In order to provide comprehensive care to persons with cancer, it is essential that nurses ground their work within a humanistic framework which encompasses and endorses the individual's experiences of stress. The transactional model of stress serves as an appropriate framework for nurses to assess, monitor, manage and evaluate stress, as it takes into account that each person is an individual with unique needs.

The transactional model was espoused by Lazarus (1966) and subsequently developed by Lazarus and Folkman (1984). They stated that stress occurs when there are demands on the person that tax or exceed their adjustive resources. Stress is viewed as an interaction between the individual and the environment. The individual is perceived as an active agent, as opposed to the passive being highlighted in the medical model and, in particular, in the response-and-stimulus theories of stress. Thus, stress may constitute a mixture of personal and environmental factors, but the central element remains the individual's perception of themselves and a particular situation. Both the response-and-stimulus-based models of stress overlook the individual and emphasize physiological factors (response model) and external life events (stimulus model), so that the person tends to be viewed almost as a machine.

The emphasis on the active role of the individual reflects the growing trend over the last decade within nursing philosophy and lay-advocate groups towards self-care and empowerment of the individual for their own health. This moves away from the traditional medical model of the patient as a passive being and healthcare professionals as 'experts' on the individual's illness.

Lazarus and Folkman (1984) argued that one must treat the person as an active agent of change on the environment as well as respondent to that environment. Thus, it is a dynamic relationship characterized by change and flux (Somerfield and Curbow, 1992). Within the psychosocial cancer literature, suffering from cancer is viewed as a type of status passage, a process involving change over time which has developed out of Glaser and Strauss' (1968) concept of the dying trajectory. Changes in an individual with cancer's stress and coping patterns occur in the context of a hospital-based, medically oriented system of intervention, often characterized by a loss of self (Cassell, 1982, 1991; Glaser and Strauss, 1968, 1971; Parker, 1985). Several nurses in my study acknowledged that living with cancer is potentially stressful for most or all of the time. One nurse commented:

> I can't pinpoint when there is any time when you can't say with cancer patients, that there isn't a stressful time – I'm not saying all patients are laid in a state of stress, constantly 24 hours – but each and every day can be stressful.

Concerning the indicators of stress within a humanistic framework, Lazarus and Folkman considered an individual's verbal reports of stress as important, the premise being that the person is the expert in matters regarding themselves. The cancer nurses in my study reiterated this view as they felt it was essential to know the person with cancer in order for them to be able to confide in the nurse. The role of intuition was explained by several nurses in relation to assessing stress in persons with cancer. For example, 'just a feeling', 'you just know – it's difficult to put into words'. This phenomenon relates to the complex role of cognition in perceiving stress, acknowledged by Lazarus and Folkman (1984). Clearly, the cancer nurse is likely to intuit an individual's stress accurately if they know the individual well, as opposed to making assumptions about the person's stress.

Lazarus and Folkman (1984) accepted that there are occasions when an individual may be unaware of the true nature of their stress due to the subconscious use of defence mechanisms such as denial. For example, in my study one nurse recalled an individual who was unaware that she was denying the stress associated with her diagnosis of cancer as she adopted a cheerful front. In this situation, Lazarus and Folkman (1984) explain that it is important to take other indicators into consideration: that is, non-verbal and behavioural cues, to explore if there are any revealing differences. Therefore, it is important that cancer nurses carry out a thorough assessment which considers a person's verbal reports of stress, but also relate these to the individual's non-verbal and behavioural cues.

In contrast to the medical model in which healthcare professionals are viewed as the experts on the cancer patient, a humanistic approach recognizes family members as an invaluable resource on the individual as, in most cases, they know the person well. This reflects the hospice/palliative care philosophy in which the patient and family are considered the unit of care. The goal of healthcare professionals working within this philosophy is to improve the quality of life of the person with cancer and reduce the stress experienced by families as they support their ill family member (Dobratz, 1990; Doyle, 1991; Kennedy, 1991).

Thus, family members are more likely to detect any subtle changes in the person's psychological well-being. This information, when relayed back to the nursing staff, provides them with a greater awareness and subsequent understanding of the individual concerned. In my study, the nurses emphasized the importance of communicating effectively with a person's family member/s to create a mutually supportive network.

If nurses are to adopt Lazarus and Folkman's transactional model of stress in which an individual's appraisal of a situation is central, it follows that they need to fulfil their psychological support role. Thus, nurses need to give due consideration to the verbal reports of persons with cancer regarding their experiences of stress in order to assess their psychological well-being. However, the following section discusses the problems surrounding the implementation of psychosocial aspects of cancer nursing care.

REVIEW OF HEALTHCARE LITERATURE RELATING TO THE PSYCHOSOCIAL CARE OF PERSONS WITH CANCER

A review of key studies of communication over the last 16 years between nurses and persons with cancer leads to the overriding criticism of the cancer nurse's ability to detect and monitor stress among persons with cancer. Bond (1978, 1982) and Maguire's (1978; Maguire, Tait and Brooke, 1980; Maguire, 1985) initial findings in this area were that nurses give a low level of attention to the social and psychological aspects of illness, as few interactions with cancer patients concerned their psychological well-being. In subsequent work, Maguire (1985) labelled this phenomenon 'distancing tactics', with nurses assuming that persons with cancer will disclose their problems. As a result, nurses rarely asked patients about their psychological state. Examples of diverting tactics include attempting to brush away the problem with premature or false reassurances; ignoring the person's words; changing the topic of conversation or avoiding conversation with them.

These techniques effectively block communication about the psychosocial aspects of a person's care. More recent empirical studies reveal that nurses in specialist and non-specialist care-settings are continuing to block communication with cancer patients (Blum and Blum, 1991; Fallowfield, 1988; Krause, Munnukka and Vaatainen, 1992; Maguire and Faulkner, 1988; Wilkinson, 1991a, 1992). Similarly, patient education and information-giving is often of an *ad hoc* nature (Agre *et al.*, 1990; Johnson, 1988; MacLeod Clark and Sims, 1988). It has been argued that these problems often have negative consequences for the patient's psychological well-being in terms of negative social and psychological outcomes (Hardman, Maguire and Crowther, 1989; Kaye and Gracely, 1993; Nichols, 1993; Spiegel, 1992).

Maguire and Faulkner (1988), Fallowfield (1991) and Wilkinson (1991b) put forward the view that some nurses, albeit subconsciously in some cases, attempt to maintain an emotional distance. Nurses may take the view that they are acting in the best interests of the person with cancer: the rationale is that the less the problem is discussed, the less upset the person will become. Thus, some nurses believe it is unwise to 'go looking for problems' by directly asking about a person's psychological well-being. This may lead to the individual with cancer asking such challenging questions as: 'Am I going to die? or 'Is the treatment really working'? Many nurses fear that the individual will reveal strong emotions which then create reciprocal distress in the nurse concerned. In order to avoid such a situation, both cancer sufferers and nurses conspire to pretend that they are coping satisfactorily. As a result, nurses have a tendency to ignore crucial verbal and non-verbal cues which persons with cancer reveal about their problems.

Thus, the conclusion from key empirical studies spanning the last 16 years is that many nurses are not able to provide emotional support to persons with cancer because they find it stressful to do so. Clearly, the stress levels of nurses is a significant factor affecting their patterns of communication (Maguire and Faulkner, 1988; Nash, 1993; Vachon, 1987). Nurses who consistently support cancer patients are at increased risk of becoming 'burnt-out', negatively affecting their personal health. It is now recognized that support is a dual-edged sword. Thus, support for the professional caregiver is essential in order to carry out their support role effectively (Crockett, 1993; Faulkner and Maguire, 1988; Firth-Cozens, 1989). Nichols (1993) advocated principles of self-care and preventive support for nurses and described the skill of receiving support. Support may be informal, such as reciprocal support with colleagues, or more formal, such as a support group consisting of nurses on a unit (Nichols, 1993).

Maguire and Faulkner (1988) and Wilkinson (1991a, b) point to the inadequacies of nurse education to provide effective training in communication and counselling skills. In the past, communication has tended not to be a subject that is taught, but is simply regarded as an accumulation of experience. In contrast, with the onset of Project 2000 in recent years, communication now forms an essential part of the education programmes for nursing students (Burnard, 1991; Faulkner, 1992).

However, problems still remain because in order to incorporate the principles of effective communication and counselling skills, it is essential that students are able to practise and develop their skills in a ward environment which offers excellent role models. Unfortunately, this currently cannot be standardized for all students, as access to continuing education for all registered nurses remains an ideal. Thus, for the present, commonsense methods are often employed within cancer-care settings, with tactics and routines learned through observation and experience. Other possible creative and innovative practices and learning strategies may only be implemented on an *ad hoc* basis dependent on the ward-learning environment and the philosophy and commitment of the sister or charge nurse (Wilkinson, 1991a).

Faulkner, Webb and Maguire (1991), Nichols (1993) and Wilkinson (1992) emphasized the importance of registered nurses working on cancer wards to receive training in the psychological aspects of cancer. They argued that the nurses would then be able to develop specialist communication skills in interviewing and assessing persons with cancer and give sufficient attention to the psychological and social areas of an individual's history.

The assessment phase of the nursing process constitutes the first crucial step in the problem-solving approach, as needs or problems must be identified at the outset before care is enacted (Burton, 1991; Faulkner, 1992; Tschudin, 1991; Webb, 1990). This may appear at first to be commonsense to the reader. However, my study revealed that some nurses, when interviewing persons with cancer, gave detailed information regarding treatment and its side effects without first exploring the individual's perceptions of their treatment and then appropriately adjusting the information. Cancer nurses must also be attentive to making judgments based on assumptions rather than deliberative assessment.

Common psychological areas of concern for persons with cancer identified by nurses from my study included perceptions of cancer as stigmatizing; perceptions of cancer as equalling a death sentence; well-being of family members; effect of cancer on their lifestyle; the treatment itself and its side-effects; feelings of loss of self; an altered body image; feelings of helplessness; fear of pain; experiences of cancer-related pain and fear of addiction to analgesia.

In keeping with Lazarus and Folkman's transactional model of stress, after exploring a person's stress experience it is important to understand their perceptions of coping and their coping patterns and factors that help to reduce stress. Thus a comprehensive picture is gained of the person's psychological status. Within this humanistic framework, the cancer nurse needs to regularly monitor the psychological well-being of the person with cancer by asking open-ended questions such as: 'How are you feeling in yourself?' Monitoring should occur around the clock and not only on day and evening shifts. My recent qualitative studies of the night-nursing care of cancer patients (Hanson, 1994b) has confirmed anecdotal evidence that persons with cancer feel particularly vulnerable at night and the cancer nurse can play a valuable role by providing empathic presence and support to patients and their family at this time.

Within the last five years, specific educational initiatives have included national education programmes, courses (Faulkner, Webb and Maguire, 1991), workshops (Corner and Wilson-Barnett, 1992; Faulkner and O'Neil, 1994), descriptions of team interventions (Blum and Blum, 1991) and the use of instruments (Pace, 1993). Initial evaluation studies of educational programmes have favoured the use of experiential methods, such as group work and role play, as opposed to more structured approaches, such as a lecture-guide approach (Corner and Wilson-Barnett, 1992; Wilkinson, 1992).

While these initiatives endeavour to redress the long-term problems described above, it is becoming more widely recognized that the issues are more complex than specific educational input and merit further empirical studies which explore the context in which psychological care is given. For example, studies which explore environmental factors that impinge on the nurse-patient helping relationship, such as the hospital's organizational structure (Wright, 1991); the method of organizing nursing care (Wright, 1991) and the ward environment created by the sister or charge nurse (Corner and Wilson-Barnett, 1992; Wilkinson, 1991a).

CONCLUSION

Within this chapter, an exploration of the main psychological perspectives of stress led to a discussion of the implications of the prevalent emphasis on the response-and-stimulus based theories. An outline of the literature has been presented about the psychological care of persons with cancer and the role of the cancer nurse. It can be seen that to date the empirical studies have not answered all the significant problems surrounding the cancer nurse's implementation of the support role. It has been argued that in order for the cancer nurse to provide a comprehensive psychological care of persons with cancer, they need to adopt a humanistic framework to guide their work. The transactional model of stress (Lazarus and Folkman, 1984) is recommended as an approach in which the individual and their perceptions of a situation remain of paramount importance and significance.

ACKNOWLEDGMENTS

The author wishes to thank the Department of Health, England, and the University of Manitoba Social Sciences and Health Research Council, Canada, for their support given to undertake the research mentioned in this chapter.

REFERENCES

Agre, P., Bookbinder, M., Cirrincione, C. and Keating, E. (1990) How much time do nurses spend teaching cancer patients? *Patient Education and Counselling*, **16**, 29–38.

Blum, D. and Blum, R. (1991) Patient-team communication. *Journal of Psychosocial Oncology*, **9**(3), 81–8.

Bond, S. (1978) Processes of communication about cancer in a radiotherapy department, unpublished PhD thesis, University of Edinburgh.

Bond, S. (1982) Communication in cancer nursing, in *Recent Advances in Cancer Nursing* (ed. M. Cahoon), Churchill Livingstone, Edinburgh, pp. 3–31.

Burnard, P. (1991) Acquiring minimal counselling skills. *Nursing Standard*, **5**(46), 37–9.

Burton, M.V. (1991) Counselling in routine care: a client-centred approach, in *Cancer Patient Care: Psychosocial Treatment Methods* (ed. M. Watson), The British Psychological Society, Cambridge, pp. 74–93.

Cassell, E.J. (1982) The nature of suffering and the goals of medicine. *New England Journal of Medicine*, **306**(11), 639–41.

Cassell, E.J. (1991) *The Nature of Suffering and the Goals of Medicine*, Oxford University Press, Oxford.

Corner, J. and Wilson-Barnett, J. (1992) The newly registered nurse and the cancer patient: an educational evaluation. *International Journal of Nursing Studies*, **29**(2),177–90.

Cox, T. (1978) *Stress*, Macmillan, London.

Cox, T. and Cox, S. (1993) Occupational health: control and monitoring of psychosocial and organisational hazards at work. *Journal of the Royal Society of Health*, **113**(4), 201–5.

Crockett, D. (1993) Supporting the care-givers in oncology. *Nursing RSA Verpleging*, **8**(1), 30–1.

Dobratz, M.C. (1990) Hospice nursing: present perspectives and future directives. *Cancer Nursing*, **13**(2), 116–22.

Doyle, D. (1991) Palliative care education and training in the United Kingdom: a review. *Death Studies*, **15**, 95–103.

Fallowfield, L.J. (1988) The psychological complications of malignant disease, in Complications of Malignant Disease, (ed. S. Kaye), *Balliere's Clinical Oncology*, **2**(2), 461–78.

Faulkner, A. (1992) *Effective interaction with patients*, Churchill Livingstone, Edinburgh.

Faulkner, A. and Maguire, P. (1988) The need for support. *Nursing* **3**(28), 1010–12.

Faulkner, A. and O'Neill, W. (1994) Bedside manner revisited: teaching effective interaction. *European Journal of Palliative Care*, **1**(2), 92–5.

Faulkner, A., Webb, P. and Maguire, P. (1991) Communication and counselling skills; educating health professionals working in cancer and palliative care. *Patient Education and Counselling*, **18**(1), 3–7.

Firth-Cozens, J. (1989) Stress in medical undergraduates and house officers. *British Journal of Hospital Medicine*, **41**(2), 161–4.

Glaser, B.G. and Strauss, A.L. (1968) *Time for Dying*, Aldine Publishing, Chicago.

Glaser, B.G. and Strauss, A.L. (1971) *Awareness of Dying*, Aldine Publishing, Chicago.

Hanson, E.J. (1994a) An exploration of the taken-for-granted world of the cancer nurse in relation to stress and the person with cancer. *Journal of Advanced Nursing*, **19**, 12–20.

Hanson, E.J. (1994b) Psychological support at night: a pilot study. *Cancer Nursing*, **7**(4), 1–6.

Hanson, E.J., McClement, S. and Kristjanson, L.J. Psychological support role of night nursing staff on an acute oncology unit: a Canadian pilot study. *Cancer Nursing* (in press).

Hardman, A., Maguire, P. and Crowther, D. (1989) The recognition of psychiatric morbidity on a medical oncology ward. *Journal of Psychosomatic Research*, **33**(2), 235–9.

Holmes, T. and Rahe, R. (1967) The social readjustment and rating scale. *Journal of Psychosomatic Research*, **11**, 213–18.

Johnson, P. (1988) Principles of cancer education, in *Oncology for Nurses and Health Care Professionals* (eds R. Tiffany and P. Webb), 2nd edn, Harper & Row, London.

Kaye, J.M. and Gracely, E.J. (1993) Psychological distress in cancer patients and their spouses. *Journal of Cancer Education*, **8**(1), 47–52.

Kennedy, M.E. (1991) Hospice care for the cancer patient. *Journal of Urological Nursing*, **10**(3), 1307–11.

Krause, K., Munnukka, T. and Vaatainen, A. (1992) Psychosocial nursing in radiotherapy cancer wards in Finland. *Scandinavian Journal of Caring Sciences*, **6**(4), 241–9.

Lazarus, R. (1966) *Psychological Stress and the Coping Process*, McGraw Hill, New York.

Lazarus, R.S. (1992) Four reasons why it is difficult to demonstrate psychosocial influences on health. *Advances*, **8**(3), 6–7.

Lazarus, R.S. and Folkman, S. (1984) *Stress, Appraisal and Coping*, Springer Publishing, New York.

McLeod Clark, J. and Sims, S. (1988) Communication with patients and relatives, in *Oncology for Nurses and Health Care Professionals* (eds R. Tiffany and P. Webbs) 2nd edn, Balliere Tindall, London.

Maguire, P. (1978) The psychological effects of cancer, in *Oncology for Nurses and Health Care Professionals*, Vol. 2 (ed. R. Tiffany), Harper & Row, London.

Maguire, P., Tait, A. and Brooke, M. (1980) Plan into practice. *Nursing Mirror*, 19–21.

Maguire, P. and Faulkner, A. (1988) The stress of communicating with seriously ill patients. *Nursing*, **3**(32), 25–7.

Maguire, P. (1985) Barriers to psychological care of the dying. *British Medical Journal*, **291**, 1711–13.

Nash, A. (1993) A stressful role. *Nursing Times*, **89**(26), 50–1.

Nichols, K.A. (1993) *Psychological Care in Physical Illness*, Chapman & Hall, London.

Pace, K. (1993) Communicating with cancer patients and families. *Caring*, **12**(2), 72–7.

Parker, J.M. (1985) Cancer passage – the change process in leukaemia, in *Long-term Care* (ed. K. King) Churchill Livingstone, New York, pp. 96, 119.

Selye, H. (1957) *The Stress of Life*, McGraw Hill, New York.

Selye, H. (1979) The stress concept and some of its implications, in *Human Stress and Cognition: an Information Processing Approach* (eds V. Hamilton and D.M. Warburton), John Wiley, Chichester, pp. 11–32.

Selye, H. (1993) History of the stress concept, in *Handbook of Stress: Theoretical and Clinical Aspects*, 2nd edn, (eds L. Goldberger and S. Breznitz), Free Press, New York.

Somerfield, M. and Curbow, B. (1992) Methodological issues and research strategies in the study of coping with cancer. *Social Science and Medicine,* **34**(11), 1203–16.

Spiegel, D. (1992) Effects of psychosocial support on patients with metastatic breast cancer. *Journal of Psychosocial Oncology*, **10**(2), 113–20.

Tache, J. and Selye, H. (1985) On stress and coping mechanisms. *Issues in Mental Health Nursing*, **7**(1–4), 3–24.

Tschudin, V. (1991) *Counselling Skills for Nurses*, Balliere Tindall, London.

Vachon, M.L.S. (1987) *Occupational Stress in the Care of the Critically Ill, the Dying and the Bereaved*, Hemisphere, New York.

Webb, P. (1990) Patient teaching, in *Oncology* (ed. A. Faulkner), Scutari Press, London, pp. 55–67.

Welford, A.T. (1975) in *Stress* (T. Cox), Macmillan, London.

Wilkinson, S. (1991a) Factors which influence how nurses communicate with cancer patients. *Journal of Advanced Nursing*, **16**, 677–88.

Wilkinson, S. (1991b) Communicating with cancer patients. *Nursing Standard*, **5**(43), 13–18.

Wilkinson, S. (1992) Good communication in cancer nursing. *Nursing Standard*, **7**(9), 35–9.

Wright, S. (1991) Facilitating therapeutic nursing and independent practice, in R. McMahon and A. Pearson (eds.), *Nursing as Therapy* (eds R. McMahon and A. Pearson), Chapman & Hall, London, pp. 85–101.

Nurses and the new industrial relations

24

Paul Bagguley

Leaders of Britain's 600,000 nurses have rejected government plans to link their pay to the performance of the National Health Service Trusts they work for. The move, days before a conference of doctors is expected to follow suit, puts health workers on course for a clash with the government over its determination to introduce performance pay next spring.

(The Guardian, 25 August 1994)

Nurses and doctors should get no national pay rise next year, ministers have told the professions' pay review bodies in a move which will inflame confrontation over the government's drive to link health workers' salaries to their performance. Pay increases should be awarded only at local level by the National Health Service Trusts which now provide 96% of hospital and community healthcare, the health departments for England, Wales and Scotland have told the review bodies.

(The Guardian, 21 September 1994)

REPRESENTING NURSES' INTERESTS

There are two types of organization that represent nurses' interests: professional organizations such as the Royal College of Nursing (RCN) and trades unions such as UNISON. What are the crucial differences between professional organizations and trades unions? In the context of nursing it is frequently noted that the difference is primarily one of attitudes towards strike action. The RCN is opposed to the use of strikes in pursuit of nurses' interests such as wage increases, while unions, such as

UNISON, are prepared to use strikes to further the claims of their membership. Social scientists, however, have developed more general models of the differences between the two types of organization. Sociologists typically see professional organizations as upholding the ethics of the profession. They control the education and qualifications for a profession and the right to practise that profession, often with the support or recognition of the state. Trade unions are seen as rather less powerful, normally seeking to protect the wages and conditions of their members through bargaining with the employers. Trade unions typically lack the control over qualifications and the rights to enter a particular occupation that are wielded by professional organizations.

While doctors and the legal professions perhaps come closest to the professional model outlined above, nursing and related professional organizations have frequently sought similar professional status. In practice, however, they have often developed into organizations akin to trade unions. Indeed, since the 1970s nurses' organizations have been seen as trades unions for legal reasons. Besides these general differences between professional and trade unionist forms of interest representation within nursing and the NHS there are more particular differences, especially in the distribution of the memberships. In a study carried out during the 1980s some significant variations in the patterns of union membership were found among professional nurses (Bagguley, 1992). Women were most frequently members of the RCN, while men were most likely to be members of the Confederation of Health Service Employees (COHSE). Those who had a break from employment in the NHS, 'middle-aged' nurses and RGNs were less likely to be members of any union. However, nursing grade and the hospital or unit of employment were the most significant determinants of union membership among professional nurses. These patterns largely reflect the history of the different organizations, with the RCN historically concentrating on general medical nurses and COHSE, for instance, having developed out of organizations that represented asylum workers.

The RCN, founded in 1916, received its royal charter in 1928 and became a registered trade union in 1977. Since the 1970s its more conventional trade-union functions, such as wage-bargaining, representing individual members' grievances and the training of stewards in industrial relations matters, have increased in importance. The Royal College of Midwives (RCM) was founded much earlier than the RCN in 1881, but only received its royal charter in 1947. The Health Visitors Association (HVA) was founded as the Women's Sanitary Inspectors' Association in 1896. The HVA has always been closely allied to the trade-union movement. It became registered as a trade union in 1918 and affiliated to the TUC in 1924. In 1990 the HVA merged with the Manufacturing, Science and Finance Union (Seifert, 1992: 89–92).

COHSE has always been a significant representative of nurses' interests and it historically developed as the union for psychiatric nurses, who account for about 70% of its members (Carpenter, 1988). Recently it joined with the National Union of Public Employees (NUPE) and the National Association of Local Government Employees (NALGO) to form the general public sector union UNISON (Seifert, 1992). In contrast to COHSE, NUPE concentrates on organizing manual workers in the NHS, although it still retained about 80,000 nurses among its membership in the late 1980s (Seifert, 1992).Together the three unions that have gone on to form UNISON can probably account for about 200,000 nurses among their total membership of around 1.4 million. Table 24.1 below summarizes the overall patterns of union membership among nurses.

Table 24.1 Membership of principal organizations representing nurses (late 1980s).

Health Visitors Association	16 435
Royal College of Midwives	33 487
Royal College of Nursing	282 000
COHSE	120 000
NUPE	80 000
GMB	7 000

Source: Seifert, 1992: 51 and 77.

Large sections of the public sector have retained a number of established features of industrial relations that have declined in recent years in the private sector (Milward et al., 1992). The NHS, for instance, retains high levels of union membership, with over 60% of employees being in unions of some kind. In addition, much of the wage-bargaining takes place in national forums known as Whitley Councils. However, even here there are exceptions and significant trends towards new forms of industrial relations. Union density[1] in hospitals, for example, has fallen from 66% to 60% between 1991 and 1992 (Bailey, 1994: 117). The merger of NALGO, NUPE and COHSE in July 1993 to form UNISON makes this new organization the largest union in the country with 1.4 million members. However, within UNISON nurses are a minority in what is very much a general union for all public sector employees. For legal purposes the RCN, like many professional organizations, registered as a trade union in the 1970s and 80% of qualified nurses are members of the RCN totalling almost 300 000 people (Bailey, 1994: 118). Many professional organizations have responded to change in the NHS and medical practice by seeking innovations in training, especially the introduction of degree-level qualifications for the nursing and related professions. Furthermore, since the mid-1980s there has been more co-operation than competition between nurses'

---

[1] Union density refers to the percentage of employees who are members of a union.

professional organizations and trade unions (Seifert, 1992:52–4). Overall, the picture is a complex one of continuities alongside major changes.

Strike action among nurses is relatively rare: there were only two significant strikes in the 1980s. In 1982, 5.3 million working days were lost (15% of the total) in a strike by nurses and ancillaries over pay and in 1988 a smaller-scale action among nurses and ancillaries occurred over privatization. Strike action among nurses was much more a feature of industrial relations in the NHS during the 1970s. In 1974 there was the first and only significant national strike of nurses. This was in demand for a national inquiry into their pay and conditions and was largely driven by COHSE. Nurses' pay had fallen by 11% in real terms between 1970 and 1973 at a time of high inflation. The RCN's response to this action was to threaten that its members would resign from the NHS and offer themselves for re-employment as agency nurses. Although this avoided breaking their no-strike rule, it proved to be an effective form of industrial action as the new Labour government relented and the resulting inquiry recommended a 30% pay increase (Lewis, 1976; Seifert, 1992: 264–5).

THE GENERAL CONTEXT OF INDUSTRIAL RELATIONS

Recent changes in the nature of industrial relations within the NHS, and for nurses in particular, cannot be fully understood without some appreciation of how industrial relations have changed more widely in Britain since 1979. One of the features of the 1980s was the experience of industrial disputes where the striking employees lost the dispute. Such instances include the steelworkers in 1980, the miners in 1984–5 and in the car industry generally during the early part of the 1980s. These very visible failures of traditional strike action by trade unions, alongside the changes in legislation, largely explain the decline in strikes in Britain since the late 1970s. During the 1970s there were on average 2600 strikes each year, but during the 1980s this annual average fell to a little over 1100 and, so far during the 1990s, this annual average has been well below 1000 (Kessler and Bayliss, 1992).

Since 1979 unions have lost around one-third of their membership due to the high levels of unemployment and the shift in employment from highly unionized, full-time, manual employment to more part-time employment in service industries, where union membership is typically much lower (Disney, 1990; Green, 1992). In addition to losing large swathes of their membership, unions have found their activities increasingly circumscribed by legislation. The closed shop – where all employees had to be members of a particular union – is pretty much illegal. Strikers can now be selectively sacked to enable employers to pick off local union leaders. Unions are required to run postal ballots for significant decisions such as strikes, electing leaders and to donate funds to political parties. Secondary action – where workers strike in support of others employed elsewhere – is now largely illegal, as are unofficial strikes which have to be adopted or repudiated by the union leadership. Finally, unions have lost their legal immunities, which means that under certain circumstances they can be sued for damages by employers (Marsh, 1992; Smith and Morton, 1994). These changes in legislation constitute a very restrictive regime for trade-union action. It is arguably the most restrictive in Europe and the most restrictive faced by unions in Britain during peacetime in the 20th century. Increasingly, unions are turning to European legislation to defend their members' rights and the European dimension of industrial relations legislation looks likely to be of increased significance for unions and their members in the future.

People at work in Britain in the 1990s face a very different situation from the 1970s. Only a minority of them are likely to be union members and have their pay decided by negotiation between unions and management, compared to a majority of the workforce 20 years ago. Most people's pay is simply decided by management. However, the NHS differs from this general set of circumstances, but it has still not been immune from these changes and some of them have affected nurses in particular.

TRUSTS AND QUASI-MARKETS: THE IMPLICATIONS OF NEW FORMS OF MANAGEMENT FOR INDUSTRIAL RELATIONS

Before the 1980s doctors were the most influential group within the NHS. However, Harrison and Pollitt (1994) have recently argued that the reforms of the 1980s and early 1990s have significantly reduced the power of the doctors and other professional groups such as nurses, in favour of managers. They suggest that in the 1970s management in the NHS was essentially reactive, responding to the demands made of them by doctors, nurses and others such as trade unions. There was no clear planning by management and change in the NHS was incremental. Harrison and Pollitt consider that much has changed since 1979 and especially in the 1990s (Harrison and Pollitt, 1994: 35–6).

Organizational change in the NHS since 1979 has taken two main forms. First, in the early 1980s general management was introduced after the Griffiths' report. This aimed to increase efficiency and accountability by employing managers from the private sector on fixed-term contracts with performance-related pay. Since many of these managers do not have nursing backgrounds, or indeed any medical background, they have little sympathy with the professional attitudes of the nurses. With the introduction of general management, Harrison and Pollitt argue, nurses lost their right within the NHS to be managed by senior members of their own profession. Indeed, only 9% of NHS general managers in 1987 came from a nursing background and only a further 16% from a medical background. The vast majority were formerly NHS administrators and managers (Harrison and Pollitt, 1994: 66–7). These kinds of changes lie behind many of the conflicts between professionals in the NHS and the management during the 1990s.

Harrison and Pollitt see a major clash developing between the NHS managers and professionals, with the managers generally winning. They point out that the roots of this conflict lie in the essential difference between professionals and managers. Professionals have autonomous styles of working where they use their own judgment to decide how they carry out their jobs. In contrast, managers are concerned with getting others to perform jobs as they think they should be done. Consequently, as managers are seeking to get whole hospitals or Trusts to perform to stringent financial and other performance criteria, they run into conflict with the professionals who see their autonomy being eroded (Harrison and Pollitt, 1994: 2–3). Since the late 1980s, there has been the more significant reforms of creating Trusts and the internal market, which have exacerbated this conflict between professionals and managers and shifted the balance of power towards the latter. These changes are fundamentally concerned with how resources are allocated within the NHS.

Resources were previously allocated with the NHS through bureaucratic formulae based on the size, age, etc. of a district or region's population. However, this has been swept away with the development of Trusts and the internal market. The consequences of these changes have led Gray and Jenkins (1993) to describe the NHS as a federation of semi-autonomous, self-managed organizations. In this new federated NHS, internal markets involve GP fund-holders and district health authorities in buying services from hospital Trusts. Within each organizational unit of the federation (the NHS as a whole) there is strong, centralized management that controls the budgets. GP fund-holders and Trusts constitute the self-managed organizations or units in Gray and Jenkins' model of market relations in the NHS. However, despite the image of a service decentralized to GP fund-holders, central government really retains overall control of the total national budget for the NHS. Consequently, this a far from perfect market: hence the term 'quasi-market'. Analysts frequently refer to it as a quasi-market for a number of reasons. The suppliers in these markets are not necessarily out to maximize profits like a private company in a normal market. Furthermore, 'vouchers' or ear-marked budgets are often used to purchase services rather than money (Le Grand and Bartlett, 1993: 10).

These changes in the management and allocation of resources within the NHS have both direct and indirect implications for industrial relations and the pay and conditions of nurses. Frequently this means that local managers will seek greater discretion over hours of work, etc. Trades unions may find that some issues are no longer up for negotiation with employers and that Trusts may introduce new kinds of employee and redesign jobs (Seifert, 1992: 361). The main reason for this is that the demand for services will feed directly into the demand for labour in the new NHS. This includes the number of nurses required. If particular hospitals or specialisms face high demand, then more staff will need to be recruited or existing staff will have to work longer hours. Conversely, if demand for a particular hospital or specialism contracts, then staff may have to be laid off. Overall it is feared that the development of Trusts will lead to flexible, locally determined, performance-related pay alongside the de-recognition of unions for bargaining over pay and conditions.

This variation in demand for health services generated by the new quasi-market is beginning to have an impact on how nurses are employed. Trusts cope with the uncertainty of demand for their health services by employing fewer qualified nurses and by relying to a much greater extent on bank and agency nurses. This means that nurses can be employed only as and when their skills are required. During 1993 to 1994, for instance, the total nursing workforce fell by 4350 or 1%, and the number of qualified nursing staff fell by 1.8% or 5450, but there was an increase in the number of unqualified nursing staff. More significantly, the number of bank nurses increased by 20%, and the number of agency nurses employed by the NHS increased by 44% in just one year. These are provisional figures submitted by the government to the nurses' pay review body in September 1994 and it was noted that the figures for London seem to be full of inaccuracies. Nevertheless, nurses' leaders complained that they signify a 'casualization' or nurses' conditions of employment that is likely to get worse as the quasi-markets develop (*The Guardian*, 22 September 1994). More obviously controversial, perhaps, are related figures on the trends in the employment of managers and nurses. Between 1989 and 1991 the number of NHS managers increased by 7610 and the number of nurses declined by 3450 (Harrison and Pollitt, 1994: 113).

NURSES AND THE NEW INDUSTRIAL RELATIONS IN THE NHS

Before the 1980s, bargaining over nurses' pay and conditions took place in Whitley Councils. These rest on three principles for their organization and activities: national negotiations between employer and employee representatives, joint agreements and formal procedures for conciliation and arbitration. However, in 1983 nurses were given their own pay-review body, rather like the one established for doctors and dentists in the 1960s. Evidence on pay levels is presented to the independent pay-review body by employee representatives, management and the Treasury. Based on this and other evidence, the pay-review body then advises the Prime

Minister on what would be an appropriate pay increase. In the case of the nurses' pay-review body, its establishment in the early 1980s was seen as a victory for the RCN's 'no-strike' policy. Other unions representing nurses, such as COHSE and NUPE, opposed the loss of rights of traditional wage-bargaining through the Whitley Councils (Bailey, 1994: 125). The government expected that nurses, midwives and other health professionals would refrain from strike action with other health service employees in the future (Bach and Winchester, 1994: 269). In other respects the creation of the nurses' pay-review body also put them on an equal status to that of doctors with respect to the way in which their pay was determined, so it may also be seen as enhancing the nurses' professional status.

The government has also been keen to introduce performance-related pay, as it believes that national pay awards are insensitive to local conditions and they restrict the ability of managers to achieve their targets (Bach and Winchester, 1994: 264). However, the practice of industrial relations in the NHS frequently departs from the rhetoric of the government. Indeed, in some instances the government seems to be pursuing incompatible policies. The desire to maintain a public sector pay norm – restricting pay rises to 1.5% in 1993, for example – seems to contradict the aim of rewarding productivity and individual performance at the local level, i.e. in individual hospitals. This latter goal, often referred to as pay flexibility, frequently leads to a larger wage bill, as pay flexibility is often only flexible in an upward direction. Such individualized forms of reward are an anathema to both unions and professional bodies in the NHS. As an attempt at a compromise, the health service management has proposed that performance-related pay be linked to the performance of the NHS Trusts that employ nurses and doctors (Bailey, 1994; Bach and Winchester, 1994).

This aim of local pay flexibility rewarding individual productivity and performance has become an issue of central concern during the mid-1990s, as the quotation from *The Guardian* at the beginning of this chapter shows. However, at the time of writing (1994) the final outcomes are still undecided, but the principles are clear. Such issues of pay determination are centrally linked to the development of Trusts and the internal market that now co-ordinates the activities of the NHS. Trusts have responsibility for the pay and conditions of their staff and effectively have the right to set wage levels and conditions of service that are not constrained by the national agreements between employer and employee representatives. By 1993, most Trusts had some staff on locally determined pay and conditions, but these only amounted to one-fifth of the workforce and most of these were agreements negotiated with local trade unions. So Trust status did not automatically lead to most Trust employees having their pay determined by the Trust. It has been identified that most Trust managers would prefer a co-operative way of deciding on pay levels through negotiating with trade unions (Bailey, 1994: 122).

Bach and Winchester (1994) have suggested a number of reasons why flexible pay has not been introduced for nurses, or indeed more generally in the NHS, in spite of Trust status becoming the norm. Nurses have a strong professional identity and high levels of union organization. This means that their unions are able to exert considerable pressure through evidence to the pay-review body and argue against performance-related pay on the basis that it would undermine professional standards. The NHS, and nurses in particular, have considerable public sympathy so any political party that is seen to be attacking them may lose public support and votes in elections. At the level of the Trust hospitals themselves, there are also a number of factors mitigating against performance-related pay. Given the determination of pay at a national level by the pay-review body, local management have little influence over national pay levels. Furthermore, they often lack the time, skills and resources to negotiate pay agreements locally. Add to this the wide range of occupations and professions within the typical Trust hospital employing over 2000 people and the negotiation of local pay wards would be a major managerial exercise consuming a large amount of resources. One of the frequently noted disadvantages of locally determined performance-related pay is that wide variations between districts and specialities may develop. One negative consequence of this is that it tends to inhibit the movement of people around the country and between specialisms. Consequently it may exacerbate or create wholly new shortages of labour (Seifert, 1992: 373). A final problem concerns how to measure the performance of health professionals such as nurses. Attempts to develop performance indicators for professional groups within the NHS have so far proved too problematic to implement and hence provide a basis for performance-related pay. The systems that have been tried have produced results that are too complex and contradictory (Harrison and Pollitt, 1994: 60).

In some respects, the creation of the pay-review body has generated political problems for the government with regard to nurses' pay. The pay-review body is only advisory and the final decision over pay levels still lies in the hands of government. Consequently any discontent about nurses' pay either among nurses themselves or the public at large is clearly aimed at the government (Bach and Winchester, 1994: 271). In the light of this reluctance by Trusts to implement performance-related pay, the government has taken a stronger line which has led to conflict with nurses' organizations and other representatives of professional employees in the NHS. In its recent statements and submissions to the pay-review bodies, the government is insisting that in 1995 there shall be no pay increase for nurses or other medical staff other than those negotiated locally and linked to individual performance (*The Guardian*, 21 September 1994).

CHANGES IN THE PATTERNS OF NURSES' PAY

Trades-union activities and industrial relations are most fundamentally concerned with pay, and pay rises might be seen as a crude measure of a union's success. Figure 24.1 shows how nurses' pay has varied in relation to the pay of all women in non-manual jobs since 1979. In general there has been a marked improvement (Bailey, 1994: 129; and Seifert, 1992: 86). The large increase in 1988–9 was due to a one-off payment to compensate for the revisions to the nurses' grades in that year. As Bailey comments: 'nurses' relative earnings in 1993 show an increase since 1979 greater than any other public service group' (Bailey, 1994: 129).

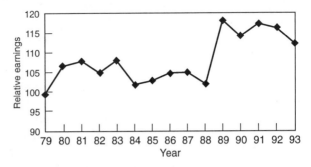

Figure 24.1 Changes in nurses' earnings relative to women's non-manual earnings: 1979–93.

However, the new grading structure introduced in 1988 caused considerable dissatisfaction among nurses. After the re-grading qualified nurses and nurse managers (grades C to G) were earning more relative to the auxiliary grades (A and B). The effect of the re-grading was to widen relative pay among nurses, i.e. there was more pay inequality among nurses. Alongside the introduction of the new job of 'healthcare assistant' these changes prompted many appeals against the re-grading (Seifert, 1992: 16). Nevertheless, this did not erupt into major strike action, as many nurses took an individual route to protest by appealing against their individual gradings, usually with the support of their unions. This illustrates quite well that there are often forms of industrial protest and conflict that do not fit the conventional stereotype of the strike.

Generally the progression of nurses up the salary scale is largely dependent on their individual performance or the state of the labour market (Seifert, 1992: 366). The largest changes have been among nurse and midwifery managers. Although their pay has increased relative to that of less well-qualified nurses, all 20 000 nurse and midwifery managers were placed on performance-related pay in 1990. Effectively this has taken them out of the 'national bargaining' of the pay-review body's recommendations, as their pay is broadly decided by the Secretary of State for Health. These developments have come on top of the Griffiths' general management reforms of the mid-1980s where the nursing profession lost much of its influence at senior management level (Seifert, 1993: 377). Consequently, the nursing profession within the NHS is now much more deeply divided, both in terms of their levels of pay and conditions and in terms of the determination of their pay and conditions than was previously the case.

CONCLUSION

I have examined the industrial relations situation facing nurses under three broad headings that focus closer and closer upon the everyday work situation of the nurse. The first heading concerns the changing nature of industrial relations in Britain as a whole, which has seen a hostile climate for unions develop especially through legislation. The second heading concerns the development of the NHS into a 'quasi-market', which encourages managers to seek flexible ways of organizing nurses' work and wages. The final heading concerns the changing relationship between the managers and the professionals, which Harrison and Pollitt (1994: 135–6) summarize as follows:

> Compared with 20 – or even 10 – years ago the average professional's work is nowadays much more likely to be costed, audited, used as an input for performance indicators, subjected to explicit budgeting or workload ceilings and/or included within the scope of patient satisfaction surveys … From 1984 to 1989 general managers were put in place and were immediately able to exert increased control over the professions allied to medicine and over nurses … And all the time the refinement of increasingly sophisticated information systems have made the amounts and types of nursing and medical work which is actually carried out more and more transparent to the managers of provider units.

However, as Harrison and Pollitt point out (1994: 137–47) there are definite limits to this increased managerial power that may become more significant over the next few years. Among these are the contingencies of the national political situation, pressure from consumers and fragmented managerial interests but, most significant perhaps, concerns about the power of the professionals themselves. The NHS or indeed any healthcare system simply cannot survive without the active consent of its doctors and nurses. Given the well-established and widely supported organizations of nurses in the NHS, the government and healthcare managers simply cannot go on ignoring their increasing protests at the impact of the current reforms.

REFERENCES

Bach, S. and Winchester, D. (1994) Opting out of pay devolution? The prospects for local pay bargaining in UK public services. *British Journal of Industrial Relations*, Vol. 32, No. 2.

Bagguley, P. (1992) Angels in red? Patterns of union membership amongst UK professional nurses in *Themes and Perspectives in Nursing*, 1st edn (eds K. Soothill *et al.*), Chapman & Hall, London.

Bailey, R. (1994) Annual review article 1993: British public sector industrial relations. *British Journal of Industrial Relations*, Vol. 32, No. 1.

Carpenter, M. (1988) *Working for Health: the History of COHSE*, Lawrence & Wishart, London.

Disney, R. (1990) Explanations of the decline in trade union density in Britain: an appraisal. *British Journal of Industrial Relations*, **28**(2).

Gray, A. and Jenkins, B. (1993) Markets, managers and the public service, in *Markets and Managers: New Issues in the Delivery of Welfare* (eds P. Taylor-Gooby and R. Lawson), Open University Press, Buckingham.

Green, F. (1992) Recent trends in British trade union density. *British Journal of Industrial Relations*, **30**(3).

Harrison, S. and Pollitt, C. (1994) *Controlling Health Professionals: the Future of Work and Organization in the NHS*, Open University Press, Buckingham.

Kessler, S. and Bayliss, F. (1992) *Contemporary British Industrial Relations*, Macmillan, London.

Le Grand, J. and Bartlett, W. (1993) 'The Theory of Quasi-Markets', in *Quasi-Markets and Social Policy*, (eds J. Le Grand and W. Bartlett), Macmillan, London.

Lewis, S. (1976) Nurses and trades unions in Britain. *International Journal of Health Services*, 6(4).

Marsh, D. (1992) *The New Politics of British Trade Unionism*, Macmillan, London.

Milward, N., Stevens, M., Smart, D. and Hawes, W.R. (1992) *Workplace Industrial Relations in Transition*, Dartmouth, Aldershot.

Seifert, R. (1992) *Industrial Relations in the NHS*, Chapman & Hall, London.

Smith, P. and Morton, G. (1994) Union exclusion in Britain – next steps. *Industrial Relations Journal*, **25**(1).

FURTHER READING

Bartlett, W. and Harrison, L. (1993) Quasi-markets and the National Health Service reforms, in *Quasi-Markets and Social Policy*, (eds J. Le Grand and W. Bartlett), Macmillan, London.

Butler, J. (1993) A case study in the National Health Service, in *Markets and Managers: New Issues in the Delivery of Welfare*, (eds P. Taylor-Gooby and R. Lawson), Open University Press, Buckingham.

25

Traditional and new management in the NHS hospital service and their effects on nursing

Stephen Ackroyd

INTRODUCTION

Traditionally, the management of public services has been a very different type of activity from management in most parts of the private sector. Because of the character of the relationship involved in the actual provision of public sector services, which in most instances are quite unlike those involved when services are supplied on the open market, management takes some quite distinct forms (Ackroyd, Hughes and Soothill, 1989). This is not a matter of inefficiency or ineffectiveness as is sometimes claimed. The patterns exhibited by public sector management have been just as viable and efficient in their own context as private sector management is when it co-ordinates and directs the supply of goods to the market. Because this is so, it is wrong to hold that public sector management should be an imitation of management in the private sector, which is the emphasis of much current thinking. Equally erroneous is the notion that the development of management must necessarily imply the extension of the market, privatization and the elimination of public service as traditionally understood (Hindess, 1987).

From this general stance on public sector management the case of the NHS hospital service will be considered. The pattern of the development of management in the service will be traced and linked with the condition of general nursing in hospitals. It will be suggested that, for much of its history, a stable and effective form of management – management by co-operating professionals, in which nurses had a central role – was in place and this secured an efficient hospital service. The problems of the service that are now apparent in shortages of resources and falling standards of provision did not arise from inadequacies in the working of the hospital system as such, or its management. In many ways they are a consequence of considerable success, in that successful and substantially free provision of hospital care has reinforced a strongly upward trend of consumption and this has produced the escalation of costs care and the need to ration provision. Indeed, it will be argued here that problems of the contemporary NHS hospitals, including such things as the drastic decline in the levels of nurse morale, can be traced to the attempt to impose on a basically effective service new and in many ways inappropriate forms of management. Contemporary problems are with us as much as anything because of the inappropriateness of proposed cures, rather than emerging from the basic sickness of the institutional body.

As a preliminary, it is necessary to discuss the development of management in the public services generally, setting out the processes that have given rise to the characteristic forms of management in this area. From this it can be seen that there are some directions in which public sector management can and should be developed and some which are far less likely to be appropriate and helpful.

HISTORICAL TYPES OF PUBLIC SECTOR MANAGEMENT

There are three types of public sector management which have been important historically, aspects of which still can be currently identified in public services. These are: producers' cooperative management, centrally directed policy management and participative management. While current services often still involve elements of these types of management the participative management pattern actually does most to preserve and promote the best aspects of public services. The active encouragement of this type of management would be beneficial as a basis for effective public service provision. It would certainly be preferable to the forms of management, modelled on private sector practice, which are actively being promoted by government policy at the present time.

Participative management in the NHS

Participative management depends on admitting relevant occupational groups and the general public to the control of services and policy-making and is taken to be effective because it provides for a close correspondence between public needs and the provisions made for them. There has been some development of this sort of system in the NHS. As we shall see, it is a part of the traditional arrangement to have high levels of co-operation between occupations within the service. To that extent, some of the elements of participative management have been in place for some time. However, for much of recent history, the public have been merely the passive recipient of what they have been given in the way of treatments and services. The need to develop participative management has been obvious for some time and has been advocated as a relevant development for more than 20 years (Heywood, 1970; Revans, 1974). Certainly, the importance of extended participation by the public is everywhere apparent, as consumers of hospital services find their individual and collective voices (Hirschman, 1970).

However, it has to be admitted that, perhaps uniquely among British public services, the prospects for the further development of participative management are not particularly good in the NHS. Essentially, the reasons for this are first, the advantages and benefits of this system are not widely acknowledged and current government policy conspicuously overlooks them in favour of extending forms of market management. Second, historically the NHS has been excessively centralized. The NHS bureaucracy has been built up over several decades and this has given any government powerful leverage – encouraging tendencies towards the central direction of policy as well as the monitoring and control of activities. Centralization and bureaucratization impede public participation, which must be local as well as regional and national to be effective.

There is a third major factor limiting the possibilities for participative management in the NHS. This is internal rather than external and stems from the presence of three powerful but distinct occupational groups in the NHS – doctors, nurses and administrators – whose involvements and interest in the service are partly divergent. It is difficult for the public to share in policy-making in a situation where no one group has firm control and can make effective decisions about resource allocation. By contrast, in education, social services and the police, there is only one relatively undifferentiated occupational group, leading members of which, in effect, monopolize the control of provision in a particular service. Although such professionals might be initially unwilling to share policy-making with their clientele, there can be effective action about such a possibility where a single group has control. In the NHS, however, divisions between professional groups exacerbate the problem of developing increased participation.

Nurses are in a position to see the potential value of participative management. They are typically the first recipients of the concerns of the public about their treatment; but because they do not control policy, they cannot necessarily do anything effective in response. By contrast, the hospital doctors, who have both more professional knowledge and more power and effective organization but who are not in direct contact with the patients much of the time, are more likely to resist attempts by the public to control and direct health outcomes. It is ironic that nurses, who are the providers of most primary medical care in hospitals and whose work profoundly affects both the quantity and quality of services, are largely excluded from those aspects of management which set the general structure of resource allocation.

More generally, while managerial functions are not in the hands of one group like this and there is also burgeoning demand for services, conflict over the use of resources will be endemic and even traditional levels and standards of services may not be met. The way forward is towards participative management. This offers a way of rationing provision within a framework of public consent. But the path towards it is effectively blocked among other things by partial failures in co-operation between groups. However, it would not be difficult to develop consultation mechanisms and to foster a new management group charged with the responsibility of the developing occupational co-operation and participative mechanisms directly involving the public. Government has certainly set its hand to produce a new managerial cadre, but it is one with a quite different policy from that which has been outlined. The ideology and practice of this group is that of divisive and coercive market management (Strong and Robinson, 1990; Pollitt, 1993). This is incongruent with the long-established patterns of working in the service and the source of many contemporary problems.

STAGES IN THE DEVELOPMENT OF MANAGEMENT OF NHS HOSPITALS

The origin of all public sector services in Britain is extremely local. Such provisions as were first made historically for relief of acute needs were made by the action and initiative of people in different localities. There is, thus, a tradition of local involvement in the provision of services. Sometimes local provision was within a framework of national legislation, as in the case of early attempts to provide relief from poverty. But even here the services provided varied a good deal according to pre-existing standards of provision.

The beginnings of medical services for the general public are in many ways a classic case of local initiatives being the basis of service. Early hospitals, first developed in a recognizably modern form in the early period of the industrial revolution (Abel-Smith, 1964), as well as personal medical services which pre-dated the hospitals, were deeply rooted in localities. The costs of these services were borne by local people and the services were for the benefit of the local community. In many ways the founding of the NHS in 1948 was not a departure from localism except in funding and administration. The founding policy of the NHS was personalized care, an individual treating an individual patient. Generally, the growth in the scale of public services resulting from the growth of population size and the concentrations of populations into urban centres did not produce any change from this basic plan.What did occur, however, was the rapid and extensive emergence of a more bureaucratized administration of services, in which extensive recording of aspects of provision developed. To some extent this was justified by the need for good clinical records, sometimes also by the perceived need for good housekeeping in respect of the cost of provision.

However, it is important to distinguish this increasing administration associated with services from the active management of services. With administered services, clerical staff simply support the activities of professionals by keeping records, accounts and recording decisions. Policy about physical development, the use of capital and consumable equipment, employment policy and employment decisions, which are the core of management concerns, were all securely retained by community leaders and senior professionals. In the health service, a curious division of professional labour grew up between doctors and nurses, with clinical and treatment decisions being retained by the doctors – together with control over all major technical expenditure – while the nurses developed an extended responsibility for all the remaining delivery of care (Abel-Smith, 1960; Davies, 1980). This role carried with it, as did that of the doctors, responsibility for many aspects of organization that would be seen today as management. For example, such things as the recruitment, training and employment of nursing staff; planning, direction and supervision of the use of nursing and ancilliary staff; the provisioning, cleaning and refurbishment of wards, as well as responsibility for the quality of clinical routine, were all areas of management that were the responsibility of nurses. The matron of a hospital, any time up to and until 20 years after the Second World War, was primarily a line-manager whose principal responsibility was practical healthcare delivery within the hospital (Davies, 1980). Although they did not think of their work in that way, management being a male occupation mainly restricted to factories, analysis of the actual activities of senior nurses shows how wide were the directing, controlling and organizing aspects of their work. During this period, when doctors and nurses shared a good deal of the organizing and directive work and arranged any necessary coordination of activities between themselves, there was actually little except record-keeping for administrators to do. The numbers of administrators in hospitals were few and their status low.

In most of the public sector services the rise of a distinct managerial cadre, drawn from professional occupations, can be traced to the emergence of increasing governmental interest in local service provision. In this case, management, which in many people's thinking is associated with the development of private industry, can be shown here to arise largely in response to the activities of central government. In point of fact, however, this view of the origin of private management is an over-simplification.

Private sector management, as a distinctive occupation and competence, was itself the product of an increasing separation between ownership and control in the maturing private enterprise economy. Private sector management emerged with large-scale industry because of the need for the co-ordination and planning of large-scale industry. The new managers were not usually owners of the firms they managed; that is, they were property-less professionals. True, they had a vested interest in the profitability and success of any business they were managing, but their concerns were not precisely the same as the owners. Professional managers have an interest in medium-term stability and profitability and relatively little in short-term returns. For career managers in private enterprise, major shareholders and their representatives on boards of directors were increasingly just one of a number of groups whose interest in a firm had to be managed. Hence a case can be made that private sector management also first emerged as a role which mediates between different parties: owners, employees and customers.

In a similar way, the rise of a developed managerial function in public service management can be traced to the time when the government began to subsidize the activities of local authorities and so acquired an interest, somewhat akin to that of a large shareholder, in the economical and efficient provision of services. However, early public services, even in their highly bureaucratized form, were administered rather than managed, in that such policy decisions as were made were largely determined by professsionals whose expertise originated from their capacities as service providers: in the case of the early hospitals, mainly senior doctors and nurses. Those who had no such occupational competences were administrative support staff. Administrators kept records of what was done and in other ways supported on-going activity; that was all. The emergence of an active managerial function, in which separate attention is given to problems of the organization and co-ordination of services and the consideration of efficiency in service delivery, was slow to develop in these circumstances. To the extent that management took place, it was largely undertaken by senior professionals as an additional function. For this reason, when it did emerge, the specialized management of public services was often slanted towards the interests and outlook of the professional groups that had been the first managers. Indeed, in many services what managers there are have been recruited from professional groups.

Professionals managing the services which they had at some time practised, naturally sought in some part to protect the autonomy of service providers and what they saw as the integrity of service provision. We may distinguish this as a stage in the development of public management which has been identified as the producers' co-operative form of management. (This notion has been derived from the writing of Rudolf Klein (1989) on the political history of the NHS, in which he defines the NHS as a producers' co-operative.) What is being asserted here is that, to a large extent, the early management of public services was subordinated to professional expertise. It is certainly true that managers in much of the public sector still do not base their role on a claim to managerial skill *per se* but on their professional skills and abilities as service providers. Chief constables and chief education officers are managers in the sense that they devote their time to organizational matters and are generally interested in performance, but they are equally if not more interested in maintaining customary types and standards of service provision. Because they have these matters at the centre of their concern, they can be thought of as custodians of the services they provide as much as managers of them. For this reason, this management orientation has been described elsewhere as 'custodial management' (Ackroyd, Hughes and Soothill, 1989). It involves active co-operation between professional groups to decide on and deliver public services.

It might be thought that, in this situation, it is only when the government begins to exert itself with such things as threats of reduced funding, do professionals see the relevance of overall rationing of supply. As professionals, managers may have little acceptance of the need for economy. Indeed, their ideas about economy might only be limited by their understanding of the limits of their expertise and their definitions of public need. In short, professionals only manage within the assumption that services, and their associated standards and levels of provision, should be preserved and developed. But when the functioning of the system is studied, there is a lack of evidence of waste. The period of the highest development of the producers' co-operative, the 1950s and 1960s, is also a period marked by high levels of satisfaction with public services. On the contrary, because the interest of the government is the limitation of expenditure, whatever the likely efficacy of new treatments and procedures, the defensive outlook of public sector management that we see with the custodial attitude is likely to be endemic. It is not *prima facie* evidence of inefficiency, and is sometimes assumed. Thus Pettigrew, Ferlie and McKee (1992: 11) suggest that the custodial attitude is necessarily indicative of poor management. However, the senior levels of educational administration, the police service and social services are still securely monopolized by people who began their service as teachers, police constables and social workers, which is not the case any longer in the NHS.

The label 'producers' co-operative' was appropriate to the hospital service in the early stages of its development up to and including the period of local authority control before nationalization. It was developed to a high level in the early decades of the NHS. Here, however, the wealth and independence of the senior doctors and the fact they shared their managerial role with senior nurses weakened the security of specifically professional control over the developing bureaucracy. The adoption of the unique form of boards of management for health authorities reflects the complex division of labour between professional groups in the service and the fact that it was actually difficult to exert effective control through direct forms of local representation.

In accounting for the rise of public service management – as a separate and more complex form of organizational co-ordination than public service administration – it is important to recognize that the interests of political paymasters at the centre and the actual providers of services in localities do not precisely correspond. Generally speaking, the former are interested in obtaining maximum benefit for minimum cost, while the latter has as its primary concern serving a particular community by supplying what are seen to be its immediate needs. While from the point of view of the political centre, there must necessarily be some limit to state expenditure, from the point of view of service providers this is much less obviously true. In contrast, for professionals, what might be done for people is limited mainly by the applicability of their experience and knowledge. Although they are still centrally involved in management, professionals no longer entirely control it. In most of its present forms, public service management can be seen as mediating between two orientations: rationing/economy and professional standards/definitions. By various means and devices, the political centre may seek to reduce the cost of public service provision but, because they cannot directly control the activities of service providers by whose changed activity any economies will be made, it is difficult to translate their economizing intentions into real economies in provision. Moreover, in devising more economical and effective ways of delivering the same – or preferably better – levels of services for the same price, the political centre is almost entirely in the hands of the professionals themselves. However, while identifying these realities, we are in fact describing here the emergence of a new form of management in which the central government has a much more formative effect. At the high points of this development, between the early 1970s and the mid-1980s, we may call this *centrally directed policy management*.

It should not be surprising that it has often been government that has taken initiatives to impose what has taken to be the best innovations of practice by progressive localities on other authorities as well as taking other initiatives for the dissemination of ideas and sponsoring research. This has often involved government directly and indirectly fostering the emergence of new kinds of local management because this is the agency through which such changes will be introduced. Indeed, much central government administration can now be seen to be implicated in the process of local management development. These processes of engineering change are just as important as straightforward ideological attempts to control policy and limit the provision of public services. However, the basic problem for government is that so much in service delivery depends on basically qualitative judgments about the appropriateness of particular treatments and services which can only be made by public sector workers themselves. For many years, doctors have successfully claimed the right to be the only party whose judgment is relevant to clinical decisions. In effect, the degree of customary control over 'clinical' decision-making is one of the main concerns of public sector management and an indicator of its custodial orientation. In a similar way, but with less conviction and less complete success, educators, social workers and policemen have made similar claims. However, that government has been the leader in forming policy and effectively ensuring that localities follow directions, suggests the relevance of the label 'centrally directed policy management'. In using this label there is no implication that management of this type is simply the tool of government policy or that elements of custodial control have entirely disappeared.

One variant of centrally directed policy is to make the supply of services responsive to economic demand. Apart from the ideological preferences recent governments have had for this, such a policy recommends itself as a way of making services in some degree responsive to the preferences of recipients. Manifestly, the partiality of such a mode of allocation is an obvious problem. However, there are other ways of making sure that the interests of the public are taken into account. Recent decades have seen the emergence of an identifiable consumer interest in patterns and standards of service. This can vary between increased willingness to complain, to express dissent either personally or through complaints machinery and tribunals, to the formation of local interest and pressure groups. Most promising of these developments is the increasing organization of public opinion through pressure groups and even mass movements expressing interest in public service provision. In many ways these are significant developments because public opinion of this kind potentially constitutes an alternative basis on which appropriate levels and kinds of service provision might be evaluated and directed. As such, public opinion stands as a clear alternative to the ideas of cost reduction, cost economy and quasi-markets with which the political centre tends to operate and which therefore tends to dominate the centrally directed mode of management. Similarly, it is an alternative to the idea that principles underlying professional judgment should be the supreme point of reference on the nature and types of service offered, which is the operative idea behind the producers' co-operative pattern of management.

It is an arresting idea but none the less probably true that, for much of their history, public sector services were provided substantially in ignorance of what their recipients thought about them. This applied not only to the standards of services, but the provision of services as such. In a sense the police are the public providers whose activity marks the extreme of this approach. Members of the public are, in certain circumstances, likely to get the attention of the police 'service' whether they want it or not. In much the same spirit – at best paternalistic, at worst authoritarian – other public services operate. So, for example, within the NHS the real therapeutic benefits of proffered treatments are often not fully discussed with patients. Indeed, there is no escaping the conclusion that public sector services have always had a coercive element (Pinker, 1971).

In a democratic and increasingly individualistic age, paternalism and authoritarianism are questioned and resisted. As a result public services have developed the capacity to take public opinion into account. To the extent that they appear to do so they can acquire increased legitimacy and security. In this sense pressure groups, and other devices by which public opinion can achieve expression so as to be taken into account by service providers, are the functional equivalent of the feedback given to producers by consumer demand in the private sector. Indeed, it seems clear that unless such devices are fostered, public sector services may well be increasingly under threat in some areas if they do not disappear entirely. What will be left will be only services provided on the market (the level of provision of which is regulated by the ability to pay) and a residue of overtly coercive state functions whose presence is necessitated by the need for public order.

In these circumstances, the significance of the development of organized public opinion about public services can hardly be exaggerated. This is because it offers a way in which the effects of public services and the needs and desires of the public can be more effectively reconciled. This is vital. Only by more closely aligning the needs of people as they perceive them with what the public services actually provide can the future of public services be effectively guaranteed. Where public opinion is taken into account, viable and responsible public sector services can survive and develop. Management which recognizes the need for this is an extension of traditional forms of participative management. An extension of co-operation between expressed public need and the organization of professional groups will indeed require, as in the early days of public service provision, little costly administration. Arguably, elements of this emergent kind of participative management are recognizable in contemporary public sector services, but their development depends on the willingness of managers to take participation seriously and on their understanding of the divisiveness and inappropriateness of market management in the public sector.

While, in many ways, the NHS has shown considerable development of public sector management, its capacity for participative management remains weak and this is very much to its detriment.

THREE TYPES OF HOSPITAL MANAGEMENT AND THE ROLE OF THE NURSE

The three patterns of public sector management distinguished in the last section have different implications for the internal organization and dynamics of the NHS hospital. Broadly speaking, the service has followed a particular path between the three patterns of management discussed here and has done so for reasons that can be clearly identified. The consequences of change for the status and role of nurses have been profound and it is important to trace out these connections.

Briefly, the sequence of change has been as follows. First, the hospital service is an example of a full development of the producers' co-operative form of management. This form of organization began to develop in the early years of the modern hospital service and continued until the advent of the NHS. For at least 20 years after the formation of the NHS, the hospital consultants were the dominant group in the hospital service. However, second, the producers' co-operative gave over very rapidly to a full development of centrally directed policy management as the centralized bureaucracy grew and the level of expenditure mounted. In the producers' co-operative arrangement, the nurses were the junior partner to the hospital doctors and acquired both a considerable role in management and significant occupational prestige. This was reflected in the adoption of a highly hierarchical occupational structure, which copied the professional hierarchy of hospital doctors. However, the emergence of centrally directed policy management re-organized the functions of management and placed increasingly effective power in other hands of administrators and bureaucrats. As hospital doctors withdrew from involvement in management, nurses found themselves increasingly subject to administrative scrutiny and control by the administration. Because of the scale of its activities, the NHS became firmly locked into the centrally directed mode of management in which administrators implement government policy. Government was strongly behind this development, being interested in controlling local activities and limiting expenditure. This has greatly added to the bureaucracy. It is not until relatively recently – the last five years or so – that government policy has tried to break this down by encouraging a new market emphasis.

The exclusion of nurses from central management functions controlling resources and their sidelining into advisory capacities was progressive under centrally directed management. This is the key to understanding the fall in the status of the profession and such things as the loss of morale among the senior grades and the rise of aggressive trades unionism among the rank and file. (See also Chapter 24). The movement of some other public sector services – for example, education and the police – towards a more decentralized form of organization, combined with increased local autonomy for managers and increased public participation, has not been observed in the NHS hospitals. Without much understanding of the importance of participative management in public service, in recent days central government has used existing centralization as a platform from which to launch new forms of management with a market orientation. This has entailed the development of a specialized and exclusive managerial cadre, mainly recruited from the adminstrative structure. By the mid-1980s, the administration was very strong and within it health professionals in general were poorly represented. It is hardly surprising that former nurses are few and far between among these new managers. As a result, nurses are not only substantially deprived of participation in management, but they are also exposed to the rising demands of the public without any effective power to change things.

Nurses today have to deal with insurgent public opinion without any possibility of mobilizing resources to deal with their own problems or those of the public concerned. In fact, a wide-ranging adoption of participative management and participative structures would be needed to deal with the present alienation of the nurses from their organizations and, increasingly, from the general public. However, before concluding with some comments on the benefits of participative management, more can be said about the way traditional forms of management have impacted on the role of the nurse.

Producers' co-operative management: nursing as an élite profession

Until the formation of the NHS and for more than a decade thereafter, the form of public sector management in the hospital service was the producers' co-operative. The hospital consultants were securely in charge of the medical services provided by the hospitals in which they worked; and nurses, as junior partners with the doctors, completed the monopoly of professional control of the clinical services provided (Abel-Smith, 1964). It is true that their control was not absolute in that they had to operate within a political structure, either in the shape of a local authority committee from 1930 or a regional hospital board after the start of the NHS. However, the power and influence of the consultants was considerable: they were often the single most concerted voice on the hospital boards, and they had an important presence at other levels. But the point to note is not simply their formal power, but the fact that their professional standing commanded great respect. In decisions about what should be done and how funds should be divided between heads, a good deal of deference was extended to medical opinion. True, in order to get their way and to achieve their ends, there had to be a degree of professional solidarity among consultants. Agreements between consultants had to be secured. But, where this occurred, professional control of the hospitals was almost absolute.

Nurses had every reason to consolidate a professional alliance with doctors. Nurses had historically identified closely with the doctors and modelled aspects of their professional organization on medicine (Davies,

1972). The steep hierarchy in nursing – hierarchy based on knowledge and ability as much as practical skill – is a key indicator of the extent of identification with the medical profession. Along with this copying of forms of organization, it is important to emphasize the symbiotic (mutually dependent) relationship between doctors and nurses in the division of labour for the provision of care. The work of doctors, in dealing effectively with large numbers of patients, was enormously facilitated by the understudy-and-support role taken by the nurses. Nurses were very much subordinated to medical control, having to discharge all the routine and distasteful aspects of care, obtaining in exchange professional autonomy and significant involvement in management. However, in career terms, in the first half of this century, nursing was one of the few professions offering the possibility of the progression to positions of considerable power and influence, specifically to women. Nursing hierarchies were steep and the number of élite positions – as the matron of a major hospital, for example – were few; but symbolically the existence of these positions were arguably much more important than their numbers.

If the tradition of managerial power for senior nurses has not persisted, one important legacy of this period for the nurse has remained. This lies in opportunities for education. One aspect of this is the high level of specialist training that the able and energetic recruit to nursing could expect to obtain. The high level of education of many recruits to nursing in the post-war years and the formalized character of knowledge on the subject allowed the emergence of degrees in nursing studies. Nurses were often much better qualified academically than many of their administrative counterparts. Nevertheless, the position of nurses in the professional division of labour depended a great deal on the continued power and influence of doctors.

The great problem with the producers' co-operative as a form of management has been the extent to which it serves the interests of the producers, as opposed to those who consume the production. Often it does this more than perhaps it should. It is not easy to provide a built-in regulatory mechanism to operate when there is abuse of professional power. However, it would be wrong to assume that only the market can constitute a mechanism to ensure the provision of excellent service. As evidence of this, it is clear that the post-war period produced some of the finest and largest hospitals in Europe and possibly the world. Renowned centres of specialist treatment, such as Christies, Addenbrookes and the Brompton hospitals, attracted first the specialized staff and then the level of capital equipment and consumable funding which allowed them to rise to importance. Nor were centres of excellence confined to specialist centres: many London and provincial urban hospitals became deservedly renowned for the range of services provided. However, the producer's co-operative form of organization will protect the inadequate to the same degree that it can empower the excellent. Indeed, part of the justification for centralized control was to tackle the wide variations in levels and standards of service throughout the country.

The rise of centralized control: nursing as a costly factor of production

The deal struck with the reforming post-war Labour administration by the hospital consultants as a condition for their participation in the NHS was, as is well known, extremely beneficial to them. It left many senior consultants with a high and secure income and perhaps the majority with the option of being employed only part-time within the new structure. This contractual arrangement certainly enhanced the professional prestige of consultants and so, in the short term, enhanced their political standing as independent advisers. However, indirectly and in the longer term, the influence of the professionals within the hospital structure was fatally compromised and gradually became weaker. It led them progressively to reduce their interest in management issues, to be concerned about resource allocation only in so far as it affected their ability to develop their own specialist aspects of medical care. To an extent this reduction in involvement is attributable to the very success of the early NHS. Under the producers' co-operative, hospitals had become large and expenditure huge. As managers everywhere in the world have discovered, logistical problems grow disproportionately with scale. Co-ordination becomes a pressing issue as scale increases. In short, the practical division of labour worked out by the doctors and nurses was not equal to the new managerial tasks that began to emerge as the hospital service grew. Bureaucracy, the extensive record-keeping and accounting work of the hospital administrators, burgeoned and this development of their role was almost entirely without function or benefit. In this pair of related processes – the rise of administration and the withdrawal of the doctors – nurses, as the weaker and more dependent partner in the old professional alliance, lost both managerial function and occupational status. The high point of the managerial involvement of the hospital nurse occurs with the Salmon Report (Ministry of Health, 1966). Not long after this, the status of the nurse began to decline.

Introducing a national system of hospital provision, the developing NHS involved a huge and growing increase in administrative functions and costs in itself. The centralized control of the system, which gradually developed, also added new tiers of bureaucracy. Some of this was concerned with monitoring the costs of the service, comparing the activities and costs from region to region and imposing policies for public health on localities. But for a long time, this increased administration had few recognizably improved attributes from a managerial point of view. There was a delay before administrative practice began to acquire significant material aspects and to become the main organizational device for co-ordination and control of the service.

It is usual for descriptions of the management of the NHS in the 1970s to emphasize the plurality of kinds of practice in the service. Smith (1978), for example, stresses the simultaneous existence of three domains – managerial, professional and political – and suggests that each is extremely influential in affecting practical outcomes. He suggests, however, that no one of these domains can be dominant and that the NHS is a strange hybrid type of organization which does not fit the available theoretical accounts of organization. Similarly, Davies and Francis (1976) suggest that neither a pure professional model of the hospital as an organization nor a bureaucratic model will do as a basic description. In their different ways these writers suggest that the hospital service of the time is best understood as an overlapping set of processes in which specifically managerial functions are dispersed among a number of groups. In fact, it is possible to interpret this as a stage in a process of transition from an organization controlled by professionals to one in which administrative control is much more evident. Crudely expressed, the pattern of change is that administrators – through their tie with the central bureaucracy and overall knowledge of expenditures – are gaining an increasing control over resources. In the emerging new arrangement, senior doctors retain some control over decision-making through a power of veto, while the nurses continue practically to organize and manage the delivery of care but lose many of their other managerial functions.

At this point, administrators increasingly see themselves as managers in the sense of having strategic control of the organization and giving direction to other groups of employees, particularly nurses, technicians and ancillary staff. Nurses fought a tentative rearguard action over their exclusion from the executive aspects of management, retaining formal recognition of their function as controllers of the activity of other nurses. By the use of the 'management team' concept and other devices, they tried to perpetuate a version of the producer's co-operative form (cf. Bellaby and Oribabar, 1980). The point to make, however, is that in the process of the emergence of a more centrally directed kind of management, in which strategic control is seen as the core function and the limitation of costs becomes the key means of exerting control, the actual managerial role nurses continued to discharge was not lost so much as devalued and overlooked. The perceived importance of their functions was vastly weakened by the absence of control over resources. The progressive alienation of senior nurses from what was now seen as basic managerial practice, increasingly consolidated in the hands of administrators turned managers, has had a number of identifiable effects.

One of the most obvious early indicators of the exclusion from key aspects of management was a drop in morale among nurses. It is no accident that the classic study of occupational morale among nurses by Revans (1964) took place in the 1960s. Since that time, concern for the morale of nurses has been recurrent (Ackroyd, 1993; Mackay, 1989). Perceiving the problem of low morale among hospital staff to be more than a matter of psychology, Revans and some colleagues later conducted a series of studies of communication in hospitals (1974). There is some substance to his suggestion that NHS hospitals suffered from problems of poor communication at this time. The involvement of many different groups of employees is one reason for this. Also, however, the hierarchies in which professionals are involved display different patterns of relationships and norms of conduct from those of administrators. Although there were some obvious areas of co-operation among occupations, the fact that these groups were actively in contention with each other over aspects of organizational control compounded communication difficulties. It would seem, then, that these problems are more than just the results of NHS hospitals being large and complex organizations.

Nurses have been extensively researched since the 1960s. Research that has looked at the way that nurses in hospitals actually organize themselves has shown that they are extremely resourceful and independent. They fit well with what have been described as autonomous or self-managing work-groups. Nurses achieve remarkable levels of care in the face of undermanning and other shortages (Anthony and Reed, 1990; Strong and Robinson, 1990). The system of self-management, the only significant area of management left to the nursing profession, was evolved by the hospital nurses in the earliest days of hospitals. It developed further with producers' co-operative management and has survived until the present day. It still provides the basis for effective, routine accomplishment of care. In some respects, then, nurses have not entirely relinquished managerial functions and a potential capacity for practical management is still present.

It is tempting to suggest that what occurred during the 1960s and 1970s with the development of centrally directed management was the proletarianization of the hospital nurse (Derber, 1983; Shaw, 1994). The gradual subordination of nurses to the administrative cadre in hospitals is a reality which ought to be acknowledged. But administrative control of the nursing profession has many features that are not symptomatic of classic proletarianization. There is no effective direction of labour to specific tasks or close supervision of quantities of work done as in the 'scientific management' applied in many industrial situations. In fact, the direct control of nursing in anything like the fashion used in scientific management would be difficult to contrive by people who have no direct experience or detailed knowledge of the work. For this reason, although even today the pressures of nursing work in hospitals are often considerable, they are not directly imposed. There is a good deal of self-pacing of work activity, with periods of remission from intense work. There is also considerable variety of task. Teamwork and other forms of co-operation are everywhere apparent. There is also some evidence that absenteeism and other kinds of time indiscipline are much higher in nursing than would be tolerated in private enterprise (Whitson and Edwards, 1990). On the other hand, it would be difficult to exaggerate the extent to which the hospital nurse has been marginalized and ignored in the organization of hospital care in recent years. To those who have acquired executive power in the hospitals, the nurse has become merely a costly and potentially troublesome factor of production – a fact that can hardly have greater symbolic importance.

The prospects for participative management in the NHS: nursing as a skilled public service

It is a considerable paradox of contemporary management that private and public sector management are moving in opposite directions. In the private sector, radical initiatives are being taken to increase the teamworking and co-operative capacities of employees in a situation where they have scarcely existed while, at the same time, public sector management often works on the assumption that it must achieve exclusive power and control over work performance in the manner assumed to be operative in the private sector. Public service managers often assume they must learn from the private sector and, working on an outdated model of practice, are at best overlooking and at at worst dissipating the results of generations of practical teamworking and co-operation.

Another way in which public and private management are directly opposed is in their attitudes towards centralization. The private sector is trying to decentralize, pushing out all managerial functions except those elements necessary for strategic control to the periphery and reducing the size of units that can be autonomous. The public sector – particularly in the NHS – seems to be obsessed with centralization and the exertion of direct control. Large-scale and excessively bureaucratic organizations cannot be responsive to the public interest and therefore decentralization of management in the NHS is a necessity. This cannot be done effectively without the participation of the main occupational groups and of the general public in policy-making. The nurse, as the person who shapes the interface between the organization and its clientele, must become the key contributor to a new system of co-operative management.

A case can be made that the private sector has as much to learn from public services as the other way about. This is because the way many public sector services are organized depends a great deal on the skills of highly knowledgeable and experienced people who are able to adapt themselves to provide high-quality services in difficult circumstances. In short, some of the key ingredients for fuller participative management are already present in our hospitals. This pattern of provision recommends itself for two reasons. First, it is highly appropriate to the provision of care in circumstances where the public is increasingly vigilant about the treatment being given. Second, this pattern actually conforms with many attributes now taken to be indicative of best practice in many parts of the private sector. The government has its own reasons for wanting a different version of private sector management to be adopted in the NHS. Hospital managers have been only too happy to take their cue from the Griffiths Report (1983) and are attempting to model their practice on this outmoded caricature of what modern private sector management is actually like. But, as nurses know well and their practice clearly shows, nursing is not a tin of beans and the retailing of baked beans and the provision of healthcare are by no means the same thing. More recent recommendations than Griffiths about the management of healthcare, for example in the government proposals for self-managing hospitals, are more obviously appropriate to the dilemmas of the health service at the present time and should be looked at more carefully and preferably not through ideological lenses (cf. Strong and Robinson, 1990). There is much in such proposals that constitute opportunities for a responsive and caring hospital service fully within the public sector.

Nurses occupy a key position in the delivery of healthcare between executive management and the patient. In a situation where the actual experience of care is a crucial one for the perpetuation and development of the service, management cannot proceed without the participation of such professionals. Nurses are in a position to make or break the NHS as a social service. Equally, managers are in a position to ensure the making of the service rather than its breaking.

REFERENCES

Abel-Smith, B. (1960) *A History of the Nursing Profession*, Heinemann, London.

Abel-Smith, B. (1964) *The Hospitals 1800–1948*, Heinemann, London.

Ackroyd, S. (1993) Towards an understanding of nurses' attachments to their work; morale amongst nurses in an acute hopsital. *Journal for Advances in Health and Nursing Care*, **2**.

Ackroyd, S., Hughes, J.A. and Soothill, K.L. (1989) Public sector services and their management. *Journal of Management Studies*, **26**.

Anthony, P.D. and Reed, M.I. (1990) Managerial roles and relationships in a district health authority. *International Journal of Health Care*, **2**.

Bellaby, P. and Oribabar, P. (1980) Determinants of occupational strategies adopted by British hospital nurses. *International Journal of Health Services*, **10**.

Davies, C. (1972) Professionals in organisations: observations on hospital consultants. *Sociological Review*, **20**.

Davies, C. (ed) (1980) Rewriting Nursing History, Croom Helm, London.

Davies, C. and Francis, A. (1976) Perceptions of structure in NHS hospitals, in *The Sociology of the NHS, Sociological Review Monograph 22* (ed. M. Stacey), University of Keele, Staffs.

Derber, C. (1983) Managing professionals: ideological proletarianisation and ideological labour. *Theory and Society*, 12.

Griffiths Report (1983) *NHS Management Inquiry*, DHSS, London.

Heywood, S. (1970) *Managing the Health Service*, Allen & Unwin, London.

Hindess, B. (1987) *Freedom, Equality and the Market: Arguments on Social Policy*, Tavistock, London.

Hirschman, A. (1970) *Exit, Voice and Loyalty*, Harvard University, Cambridge, Mass.

Klein, R. (1989) *The Politics of the NHS*, (2nd edn) Longman, London.

Mackay, L. (1989) *Nursing a Problem London*, Open University Press, Buckingham.

Ministry of Health, Scottish Home and Health Department (1966) *Report of the Committee on Senior Nursing Staff Structure (the Salmon Report)*, HMSO, London.

Pettigrew, A., Ferlie, E. and McKee, L. (1992) *Shaping Strategic Change: The Case of the National Health Service*, Sage, London.

Pinker, R. (1971) *Social Theory and Social Policy*, Heinemann, London.

Pollitt, C. (1993) *Managerialism and the Public Services*, Basil Blackwell, Oxford.

Revans, R. (1964) *Standards for Morale*, Oxford University Press, London.

Revans, R. (1974) *Hospital Communication – Choice and Change*, Tavistock, London.

Shaw, I. (1994) Deregulation and the professions: the road to proletarianisation? Paper to the 12th International Labour Process Conference, Aston.

Smith, G.W. (1978) Towards an organisation theory for the NHS, Unpublished Organisational Development Conference Paper.

Strong, P. and Robinson, J. (1990) *The NHS: Under New Management*, Oxford University Press, Oxford.

Whitson, C. and Edwards, P. (1990) Managing absenteeism in an NHS hospital. *Industrial Relations Journal*, **21**.

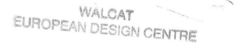

Index

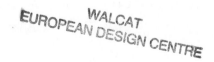